Access the web site at
vannoortdentalmaterials.com

Commissioning Editor: *Alison Taylor*
Development Editor: *Fiona Conn*
Project Manager: *Louisa Talbott*
Design Direction: *Christian Bilbow*
Illustration Manager: *Jennifer Rose*
Illustrator: *Kinesis Illustration*

Introduction to
Dental Materials

Fourth Edition

Richard van Noort BSc, DPhil, DSc

Professor in Dental Materials Science, Department of Restorative Dentistry, University of Sheffield, Sheffield, UK

With contributions by

Michele E. Barbour MPhys, PhD, PGCHE

Senior Lecturer in Dental Biomaterials, School of Oral and Dental Sciences, University of Bristol, Bristol, UK

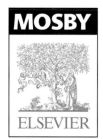

Edinburgh   London   New York   Oxford   Philadelphia   St Louis   Sydney   Toronto   2013

First edition 1994 Times Mirror International Publishers Limited
Second edition 2002 Elsevier Science Limited
Third edition 2007 Elsevier Limited
Fourth edition 2013 Elsevier Limited
 Reprinted 2013

ISBN: 978-0-7234-3659-1
Ebook ISBN: 978-0-7234-3781-9

British Library Cataloguing in Publication Data
A catalogue record for this book is available from the British Library

Library of Congress Cataloging in Publication Data
A catalog record for this book is available from the Library of Congress

Notices
Knowledge and best practice in this field are constantly changing. As new research and experience broaden our understanding, changes in research methods, professional practices, or medical treatment may become necessary.

Practitioners and researchers must always rely on their own experience and knowledge in evaluating and using any information, methods, compounds, or experiments described herein. In using such information or methods they should be mindful of their own safety and the safety of others, including parties for whom they have a professional responsibility.

With respect to any drug or pharmaceutical products identified, readers are advised to check the most current information provided (i) on procedures featured or (ii) by the manufacturer of each product to be administered, to verify the recommended dose or formula, the method and duration of administration, and contraindications. It is the responsibility of practitioners, relying on their own experience and knowledge of their patients, to make diagnoses, to determine dosages and the best treatment for each individual patient, and to take all appropriate safety precautions.

To the fullest extent of the law, neither the Publisher nor the authors, contributors, or editors, assume any liability for any injury and/or damage to persons or property as a matter of products liability, negligence or otherwise, or from any use or operation of any methods, products, instructions, or ideas contained in the material herein.

 your source for books,
journals and multimedia
in the health sciences
www.elsevierhealth.com

Working together to grow
libraries in developing countries

www.elsevier.com | www.bookaid.org | www.sabre.org

ELSEVIER   BOOK AID International   Sabre Foundation

The publisher's policy is to use paper manufactured from sustainable forests

Printed in China

Contents

Preface

There is scarcely a dental restorative procedure that does not make use of a dental material in one way or another. In these days of rapid developments in dental materials, the typical lifespan of a material, before it is modified or replaced, can sometimes be as little as 3 years. Consequently, within a very short space of time, many materials in use today will be superseded by new ones. We have seen the introduction of new restorative materials such as resin-modified glass–ionomer cements and compomers, and new resin technologies, such as ormocers and siloranes. Adhesive procedures have evolved further with the introduction of self-adhesive resin cements, and new bonding procedures to base metal alloys and gold alloys have been developed. The need for a fourth edition of this book so soon after the third is testimony to the fact that the rapid changes taking place in dental materials are continuing apace. Thus, many of the materials that an undergraduate dental student learns about will be altered or replaced when that student is a practising dentist. To cope with the rapid advances, the dentist needs the ability to assess the potential of new dental materials, which requires more than a superficial knowledge of the materials used. A thorough understanding and appreciation of their composition, chemistry and properties will provide the necessary springboard for achieving this. The dentist has ultimate responsibility for what is placed in the patient's mouth and thus needs to have a sound knowledge of the materials used.

The book is set out in three sections, each covering a different aspect of dental materials science.

SECTION ONE: BASIC SCIENCE FOR DENTAL MATERIALS

This section describes the structure of materials, with chapters on atomic bonding, metals, ceramics and polymers. The first chapter has been revised to reflect the growing need to be aware of the safety aspects of dental materials and the care that has to be taken when sourcing materials from across the world. Further chapters explain the necessary terminology used in the description of the physical, chemical and mechanical behaviour of materials. A separate chapter is devoted to the principles of adhesion.

SECTION TWO: CLINICAL DENTAL MATERIALS

This section deals with those materials commonly used in the dental surgery, including dental amalgam, composite resin and compomers, glass–ionomer cements and resin-modified glass–ionomer cements. The composition, chemistry, handling characteristics and properties relevant to their clinical use are discussed. The chapter on intermediate materials considers issues relating to pulpal protection, which is also taken up in the chapter on endodontic materials. The latter has been extended to include information on the wide variety of post-core systems. Resin bonding to enamel and dentine is covered in a separate chapter, reflecting the high importance of this subject in clinical dentistry. Impression materials are also covered in this section. A further chapter has been added that explores the recent developments in nanotechnology and how this has affected dental materials.

SECTION THREE: LABORATORY AND RELATED DENTAL MATERIALS

In this section, the student of dental materials science is introduced to the materials used by dental technicians in the construction of fixed and removable prostheses. A sound knowledge of the materials available and how they are used will help towards developing an understanding of the work of the dental technician and assist in communication with him or her. Also included in this section is a chapter on cementation, describing the wide variety of materials and procedures used in the dental surgery when providing patients with indirect restorations.

The philosophy in the earlier editions of this book was to make dental materials science readily accessible to the dental student. Although there is a tendency to use the opportunity of a new edition to change everything, I have resisted this as much as possible. I wanted to retain the simplicity and clarity that I feel had been achieved in the previous editions. Nevertheless, those who are familiar with the previous edition will notice that much has been added to reflect the changes in clinical dental materials. I have retained the comment boxes throughout the text in order to highlight issues of clinical significance, which I hope the reader will continue to find helpful.

It should be appreciated that this book was written on a need-to-know basis and is only the first step towards that process of independent learning and critical appraisal of dental materials. As the title suggests, the book represents only an introduction to dental materials and there is obviously much, much more that can be learnt. The list of suggested further reading at the end of each chapter has again been updated and the reader is urged to take advantage of the better knowledge and understanding that can be gained from reading widely around the subject.

The aim of this textbook is to guide readers down the long road to becoming informed practitioners who not only know what should be done and how it should be done, but also why it should be done. I believe that the student of dental materials science will find this book a useful first step in the right direction.

R. van Noort
2013

Self-assessment

The 4th edition of this textbook is enhanced by the addition of a new online self-assessment resource. This contains over 450 questions grouped by chapter and level of difficulty, from which the reader can create their own electronic assessments, customised to their needs, at any time.

The self-assessment resource comprises questions of five different styles, selected and designed with reference to methods commonly employed in undergraduate dental programmes. As well as allowing the student to check their knowledge and understanding, this resource will provide an invaluable opportunity to aid revision and practice for exams.

**Access the web site at
vannoortdentalmaterials.com**

A historical perspective

Introduction

Poor dentition is often thought of as being a modern-day problem, arising as a consequence of overindulgence in all things considered 'naughty, but nice'! At first glance, the diet of years gone by, consisting of raw meat, fish, rye bread and nuts, would be considered better for the dentition than the cooked food and high sugar intake foods consumed today. However, the food was not washed as diligently then as it is now, meaning that it contained grit in the form of sand, flint and shells, which had the effect of wearing away the grinding surfaces of the teeth. The surface protective layer of enamel is only thin, and the underlying dentine is worn away rapidly. Eventually, the pulp is exposed and will be invaded by bacteria, which, before long, will cause the formation of an abscess, leaving no other recourse than to have the offending tooth extracted. The problems this presented were formidable, and we will return to these at a later stage.

Thus, the loss of teeth is by no means a new problem, and has been with man for time for as long as can be remembered.

Etruscans (1000–600 BC)

For some of the earliest records of the treatment of dental disease, one has to go back well before the time of Christ. While much is lost with the passage of time, the Etruscans did leave behind a legacy of some very high-quality dentistry.

The Etruscans were a people that came from the near East and established themselves in the leg of Italy. They were the forebears of the Romans (upon whom they had a great influence) and laid the basis for the formation of the Roman Empire. The quality of their craftsmanship was outstanding. Their skills were put to good use, as they fashioned artificial teeth from cadaver teeth using gold to hold the tooth in place. Gold had the two advantages of being aesthetically acceptable, and of being one of the few metals available to them with the necessary malleability for the production of intricate shapes.

The Romans must have inherited at least some of their interest in teeth, as made evident by one of their articles of law of the Twelve Tables, which states that:

> To cause the loss of a tooth of a free man will result in a fine of 300 As.

More remarkable, perhaps, is the fact that the slaves too were offered some protection, but in their case the fine was only 100 As. Although no physical evidence remains that false teeth were worn, it may be inferred from the written records that this was the case. Horace (65 BC), wrote of 'witches being chased and running so fast that one lost her teeth', and later still Martial (AD 40–100), referred to ivory and wooden teeth.

The Dark Ages

Little is known of what happened in dentistry from Martial's time until the 16th century, and this period must be considered as being the 'Dark Age of Dentistry'. We owe our patron saint of dental diseases, Saint Apollonia, to this period. She was 'encouraged' to speak ungodly words by having her teeth extracted or else be burnt on the pyre. She chose to burn! This did leave the church with somewhat of a dilemma, because suicide was not allowed, but in this case the problem was overcome by considering this as divine will.

There are odd records scattered about throughout this period showing that toothache was a persistent problem. For example, one important person was known to pad out her face with cloth in order to hide the loss of teeth, whenever there was an important function to attend. This was none other than Queen Elizabeth I. Then there was Louis XIV, the 'Sun King', who suffered terribly from toothache and had to make many momentous decisions, such as the revocation of the Edict of Nantes (in 1642), while suffering excruciating pain. Possibly this clouded his judgement.

The first dentures (18th century)

In the 18th century, it became possible to produce reasonably accurate models of the mouth by the use of wax. These models were then used as templates from which ivory dentures were carved to the required shape. By the latter part of the 18th century, various craftsmen produced finely carved ivory teeth. They set up in business solely to supply false teeth to the rich. Of course, this type of dentistry was not available for the masses.

Lower dentures made of ivory and inset with cadaver teeth worked reasonably well and managed to stay in place without too much difficulty, especially if weighted with some lead. The difficulties really came to the fore with the upper denture, which refused to stay in place due both to the heavy weight and the poor fit. In order to overcome this problem, upper dentures were fashioned onto the lower denture by means of springs or hinges. This technique would ensure that the upper denture would always be pushed up against the roof of the mouth, but, as can be imagined, they were large, cumbersome and very heavy.

Clearly, the use of cadaver teeth could hardly have been hygienic. Similarly, ivory is slightly porous and thus presented an ideal substrate for the accumulation of bacteria. In fact, George Washington regularly soaked his dentures in port, ostensibly to overcome the bad taste and to mask the smell.

In 1728, Fauchard suggested that dentures should be made from porcelain instead of ivory inset with cadaver teeth, arguing that porcelain would be more attractive (as it could be coloured as required) and would be considerably more hygienic. What made this suggestion possible was the introduction into Europe of the secret of making porcelain by Father d'Entrecolle, a Jesuit priest who had spent many years in China. Given the problems of the high shrinkage of porcelain during firing, it is perhaps not surprising that we had to wait until 1744 for the first recorded case of a porcelain denture, made by a man called Duchateau.

The Victorian Age

The Victorians frowned on the wearing of dentures as a terrible vanity, more so because all of these false teeth were absolutely useless for eating with! Nevertheless, false teeth were still worn extensively by the rich. The fact that they were non-functional, combined with Victorian prudishness, is said to lie behind the custom that developed during that time of eating in the bedroom just prior to going to dinner – a custom that insured against any possible disaster at the dinner table as well as making possible the romantic affectation that young ladies lived on air.

A number of important discoveries were made during the 19th century that had a profound effect on the treatment of dental disease. The first of these was made in about 1800 by a 'dentist' from Philadelphia by the name of James Gardette.

He had carved a full set of ivory dentures for a woman patient, and had delivered these to the woman saying that he did not have time to fit the springs there and then, but that he would return to do so as soon as he possibly could. (It was the custom in those days for the dentist to visit the patient!) As it turned out, it was some months before he returned to the woman patient, and he was astonished to find that on asking her to fetch the dentures, the woman replied that she had been wearing them ever since he had delivered them. She had found the dentures a little uncomfortable at first but had persevered, and, after a little while, had found them to be quite comfortable and had no need for the springs.

Upon examination of the dentures, he realized immediately that the retention of the dentures was due to a combination of a suction effect arising from the different pressure of the atmosphere and the fluid film, and the surface tension effects of the fluid. This retention was attained because of the close fit of the denture, so it was possible to do without springs altogether, if only the denture could be made to fit as closely as possible to the contours of the oral structures. Unfortunately, the production of close-fitting dentures still presented a serious problem, which we will return to in a moment.

At this time, the extraction of diseased teeth presented a formidable problem, because there was no painless means of accomplishing the extraction. This situation was to change dramatically in 1844 due to the astuteness of a young dentist called Horace Wells, who discovered the anaesthetic effects of nitrous oxide, more commonly known as 'laughing gas'. One evening, he found himself present at a public entertainment on the amusing effects of laughing gas. A friend who subjected himself to the gas became very violent while under the influence, and in the ensuing fracas stumbled and badly gashed his leg. He had no knowledge of this wound until Wells pointed to the bloodstained leg, upon which his friend responded that he had not felt a thing. Wells realized immediately the importance of this discovery, and the next day subjected himself to the removal of one of his own teeth with the aid of the gas. This turned out to be highly successful, and before long many sufferers of toothache had the offending teeth painlessly extracted.

Unfortunately, Wells did not live to see the benefit of his discovery for long, as he committed suicide 3 years later after becoming addicted to chloroform. As a consequence of Wells's discovery, there were many people who had their teeth painlessly extracted.

At that time, few were in the position of being able to afford dentures of either carved ivory or porcelain. Other techniques had been developed, whereby it was possible to obtain accurate impressions of the oral structures, and much of the ivory was replaced by swaged gold, beaten to a thin plate on a model. The fixing of the artificial teeth to the gold was a difficult and lengthy process, and, like dentures, was also expensive.

This situation was to change dramatically with the invention, by Charles Goodyear (in about 1850), of the process of vulcanization. In this process, rubber was hardened in the presence of sulphur to produce a material called vulcanite. This material was not only cheap but was also easy to work with; it could be moulded to provide an accurate fit to the model and hence to the oral structures. It did not take off as quickly as might have been expected however, because the Goodyear Rubber Company held all the patents on the process and charged dentists up to $100 a year to use it, with a royalty of $2 per denture on top of this. The situation changed when the patent expired in 1881, and cheap dentures could be made available to the masses of people in need of them.

Nowadays, vulcanite has been replaced by acrylic resins, which came with the discovery of synthetic polymers, first made between the two World Wars. Also, wax has been replaced by a wide range of oral impression materials with far superior qualities; this has made possible the construction of very close fitting, complex prostheses.

Tooth conservation

If the 19th century was the time for tooth replacement, then the 20th century must be considered the time of tooth preservation. For example, in 1938, 60% of dental treatment was still concerned with the provision of dentures, but by 1976 this had dropped to 7%, with the rest consisting essentially of tooth preservation procedures.

Of course, the idea of preserving a decayed tooth was by no means new. As far back as the 11th century, Rhazes suggested that cavities in teeth could be filled with a mixture of alum, ground mastic and honey. Oil of cloves was promoted by Ambrose Pare (1562) to alleviate toothache, and Giovanni de Vigo (1460–1520) suggested the use of gold leaf to fill cavities. Pierre Fauchard (1728), considered by many to be the father of dentistry, discussed many aspects of dentistry, including operative and prosthetic procedures, and mentioned lead, tin and gold as possible filling materials.

However, there were a number of important gaps in the knowledge of the dentition that held back the development of conservative dental techniques.

There was a lack of understanding of the reasons for tooth decay, which was originally thought to be due to some evil spirit invading the tooth. Some thought it was due to a worm of sorts, and promoted various nasty tinctures with the objective of killing it.

The first serious conservative dental procedures did not come into use until the second half of the 19th century. By then, it was possible to work on people's teeth without causing severe pain and discomfort, thanks to the discovery of anaesthetics. This discovery made the use of the dental drill feasible.

The first such drill only became available in about 1870, but this is not too surprising, given that the drilling of teeth without an anaesthetic would have been unthinkable. Now that the preparation of teeth could be carried out, it was possible to undertake some more adventurous procedures than the wholesale extraction of decayed teeth.

Crowns and bridges

By the turn of the century, some highly advanced dental work was carried out in which badly broken-down teeth were reconstructed with porcelain crowns. This procedure was aided by the invention of a cement that would set in the mouth (i.e. zinc phosphate cement), and which is still widely used to this day. That this could give a great deal of satisfaction can be illustrated from the letters of President Roosevelt of the United States of America to his parents when still a young man:

> After lunch I went to the dentist, and am now minus my front tooth. He cut it off very neatly and painlessly, took impressions of the root and space, and is having the porcelain tip baked. I hope to have it put in next Friday, and in the meantime I shall avoid all society, as I talk with a lithp and look a thight.

May 19, 1902

This was followed by a letter a week later in which he writes:

> My tooth is no longer a dream, it is an accomplished fact. It was put in on Friday and is perfect in form, colour, lustre, texture, etc. I feel like a new person and have already been proposed to by three girls.

Obviously a delighted customer!

As is often the case with these rapid developments, there were to be some problems ahead. One of these was highlighted by an English physician, William Hunter, who accused what was then called 'American Dentistry' of contributing to the ill health of many of his patients. He had a number of patients with ailments he was at a loss to diagnose until he noticed the extensive restorative work in their mouths. These bridges and crowns appeared dirty, and were surrounded by unhealthy looking tissue, which would have been particularly bad, as oral hygiene was virtually non-existent. At that time, root canal treatment was unheard of, so the roots of teeth readily became infected. On many occasions, crowns and bridges would have been constructed on badly diseased teeth. He suggested that these crowns and bridges be removed and the teeth extracted, in response to which he received considerable objection from the patients because of the cost of the dental treatment. But, for those who agreed to have the bridgework removed, a significant number showed an immediate improvement in their health. This led Hunter to describe American Dentistry as 'mausoleums of gold over a mass of sepsis'. Consequently, teeth were blamed for all manner of illnesses that could not be readily diagnosed, and this led to many perfectly sound teeth being extracted unnecessarily.

Eventually, sanity prevailed with the introduction in 1913 of X-ray equipment by C. Edmund Kells. It could now be shown whether a tooth with a dead root was healthy or diseased. If healthy, it could be kept, and only if diseased would it be removed.

These days we take the provision of crowns and bridges for granted. Yet new developments can still excite us such as the introduction of ceramic veneers in the 1980s and the rapid developments in CAD–CAM technology that have opened up new opportunities with new materials such as pure alumina and zirconia, which give the promise of all-ceramic bridges.

Filling materials

The middle of the 19th century saw the organization of dentistry into a profession, and many dental societies came into existence, as well as numerous dental journals. One of the first acts of the American Society of Dental Surgeons was to forbid its members to use silver amalgam, resulting in the 'amalgam war'.

Amalgam is a mixture of silver, tin and mercury, and was one of the first filling materials used by the dental profession. However, many problems arose with the use of this material because of a lack of understanding of its qualities. It was not until the work of G. V. Black that some order was created out of the chaos.

He published two volumes on operative dentistry in 1895, which became the world standard for restorative dentistry. Until he had studied both the behaviour of amalgam in detail and how best to use it, amalgam did not have a very good reputation. Since then, however, and up until this very day, amalgam has become one of the most important restorative materials used by the dental profession.

It is a great credit to his intellect and ability that some of his philosophy is only now being challenged; especially in the light of what we know now compared to 1900. It is a lesson the dental profession

Table 1 Milestones in the history of dental materials

600 BC	Etruscan gold bridge work
AD1480	First authentic record of gold fillings in human teeth by Johannes Arculanus, University of Bologna
1500s	Ivory dentures began to be carved from wax models
1728	Fauchard proposed the use of porcelain
1744	Duchateau makes the first recorded porcelain denture
1826	Taveau of Paris suggests the use of silver and mercury to make a paste for filling teeth
1839	The first dental journal is published: *American Journal of Dental Science*
1840s	'Amalgam war' – the use of silver amalgam is forbidden
1850	Charles Goodyear invented vulcanite – sulphur-hardened rubber
1879	The first cement to set in the mouth, zinc phosphate, is introduced
1880s	Silicate cements developed
1895	G.V. Black publishes the first detailed study of the properties of amalgams
1907	W.H. Taggart of Chicago invented a practical method of casting gold inlays
1950s	Introduction of acrylic resin for fillings and dentures
1955	Buonacore discovered the acid-etch technique for bonding to enamel
1970	Composites began to replace silicate cements
1976	Glass ionomer cements are invented by A. Wilson
1978	Light-activated composites appear on the market
1983	Horn introduced the resin-bonded ceramic veneer
1985	Development of dentine-bonding agents
1988	Introduction of resin-modified glass–ionomer cements
1994	First compomer appears on the market

will have to learn over and over again as new materials are brought onto the market (Table 1).

Summary

As can be noted from the preceding discussion, there are numerous restorative techniques that the dentist needs to learn. In addition, dentists use a wide variety of different materials, some being hard and stiff and others being soft and flexible.

It is important that the dentist fully appreciates the various features of these materials, what it is that makes them so useful for dental applications, and what their limitations are. Only then will the dentist be able to select the most appropriate material for a particular application.

FURTHER READING

Greener EH (1979) Amalgam: yesterday, today and tomorrow. Oper Dent 4: 24

Hyson Jr JM (2003) History of the toothbrush. J Hist Dent 51: 73–80

Irish JDA (2004) 5,500 year old artificial human tooth from Egypt: a historical note. Int J Oral Maxillofac Implants 19: 645–647

Little DA (1982) The relevance of prosthodontics and the science of dental materials to the practice of dentistry. J Dent 10: 300–310

Phillips RW (1976) Future role of biomaterials in dentistry and dental education. J Dent Educ 40: 752–756

van Noort R (1985) In defence of dental materials. Brit Dent J 158: 358–360

Wildgoose DG, Johnson A, Winstanley RB (2004) Glass/ceramic/refractory techniques, their development and introduction into dentistry: a historical literature review. J Prosthet Dent 91: 136–143

Williams HA (1976) The challenge tomorrow in dental care delivery. J Dent Educ 40: 587

Woodforde J (1971) The strange story of false teeth. Universal-Tandom Publ. Co., London

Section | 1 |

Basic science for dental materials

This section addresses the relationship between the microstructure and the properties of materials.

In order to understand why different materials should have different properties and what these properties mean in relation to their use, it is necessary to understand something about the science of materials.

As this book is not intended for would-be materials scientists but rather for dentists with a good foundation in dental materials, only those aspects of the behaviour of materials that are pertinent to dental applications will be considered.

The questions to be addressed in this section will be:

- What are the microstructural features of materials?
- How do we describe the behavioural characteristics of different materials?

Chapter | 1.1 |

Biomaterials, safety and biocompatibility

BIOMATERIALS

The dental restorative materials described in this textbook are a special subgroup of what are more generally known as biomaterials. When a material is placed in, or in contact with, the human body, it is generally referred to as a biomaterial. A biomaterial may be defined as a non-living material designed to interact with biological systems.

The three main areas of use of biomaterials are:

- dental restorative materials, e.g. metallic and composite filling materials, and casting alloys and ceramics for fixed and removable intra-oral prostheses
- skeletal implants, e.g. oral and maxillofacial implants and joint prostheses
- cardiovascular implants, e.g. catheters, prosthetic heart valves and blood vessels, and dialysis and oxygenator membranes.

The latter part of the 20th century saw a remarkable development in new dental materials and technologies. At the beginning of the century, the choice of dental materials on offer was virtually limited to amalgam for posterior teeth, silicate cements for anterior teeth and vulcanite for dentures. At the start of the 21st century, the situation is really quite different and there is so much choice that the process of selecting the best materials for a particular clinical situation has become much more complex (Figure 1.1.1).

To make matters yet more complicated, there is now considerable pressure to make a move towards evidence-based dental practice and, by corollary, evidence-based dental material selection. However, it is not at all clear what constitutes evidence-based dental material selection, or even what constitutes evidence. If one were to start from the basis that only double-blind, randomized, controlled clinical trials constitute evidence, then with respect to dental materials we have a serious problem, as such evidence simply does not exist. So the first thing we need to do is to explore our understanding of what constitutes evidence-based dentistry more fully.

EVIDENCE-BASED DENTISTRY

There are many potential definitions of evidence-based medicine, but the one I wish to suggest as being a reasonable starting point for any discussion on this topic is that of the Centre for Evidence-Based Medicine at the University of Toronto (www.cebm.utoronto.ca), who define evidence-based medicine in the following way:

> *Evidence-based medicine (EBM) is the integration of best research evidence with clinical expertise and patient values.*

What I like about this definition is the fact that it encompasses all aspects of the delivery of health care: namely, the evidence of research, the evidence of clinical ability, and the evidence of patient need and choice. The value of clinical ability and patient choice are reasonably easy to understand, whereas the evidence of research requires a more in-depth exploration. This is provided in the supplementary parts of the definition, which state what best research evidence is:

> *Clinically relevant research, often from the basic sciences of medicine, but especially from patient centered clinical research into the accuracy and precision of diagnostic tests (including the clinical examination), the power of prognostic markers, and the efficacy and safety of therapeutic, rehabilitative, and preventive regimens.*
>
> *New evidence from clinical research both invalidates previously accepted diagnostic tests and treatments and replaces them with new ones that are more powerful, more accurate, more efficacious, and safer.*

The important thing to point out here is the recurring theme of safety. In this book, we will concern ourselves with dental restorative materials, and a great deal of space is devoted to two important aspects of their use: their composition and their characteristic properties. However, as the evidence-based statement above clearly indicates, we must also consider the safety of patients and of dental professionals when handling dental materials.

SAFETY

When a biomaterial is placed in contact with the tissues and fluids of the human body, there is invariably some form of interaction between the material and the biological environment. Thus, it is quite reasonable for patients to ask their dental practitioner what evidence there is to show that the material about to be put in their mouth is safe. This does rather beg the question: 'How do we know if a material is

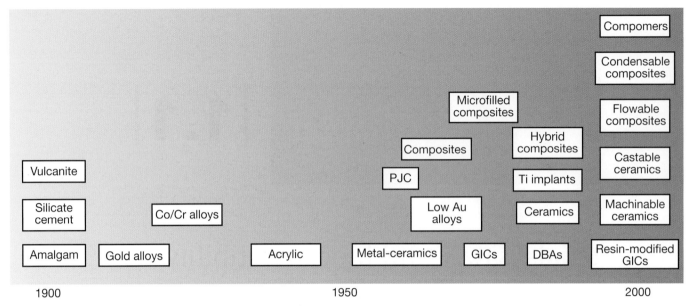

		Compomers
		Condensable composites
	Microfilled composites	Flowable composites
	Composites	Hybrid composites	Castable ceramics
Vulcanite	PJC	Ti implants	
Silicate cement	Co/Cr alloys	Low Au alloys	Ceramics	Machinable ceramics
Amalgam	Gold alloys	Acrylic	Metal-ceramics	GICs	DBAs	Resin-modified GICs

| 1900 | 1950 | 2000 |

Figure 1.1.1 The changing face of dentistry. DBA, dentine-bonding agents; GIC, glass–ionomer cements; PJC, porcelain jacket crowns

safe to use?' Besides, what do we mean by 'safe'? The most straight-forward definition of safety in this context is to suggest that dental materials should not cause any local or systemic adverse reactions, either in patients or in the dental personnel handling the materials. How we might seek evidence to support the contention that the dental materials we use will not cause any adverse reactions can be gleaned from two sources, namely:

1. basic research using methods of pre-market testing
2. clinical research via post-market surveillance.

The first of these involves putting the material through a battery of laboratory experiments and testing it for cytotoxicity, mutagenicity etc., according to well-established ISO 10993 guidelines (van Loon and Mars, 1997). But that is not all, as it is important to remember that many materials have the potential to be toxic and yet can also be beneficial. For example, many chemicals used in dental materials in their raw state would be considered highly toxic (Figure 1.1.2).

However, it should be pointed out that safety testing is not about whether or not a material is toxic; rather, it is about risk assessment. Whether or not a material can be used depends on the risk it poses, relative to the benefit it brings. Many dental materials are cytotoxic, yet this does not preclude them from being used. For example, zinc oxide–eugenol cements have been used for over 100 years, yet eugenol would not pass any cytotoxicity test. Nevertheless, what makes it effective as a temporary filling material is its ability to kill bacteria, providing its obtunding effect; if allowed to come in contact with the pulp, however, its effect can be devastating. Thus this material carries the risk of killing the pulp but, if used correctly, can save many a pulp from dying by removing the bacterial antagonist and giving the pulp the opportunity to recover from the onslaught.

In Europe, once materials have undergone a risk assessment and are considered to carry an acceptable risk, they are eligible for being awarded a CE ('European conformity') mark, assuming the material is also 'fit for purpose'. In this context, 'fit for purpose' indicates that the material is able to perform the functions for which it has been approved. In effect, all this means is that, where a material has been approved for use as, say, an anterior filling material, then it must be able to perform that function. It should be clearly understood that this does not mean that the material is efficacious. Evidence of efficacy is not a requirement for the CE approval process. It also means that

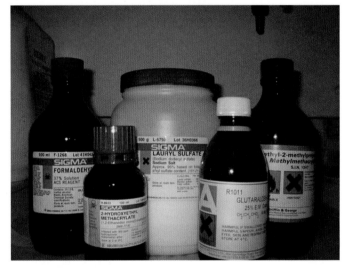

Figure 1.1.2 A range of widely used chemicals, which can be considered toxic to varying degrees

the material cannot and must not be employed in situations for which its use has not been approved.

However, there are many other potentially adverse reactions besides toxicity, such as:

- irritant contact dermatitis
  - acute toxic reaction
  - cumulative insult dermatitis
  - paraesthesia
- allergic contact dermatitis
- oral lichenoid reactions
- anaphylactoid reactions
- contact urticaria
- intolerance reactions.

Biological reactions can take place either at a local level or far removed from the site of contact (i.e. systemically). The latter is a very important consideration because it may not always be readily

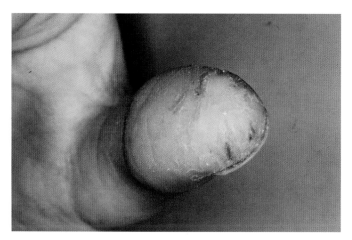

Figure 1.1.3 Irritant contact dermatitis due to resin contact

apparent that clinical symptoms, such as dermatological, rheumatic or neural reactions, could be associated with a biomaterial. Both the patient and the dental personnel are exposed to these interactions and the potential risks, with the patient being the recipient of the restorative materials and the dental personnel handling many of the materials on a daily basis.

There are therefore many aspects to risk assessment, such as making sure that any unnecessary contact with dental materials that may cause irritant contact dermatitis is avoided (Figure 1.1.3), especially amongst dentists and dental auxiliaries who will be working with these materials every day. This is often just a matter of common sense, combined with sensible packaging of the materials to be handled. There is no doubt that manufacturers have become much more aware of these issues in recent years, paying a lot more attention to how they present their materials and doing it in such a way as to minimize contact (Figure 1.1.4).

It is estimated that there are some 140 ingredients in dental materials that can cause an allergic adverse reaction (Kanerva et al. 1995). The question then is: 'How do we know if the materials used might cause any one of these adverse reactions?' Tests to assess the potential of a dental material to cause an allergic adverse reaction are very difficult since they involve the patient's immune system and we are all different in this respect. Some studies suggest that the frequency of adverse reactions to dental materials can be anything from 1 : 700 to 1 : 10 000 (Jacobsen N et al. 1991; Kallus and Mjör 1991; van Noort et al. 2004). Experience tells us that some materials are particularly likely to cause an allergic adverse reaction; these include the poly (methyl methacrylate) used in dentures or latex rubber in surgical gloves. Much of this information is anecdotal, although a limited amount of knowledge has been acquired via post-market surveillance (Scott et al. 2003). Unfortunately, there is only one centre in the world that has a track record of many years of sustained post-market surveillance of dental materials; it is the Dental Biomaterials: Adverse Reaction Unit at the University of Bergen in Norway (Lygre et al. 2004) (www.uib.no/bivirkningsgruppen/ebivirk.htm). Both the European Union (EU) and the United States of America (USA) have systems in place for the reporting of adverse events. In the EU, this is done via the competent national authority (e.g. the Medicines and Healthcare Products Regulatory Agency (MHRA) in the United Kingdom), while in the USA the reporting procedure is the responsibility of the US Food and Drug Administration (FDA) via the MedWatch programme (van Noort et al. 2004). Despite the wide use of dental materials, information on their clinical safety is not particularly abundant, although, from the little evidence that is available, it would appear that adverse reactions to dental materials are fairly rare and that severe

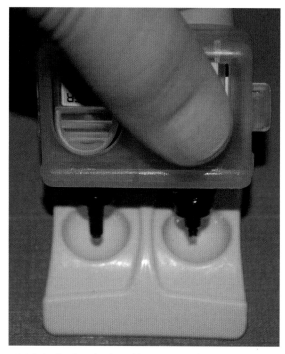

Figure 1.1.4 Packaging developed by one manufacturer to ensure there is no contact between the practitioner's hands and the resins used in a dentine-bonding agent

adverse reactions are even more so (Scott et al. 2004; Hensten-Pettersen 1998).

BIOCOMPATIBILITY

There is a subtle distinction between safety and biocompatibility. Safety is concerned primarily with the fact that materials in contact with the human body should not cause an adverse reaction. A material may be said to be *biocompatible* when it has the quality of being non-destructive in the biological environment but must also interact to the benefit of the patient. It is important to appreciate that this interaction works both ways. That is, the material may be affected in some way by the biological environment, and, equally, the biological environment may be affected by the material. Thus, to be safe is not sufficient in the context of biocompatibility; the material must also have a beneficial effect.

For example, postoperative sensitivity is a local reaction to a restorative procedure. It is often associated with the placement of filling materials, where there is an adverse pulpal reaction following the operative procedure. Although, at one time, this was thought to be due to a lack of biocompatibility of the restorative material itself, it has now become well accepted that a significant role is played by the ingress of bacteria down the gap between the restorative material and the tooth tissues. If the restorative material were able to provide a hermetic seal, which would prevent bacterial ingress, then postoperative sensitivity from this source would be far less likely. A pulpal reaction could still arise if the restorative material itself were found to be toxic to the pulp. Prevention of bacterial invasion has become an important consideration in the development of adhesive restorative materials. Some materials have a distinctly positive effect on the pulp: for example, calcium hydroxide induces secondary dentine formation by the pulp. This highlights the fact that the requirement for a biomaterial to be biocompatible does not mean that it is inert in the biological environment (i.e. that it elicits no reaction), but that it should, ideally, induce a response that is both appropriate to the situation and highly beneficial.

Corrosion is an unwanted interaction between the biological environment and the biomaterial. One of the better-known dental examples is the corrosion of dental amalgams. This corrosion causes discoloration of the tooth tissues and has been implicated in the common observation of marginal breakdown of amalgam restorations. Composite restorative materials are known to discolour in the mouth due to the corrosive action of the environment, and this causes many to be replaced when the aesthetics become unacceptable. The corrosive effects of the biological environment on the casting alloys used in the construction of fixed and removable intra-oral prostheses are also a matter of concern. When a material is susceptible to corrosion in the biological environment it tends to release large amounts of corrosion products into the local biological tissues; this may cause an adverse reaction either locally or systemically.

Some patients can develop allergic or hypersensitive reactions to even very small quantities of metals, such as mercury, nickel and cobalt, that may be released due to the corrosion process. Hence it is important that biomaterials are highly resistant to corrosion.

From the above, it should be clear that it is very important for the dentist to know the composition and chemistry of the materials to be used in the oral cavity and how these materials may interact with the biological environment.

CLINICAL SIGNIFICANCE

Dental practitioners are ultimately responsible for the materials to which a patient will be exposed. They must have a knowledge and understanding of the composition of the materials to be used and how these might affect the patient.

SUMMARY

The main objective of good design in restorative dentistry is to avoid failure of the restoration. However, it is important to appreciate that failure can come in many guises. Some failures may be due to unacceptable aesthetics. A clear example of this is the discoloration of composite restorative materials, and this points to a lack of chemical stability in the biological environment. A material may need to be removed because it elicits an allergic reaction or corrodes excessively. These are aspects of the biocompatibility of the material. Equally, a restoration may fail mechanically because it fractures or shows excessive wear, possibly because the design was poor or because the material was used in circumstances unsuited for its properties.

Thus the clinical performance of dental restorations depends on:

- appropriate material selection, based on a knowledge of each material's properties
- the optimum design of the restoration
- a knowledge of how the material will interact with the biological environment.

Aspects of the function of dental materials will be covered where appropriate.

FURTHER READING

Hensten-Pettersen A (1998) Skin and mucosal reactions associated with dental materials. Eur J Oral Sci **106(2 Pt 2)**: 707–712

Jacobsen N, Aasenden R, Hensten-Pettersen A (1991) Occupational health complaints and adverse patient reactions as perceived by personnel in public dentistry. Community Dent Oral Epidemiol **19(3)**: 155–159

Kallus T, Mjör IA (1991) Incidence of adverse effects of dental materials. Scand J Dent Res **99(3)**: 236–240

Kanerva L, Estlander T, Jolanki R (1995) Dental problems. In Guin JD (ed.) Practical contact dermatitis: a handbook for the practitioner. McGraw-Hill, New York: 397–432

Lygre GB, Gjerdet NR, Björkman L (2004) Patients' choice of dental treatment following examination at a specialty unit for adverse reactions to dental materials. Acta Odontol Scand **62(5)**: 258–263

Scott A, Gawkroger DJ, Yeoman C et al (2003) Adverse reactions of protective gloves used in the dental profession: experience of the UK Adverse Reaction Reporting Project. Brit Dent J **195**: 686–690

Scott A, Egner W, Gawkroger DJ et al (2004) The national survey of adverse reactions to dental materials in the UK: a preliminary study by the UK Adverse Reaction Reporting Project. Brit Dent J **196(8)**: 471–477

van Loon J, Mars P (1997) Biocompatibility: the latest developments. Med Device Technol **8**: 20–24

van Noort R, Gjerdet NR, Schedle A et al (2004) An overview of the current status of national reporting systems for adverse reactions to dental materials. J Dent **32(5)**: 351–358

Atomic building blocks

INTRODUCTION

All materials are built up from atoms and molecules, so it is not really surprising that there is a close relationship between the atomic basis of a material and its properties. Important in this context are the nature of the atoms and the ways in which they are arranged. The atoms combine to determine the microstructure of the solid, and, as a consequence, determine its properties. Therefore, if we are to understand the properties of materials, we need to have an understanding of the way atoms can combine to make solids.

JOINING ATOMS TOGETHER

When two atoms are brought together, they may link to form a molecule; any bonds that form are called *primary bonds*. Alternatively, they may move apart and so retain their individual identity. Depending on the degree of interaction between the atoms, one of three states can form, these being gases, liquids or solids. These are referred to as the three main *phases* of matter, where a phase is defined as a structurally homogeneous part of the system and each phase will have its own distinct structure and associated properties. In the gaseous state there is little or no resistance to the relative movement of atoms or molecules, while in the liquid state the resistance to movement is considerably greater, but molecules can still flow past each other with great ease. In solids the movement of atoms and molecules is restricted to a local vibration, although some movement at the atomic level is possible through diffusion.

The controlling factor in bond formation is energy, and a bond will only form if it results in a lowering of the total energy of the atoms being joined. This means that the total energy of the molecule must be less than the sum of the energies of the separate atoms, irrespective of the type of bond being formed. A simple way of visualizing this is the energy-separation diagram, which considers what effect moving two atoms closer together will have on their total energy. A typical energy-separation curve is shown in Figure 1.2.1.

When the two atoms are far apart, the total energy is $2E_a$, where E_a is the total energy of one atom. As they are brought closer together, the total energy begins to fall, until it reaches a minimum, E_m, at a distance a_o. Thereafter, as the atoms are brought more closely together, the total energy increases due to repulsion between their clouds of electrons. As the atoms are brought even closer together, their nuclei begin to repel each other as well, but such proximity is not usually achieved in normal circumstances. Thus, we have attraction at long range, and repulsion at short range.

The conditions under which two atoms will bond together depend on the atoms' electron configurations, which completely determine their chemical reactivity. The more stable the electron configuration, the less reactive the atom; the extremes of stability are the 'inert gases', such as argon, helium and neon, which are almost totally non-reactive. Their near-inertness is caused by their having complete outermost electron orbitals, with no opportunity for more electrons to 'join' the atom, and no 'spare' or 'loose' electrons to leave the atom.

All atoms try to reach their lowest energy state, and this is tantamount to having a complete outermost electron orbital, as the inert gases have. The atoms of some elements have 'gaps' for electrons in their outermost orbits, whereas the atoms of other elements have 'spare' electrons in their outermost orbits. By combining with each other, these two different types of atoms can both achieve complete outermost orbitals. The formation of bonds, therefore, involves only the outermost *valence* electrons.

TYPES OF PRIMARY BONDS

There are three types of primary bond: *covalent, ionic* and *metallic*.

Covalent bonds

The covalent bond is the simplest and strongest bond, and arises when atoms share their electrons so that each electron shell achieves an inert gas structure. The formation of such a bond for two hydrogen atoms is shown in Figure 1.2.2.

As the two atoms approach one another and the orbitals of the electrons begin to overlap, a molecular orbital is formed where the two electrons are shared between the two nuclei. Since the electrons

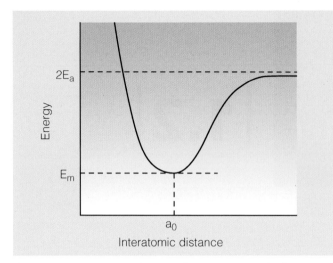

Figure 1.2.1 Energy separation curve for two atoms, each of energy E_a

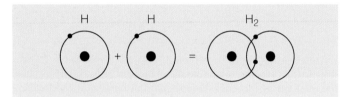

Figure 1.2.2 Two hydrogen atoms combine through covalent bonding to form hydrogen gas

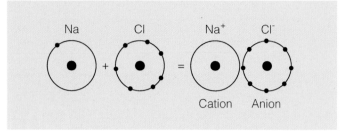

Figure 1.2.3 Formation of an ionic bond between sodium and chlorine

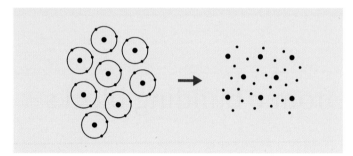

Figure 1.2.4 Formation of a metallic bond, showing a cloud of electrons surrounding the nuclei

Table 1.2.1 Typical bond energies for the three bond types

Atoms bonded	Bond type	Bond energy (eV)
C–C	Covalent	6.3
C–F		5.6
H–H		4.5
H–O		4.4
C–Cl		4.0
Na–Cl	Ionic	4.2
K–Br		3.9
Na–I		3.2
Au–Au	Metallic	2.3
Cu–Cu		2.0
Ag–Ag		1.8
Pb–Pb		0.8
Hg–Hg		0.2

will spend most of their time in the region where the orbitals overlap, the bond is highly directional.

Ionic bonds

An atom such as sodium would like to lose its single valence electron, as this would give it a configuration similar to that of neon. Naturally, it cannot do so unless there is another atom nearby which will readily accept the electron.

Elements, which can attain an inert gas structure by acquiring a single extra electron, are fluorine, chlorine, bromine and iodine, collectively known as the halogens. Thus, if a sodium and a chlorine atom are allowed to interact, there is a complete transfer of the valence electron from the sodium atom to the chlorine atom. Both attain an inert gas structure, with sodium having a positive charge due to loss of a negative electron, and chlorine a negative charge due to its acquisition of the extra electron. These two ions will be attracted to one another because of their opposite electrical charges, and there is a reduction in the total energy of the pair as they approach. This is shown in the model in Figure 1.2.3; such bonds are called ionic bonds.

An important difference between the covalent bond and the ionic bond is that the latter is not directional. This is because ionic bonds are a result of the electrostatic fields that surround ions, and these fields will interact with any other ions in the vicinity.

Metallic bonds

The third primary bond is the metallic bond. It occurs when there is a large aggregate of atoms, usually in a solid, which readily give up the electrons in their valence shells. In such a situation, the electrons can move about quite freely through the solid, spending their time

moving from atom to atom. The electron orbitals in the metallic bond have a lower energy than the electron orbitals of the individual atoms. This is because the valence electrons are always closer to one or other nucleus than would be the case in an isolated atom. A cloud of electrons, as shown in Figure 1.2.4, surrounds the atoms. Like the ionic bond, this bond is non-directional.

Bond energies

An important feature of a bond is the *bond energy*. This is the amount of energy that has to be supplied to separate the two atoms, and is equal to $2E_a - E_m$, as defined in Figure 1.2.1. Typical bond energies for each of the three types of bond are given in Table 1.2.1.

A general feature that can be seen from the bond energies is that the covalent bonds tend to be the strongest, followed by the ionic bonds, and then finally the metallic bonds. For the metallic bonds, there is a wide range of bond energies, with some approaching that of ionic bonds, and some being very low. Mercury has a very low bond energy, giving a bond that is not even strong enough to hold the atoms in place at room temperature, resulting in mercury's liquidity at this temperature.

THE FORMATION OF BULK SOLIDS

Ionic solids

Ions are surrounded by non-directional electrostatic fields, and it is possible that the positively and negatively charged ions can find positional arrangements that are mutually beneficial, from the point of view of reaching a lower energy. The ions can form a regular, three-dimensional network, with the example of sodium chloride being shown in Figure 1.2.5.

Ionic substances such as chlorides, nitrides and oxides of metals are the basic building blocks of a group of materials known as *ceramics*, of which a rather special group are the *glasses* (see Chapter 1.3). These materials are very stable because of their high ionic bond strengths.

Metallic solids

A similar arrangement to that of the ionic solids is possible with the metallic bond. In this case, there is no strong electrostatic attraction between the individual atoms (as there was between the ions in the ionic solids), as they are held together by the cloud of electrons; this cloud forms the basis of the *metals*, which are discussed in Chapter 1.4.

Covalent solids

There are only a few instances in which atoms of the same element join by covalent bonds to form a solid; these are carbon, silicon and germanium. It is the directionality of the covalent bond that is the essential difference between it and the other two primary bonds. This directionality places severe constraints on the possible arrangements of the atoms.

An example of a covalently bonded solid is diamond, which is a form of carbon. Carbon has an arrangement of electrons in its outer shell such that it needs four more electrons to obtain a configuration similar to neon; in the case of diamond, it achieves this by sharing electrons with neighbouring carbon atoms. The direction of these bonds is such that they are directed towards the four corners of a tetrahedron with the carbon atom's nucleus at its centre. The three-dimensional structure of diamond can be built up as shown in Figure 1.2.6.

Covalent solids consisting of a single element tend to be very rare. Covalent bonds are more usually formed between dissimilar elements where each takes up an inert gas configuration. Once the elements have reacted to form these bonds, the created molecule becomes highly non-reactive towards molecules of the same type, and does not provide a basis for the formation of a three-dimensional network.

The electron orbitals overlap and the electrons are shared, resulting in a filled orbital which is very stable. In this configuration, there are no partially filled orbitals available for further bonding by primary bonding mechanisms. Thus, covalently bonded elements result in stable molecules, and most elements, which join by covalent bonding, tend to be gases or liquids, e.g. water, oxygen and hydrogen. Of these examples, water will solidify at $0\,^{\circ}C$, and for this to be possible there must be some additional attraction between the water molecules; something must hold these molecules together, but it is not primary bonding.

Secondary bonding

A consequence of the sharing of electrons by two or more atomic nuclei is that the electrons will spend a disproportionately longer time in one particular position. The effect of this is that one end of the molecule may acquire a slight positive charge and the other end a slight negative charge, resulting in an electrical imbalance known as an *electric dipole*. These dipoles allow molecules to interact with one another, and to form weak bonds called *van der Waals bonds*.

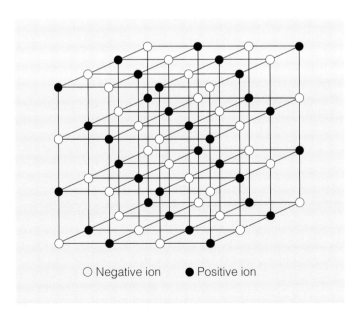

○ Negative ion   ● Positive ion

Figure 1.2.5 Formation of a bulk solid, through the ionic bonding of sodium (●) and chlorine ions (○).

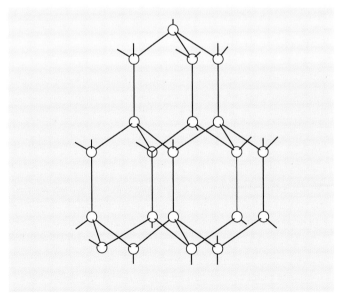

Figure 1.2.6 The structure of diamond, showing the three-dimensional network built up from the tetrahedral arrangement of the carbon bonds

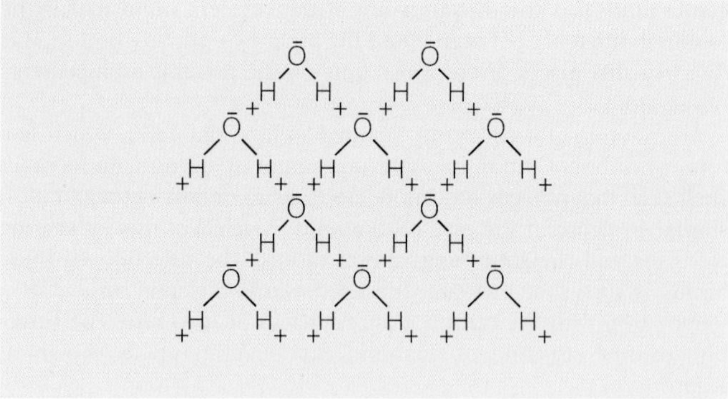

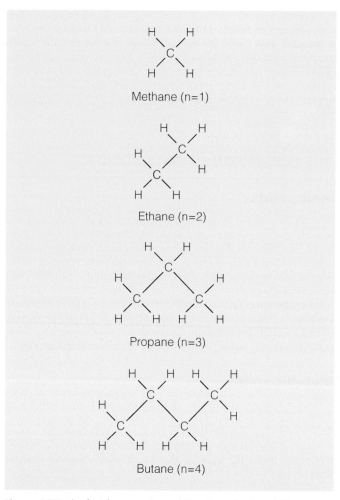

Figure 1.2.7 Hydrogen bond formation in ice

The three main factors that contribute to these relatively weak interactions are:

- interactions between permanent dipoles
- interactions between induced dipoles
- interactions between instantaneous dipoles.

The latter, known as the *London dispersion effect*, is completely general, and operates whenever two molecules, ions or atoms are in close contact. It is the result of an interaction between random motions of the electrons in the two species.

A special case of the dipole–dipole interaction is the hydrogen bond. The hydrogen atom can be imagined as a proton on the end of a covalent bond, but, unlike other atoms, the positive charge of the proton is not shielded by surrounding electrons. Therefore, it will have a positive charge and will be attracted to the electrons of atoms in other molecules. A necessary condition for the formation of a hydrogen bond is that an electronegative atom should be in the neighbourhood of the hydrogen atom, which is itself bonded to an electronegative atom. An example of this is ice, where there is an interaction between the hydrogen atom in one molecule and the oxygen atom in another molecule, shown schematically in Figure 1.2.7.

The bond strength is only about 0.4 eV, and is readily overcome by heating above $0\,°C$. The hydrogen bond is important because it accounts for the extensive adsorption possible by organic molecules, including proteins, and is therefore considered essential to the life processes. Secondary bonding forms the basis of the molecular attraction in molecular solids.

Molecular solids

It is possible to create a wide variety of different molecules, some of which can be solid at room temperature. If the molecules are sufficiently large, they are bonded together due to numerous dipole–dipole interactions. The low bond strength means that such solids will have a very low melting temperature and the upper limit for molecular solids is approximately $100\,°C$.

The best way to appreciate how these solids are formed is through a group of molecules known as the linear alkanes. These are based on a straight chain of hydrocarbons, with the general formula C_nH_{2n+2}, where n can be any positive integer. The simplest of these is methane (CH_4) which has $n = 1$. If we strip one of the hydrogen atoms from each of two methane molecules and join the molecules together through a carbon–carbon bond, we get ethane. We can continue to repeat this process and obtain very large molecules indeed (Figure 1.2.8).

Once the number of $-CH_2-$ groups becomes very large, there is very little change in the properties of these materials, which are known collectively as *polymethylene*. This name is derived from the word *poly* meaning *many* and the basic structural unit on which it is

Figure 1.2.8 The first four members of the alkane family, which are straight-chain hydrocarbons, following the general formula C_nH_{2n+2}

based, *methylene*. A material with this type of structure is known as a *polymer* since it consists of many repeat units called *mers*. How polymers can form a variety of solid structures will be discussed in detail in Chapter 1.6.

THE STRUCTURAL ARRANGEMENT OF ATOMS IN SOLIDS

Whereas the forces of attraction hold atoms close together, the mutual repulsion of the nuclei means that an equilibrium spacing is attained at which these forces balance. This interatomic spacing is presented as a_o in Figure 1.2.1.

An external force is needed to move the atoms closer together or further apart. This interatomic spacing is the configuration of minimum energy, and in order to achieve this there is a tendency for the atoms to adopt a regular close-packed arrangement. If one considers atoms to be spheres, it is possible to use the analogy of ball bearings packed in a box. The densest packing of the ball bearings is obtained when they are arranged in a regular symmetrical manner, as is shown in Figure 1.2.9. When atoms are arranged like this, the material is said to be *crystalline*.

The important feature of a crystalline structure is that, from the viewpoint of any atom in the structure, the arrangement of its neighbouring atoms is identical. Metals and ionic solids are usually crystalline at room temperature. Any solid in which there is no symmetry of the atoms is said to be *amorphous*.

Crystal structures

One of the simplest arrangements of atoms is the simple cube, in which the atoms occupy the eight corner positions.

Using the model of spheres for atoms again, this arrangement is shown in Figure 1.2.10a. Each sphere touches its nearest neighbour, such that the length of the side of the cube is equal to the diameter of the atom. If we consider a simple cube, containing only a portion of the atoms within it, as shown in Figure 1.2.10b, we get what is known as the *structural cell*. By stacking these structural cells one on top of the other, a whole three-dimensional solid can be built up.

The atoms do not occupy all of the space of the structural unit. The fraction of space occupied by the atoms is called the *packing factor* and is easily calculated.

If we assume that each side of the cube is of length 2a, then the volume of the structural cell is $8a^3$. Correspondingly, the radius of

each sphere must be a, and its volume will be given by $4/3\pi a^3$. Each sphere actually only contributes 1/8 of its volume to the structural cell, but since there are eight such segments, the spheres within the cube occupy a total volume of $4/3\pi a^3$. Thus, the packing factor for a simple cube is given by:

$$\text{packing factor} = \text{volume of atoms inside the cube}/$$
$$\text{volume of cube}$$
$$= 4/3\pi a^3/(2a)^3$$
$$= \pi/6 = 0.54$$

This indicates that nearly 50% of the space is unfilled.

It is, in fact, possible for other smaller atoms to occupy this free space without causing too much disruption to the crystalline structure, and this is something which we will return to later when discussing alloys. Given the large amount of free space in this simple structure, it is perhaps not surprising that there are other atomic arrangements where the packing factor is higher.

Two such arrangements that commonly occur in metals, are the body-centred cubic (BCC) and the face-centred cubic (FCC) configurations, which are shown in Figure 1.2.11. The packing factors for these two structures are 0.68 and 0.74 for the BCC and FCC structures respectively. With these larger packing factors, it is of course more difficult for smaller atoms to occupy the free space without upsetting the structure.

SUMMARY

In a sense, it is not surprising to find that there are three main groups of solids based on the three types of primary bonding, namely:

- ceramics – based on the ionic bond, which can exist in the crystalline and amorphous form, the latter being *glasses*
- metals – based on the metallic bond
- molecular solids – based on the covalent and secondary bonds, and including an important group of materials known as polymers.

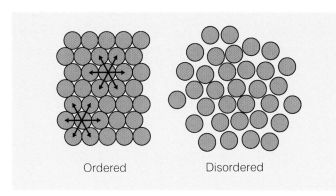

Ordered   Disordered

Figure 1.2.9 Ordered and disordered arrangements of atoms

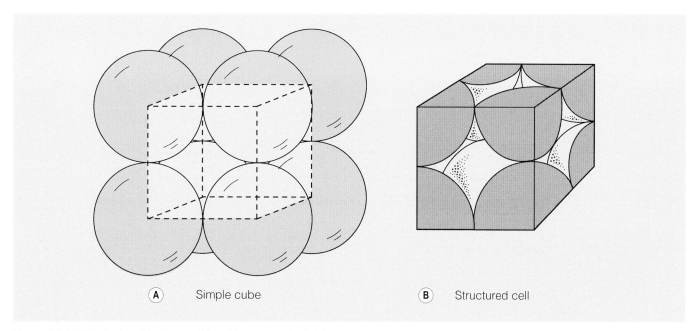

(A) Simple cube   (B) Structured cell

Figure 1.2.10 The simple cubic structure (a) and its structured cell (b)

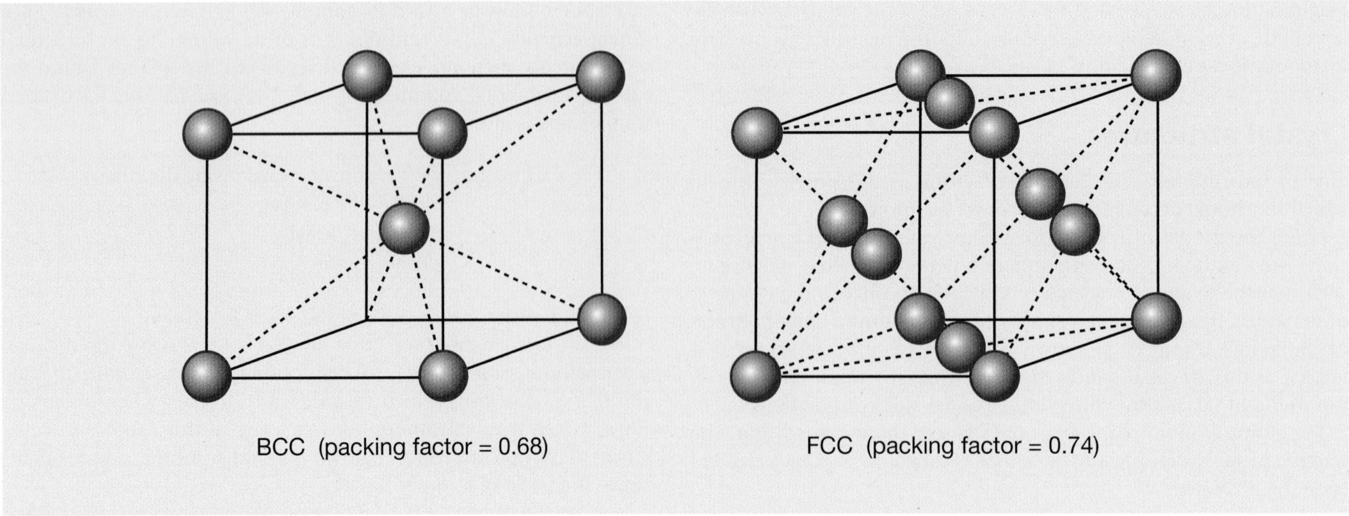

BCC (packing factor = 0.68)   FCC (packing factor = 0.74)

Figure 1.2.11 Atomic arrangements for body-centred cubic (BCC) and face-centred cubic (FCC) structures

There is one other important group of materials that has not yet been mentioned. These are the *composites*, which are based on a combination of two or more of the above solids.

There are many examples of composite materials, both natural and synthetic. Bone and dentine are natural composites, whose main constituents are collagen (a polymer) and apatite (a ceramic). Synthetic composites include glass fibre reinforced polymers, and polymers containing ceramic particles. A dental example of the latter is the composite restorative materials discussed in Chapter 2.2. Another dental example of a composite structure is the cermet, which is the filler particle used in some glass–ionomer cements (see Chapter 2.3). Its name is derived from the two components; cer(amic) and met(al).

Chapter | **1.3**

Structure of ceramics

INTRODUCTION

Ceramics are compounds of metallic elements and non-metallic substances such as oxides, nitrides and silicates. Ceramics can appear as either crystalline or amorphous solids, the latter group being called glasses.

In ceramics, the negatively charged ions (*anions*) are often significantly different in size from the positively charged ions (*cations*). An example already considered is that of sodium chloride, which has a face-centred cubic structure.

The chlorine ions take up positions at the lattice points of the FCC arrangement, with the sodium ions adopting positions between the chlorine ions, in what are called *interstitial positions*. The sodium ions are able to do this because they are considerably smaller than the chlorine ions, and fit into the free space left between them. The exact lattice structure is shown in Figure 1.3.1. Another example of this type of structure is zinc oxide, which is widely used in dentistry. There are many other applications of ceramics in dentistry; they are used as fillers for composite resins, in glass–ionomer cements, and in investments and porcelains.

CERAMIC RAW MATERIALS

Silica (SiO_2) forms the basis of many ceramics. Although it has a simple chemical formula, it is a versatile material and can exist in many different forms.

Silica occurs as a crystalline material in the forms of quartz, crystobalite and tridymite, or as a glass as in the example of fused silica. This ability of a compound such as silica to exist in different forms with distinctly different characteristics is known as *polymorphism*.

Silica is used as the basis for the formation of many complex ceramic formulations, particularly in combination with aluminium oxide with which it forms alumino-silicate glasses as used in glass–ionomer cements. Similarly, feldspathic glasses are used in ceramic restorations, and are compounds containing oxides of aluminium and silicon in combination with potassium, sodium or calcium (e.g. $NaAlSi_3O_8$).

CRYSTALLINE AND AMORPHOUS CERAMICS

Crystal transitions

When a solid is heated, it can undergo a number of transformations, the most easily recognizable of which is when the solid melts. This change of a crystal from solid to liquid is known as the *crystal melting transition*, and is accompanied by a change in the volume of the material. The volume change can be monitored to allow such transformations to be detected.

A simple means of representing this change is to plot the specific volume of the material (i.e. the volume of a unit mass of the material) against the temperature. A curve such as that shown in Figure 1.3.2 results, and at the melting point of the crystal, there is a discrete (i.e. at a specific temperature) discontinuity in the specific volume.

The specific volume is effectively the inverse of the density. This specific volume–temperature curve shows that one effect of the melting of the crystal is an increase in the volume. This is not surprising when one thinks that this transition is one from an ordered crystalline structure to that of a disordered liquid; the packing density of the atoms in the liquid will be considerably less than that in the crystalline solid.

The specific volume–temperature curve for crystalline silica is as shown in Figure 1.3.3. In this example, there are a number of solid–solid transitions, as well as the usual transition from solid to liquid. Silica is in the form of quartz at room temperature, which changes into tridymite at 870°C. A further transformation takes place at 1471°C, where tridymite changes to crystobalite and the crystobalite finally melts at 1713°C. Thus, it is possible to detect both solid–solid and solid–liquid transitions in crystalline silica.

Glass transitions

When an amorphous solid such as a glass is heated, it does not show a discrete solid–liquid transition as the material is not crystalline. Instead, what happens is that, at some point, there is an increase in the rate of change of the specific volume, as shown in Figure 1.3.4. The temperature at which this change in the slope of the specific volume occurs is known as the *glass transition temperature*, T_g. This is generally (although not always) the case for molecular solids as well.

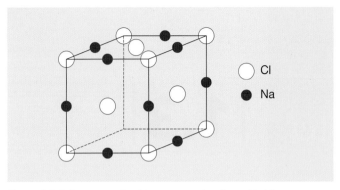

Figure 1.3.1 Face-centred cubic structure of sodium chloride

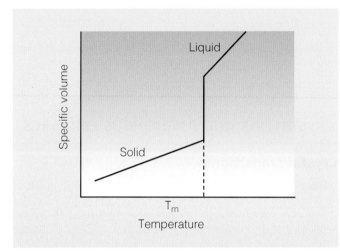

Figure 1.3.2 Transition from a solid to a liquid, where T_m is the melting temperature

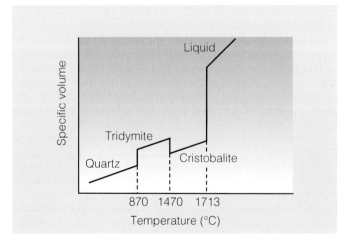

Figure 1.3.3 Solid–solid transitions for silica (SiO_2)

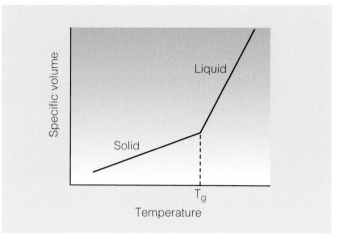

Figure 1.3.4 The variation of specific volume with temperature for an amorphous solid

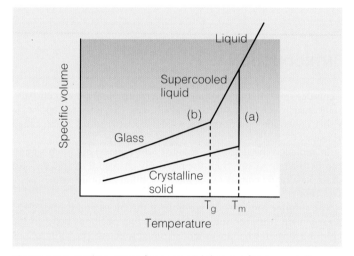

Figure 1.3.5 Cooling curves for a material that can form a crystalline solid (a) or a glass (b)

A consequence of this is that there is no *sudden* increase in the volume (and hence the unoccupied volume). Instead, there is a *gradual* increase in the volume, with the rate of increase becoming more rapid above the glass transition temperature.

The converse of this is that a liquid, which cools without forming a crystalline structure, will contain a large amount of unoccupied volume. Solids, which are formed by moving through a glass transition rather than a crystal melting transition, will be amorphous, and are referred to as *glasses*. Glasses are an important group of materials and warrant some special attention.

THE FORMATION OF A GLASS

Given their regular shapes, atoms tend to form ordered structures. Small molecules, such as methane, are able to form crystal structures easily, and even some of the higher-order linear alkanes can form crystalline structures if the molecule is regarded as a rigid rod. Once we arrive at larger, more complex molecules, however, regular arrangements become more difficult to achieve. Thus, large irregular molecules have a high probability of forming a glass on solidification.

For crystal growth to occur, *nuclei of crystallization* must be present. These are usually in the form of impurities, such as dust particles, that are virtually impossible to exclude. Thus, if there is any chance that the material can take up an ordered crystalline arrangement, it will usually do so.

Silica can form either glasses or crystalline solids, and their specific volume–temperature curves are shown in Figure 1.3.5. When crystallization occurs on cooling (curve a), there is a sharp, discrete reduction in the specific volume. This contraction is due to 'configurational contraction', as there is a large increase in the packing fraction when changing from a disordered liquid to an ordered crystalline solid. Once this sharp contraction has been completed, the material continues to contract by normal thermal contraction.

If crystallization did not occur, the material would follow curve b; the liquid continues to contract, partly by normal thermal contraction and partly by configurational contraction. The liquid takes up a less open structure, but there is no discrete jump in the specific volume. Below T_m, it forms an unstable *supercooled* liquid. This contraction continues as the temperature drops, until T_g, the glass transition temperature, is reached, whereupon the rate of contraction slows down markedly. At this point, the configurational contraction has stopped and only normal thermal contraction is taking place.

What happens at the glass transition temperature is that the supercooled liquid has become so viscous that configurational changes can no longer take place, and the liquid structure has been frozen in. The temperature at which this occurs is not a sharply defined point, but is a range of temperatures of some 50°C, represented by the bend in the curve.

Once the supercooled liquid has cooled to below its glass transition temperature, it is now described as a *glass*. It is interesting to note that the viscosity at which this occurs is roughly the same for all glasses, about 10^{12} Pa.s, although the temperature at which this happens can vary from –89°C for glycerine to over 1500°C for pure silica glass. The distinction between a supercooled liquid and a glass is that the latter has a viscosity greater than 10^{12} Pa.s.

The term *transformation temperature* is somewhat of a misnomer, since no transformation actually occurs at this temperature. The configurational changes are still taking place at temperatures below T_g; it is just that the rate of change is now so small, because of the high viscosity, that to all intents and purposes it has stopped. The glass transition temperature, i.e. the temperature at which a glass that is being cooled effectively ceases to undergo configurational changes, is sometimes referred to as the *fictive temperature* of the glass. It is the temperature below which there is no spontaneous tendency for the glass to become more dense.

The question is: 'What happens at T_m that determines whether the crystal- or glass-forming route is followed?'

When silica melts, it produces an extremely viscous liquid, which means that the molecules can only move past one another very slowly. This is not conducive to the formation of a crystalline solid, since crystallization requires a substantial and rapid rearrangement of the molecules. Any crystal nuclei present will therefore tend to grow very slowly, especially given the complex structure of crystalline silica, which is similar to that of diamond. Thus, if the liquid is cooled quickly, the solid formed is likely to be a glass. The process of forming a glass is called *vitrification*.

Glass formers

The essential component that allows the formation of glass is silica, which can itself become either a glass or a crystalline solid on cooling. Cristobalite, one of the crystalline forms of silica, has a tetrahedron as its basic unit, with an oxygen atom at each corner and a silicon atom in the centre, as shown in Figure 1.3.6.

This is a rather complex structure to use when visualizing the development of a glass, and the formation process can be understood more simply by considering a two-dimensional representation, in which one bond is missing from each of the atoms in the silica (Figure 1.3.7).

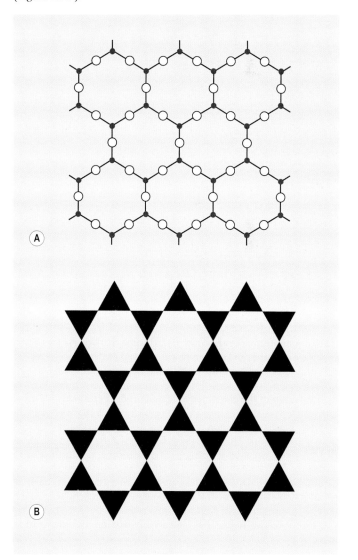

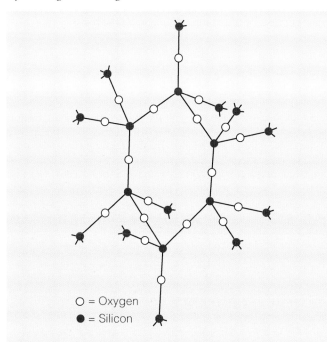

O = Oxygen
● = Silicon

Figure 1.3.6 Crystalline structure of cristobalite

Figure 1.3.7 Two-dimensional representation of crystalline silica: (a) position of atoms, (b) oxygen triangles

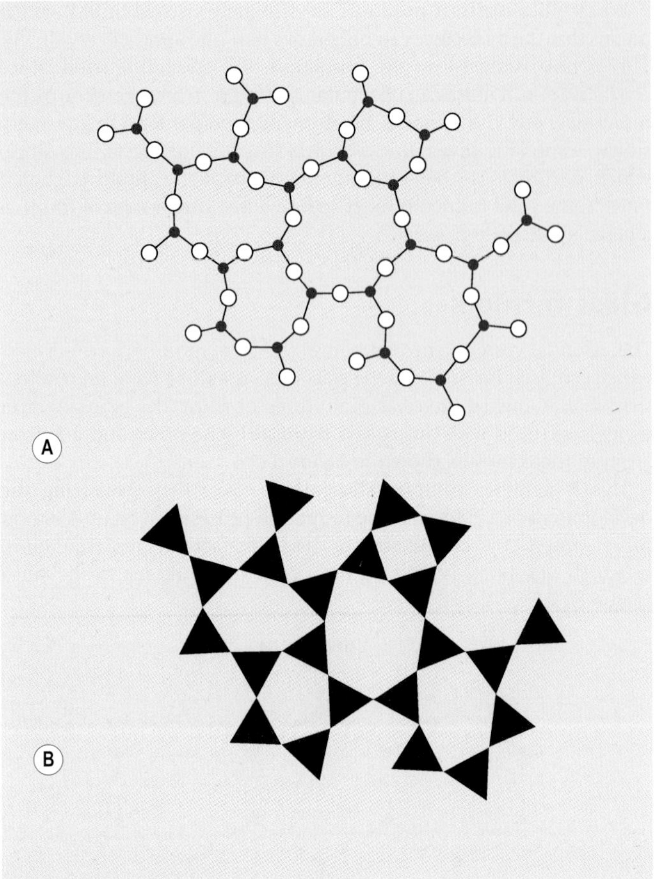

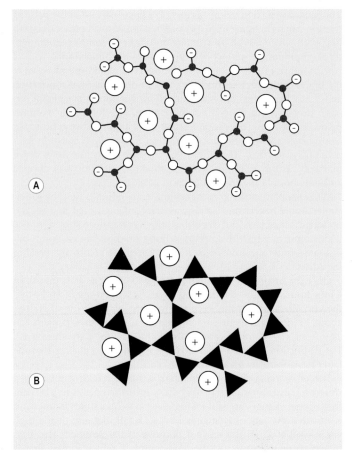

Figure 1.3.8 Two-dimensional representation of a pure silica glass: (a) position of atoms, (b) oxygen triangles

Figure 1.3.9 Two-dimensional representation of a mixed oxide glass: (a) position of atoms, (b) oxygen triangles

When molten silica is cooled rapidly, the crystalline structure does not have time to form so the silica solidifies as a glass, which is called fused quartz (Figure 1.3.8). The high melting point of this material, 1713°C, makes it too expensive for general use. If certain metal oxides are mixed with the silica, the melting temperature is greatly reduced.

As an example, a composition of three-quarters silica and one-quarter sodium oxide will melt at only 1339°C. Such glasses are called *mixed oxide glasses* and their structure is shown in Figure 1.3.9. The metal atoms form positive ions that disrupt the oxygen tetrahedra such that not all of the oxygen atoms are shared. The silica plays the role of a *glass former* and the metal oxide acts as a *glass modifier*.

Oxides of titanium, zinc, lead and aluminium can all take part in the formation of the glassy network, and produce stiff network structures. Soda (Na_2O) and lime (CaO) considerably lower the viscosity, and thus the glass transition temperature, by causing extensive disruption of the network. This eases the production of the glass. Boric oxide (B_2O_3) is also capable of acting as a glass former, producing boron glasses.

Although it is possible to make glasses from mixtures of crystalline silica and metal oxides, this is an expensive approach. It is much cheaper to use naturally occurring minerals with the required glassy structure, because nature has already carried out the vitrification process.

At one time, only naturally occurring feldspars were used by manufacturers, and these were modified with other metallic oxides to produce fillers and dental porcelains with the required properties.

Nowadays, many glasses are produced synthetically, as this allows greater control over the composition and properties.

DEVITRIFICATION

It is possible that a small amount of crystallization will occur in the production of a glass, although the rate of the crystals' growth is very low.

When a glass begins to crystallize, the process is called *devitrification*. It may happen when the glass is kept at an elevated temperature for a long time, allowing some reorganization of the molecules. The glass will tend to take on a translucent appearance, due to the scattering of light from the surfaces of the small crystals. This is the basis of the formation of glass ceramics (see Chapter 3.4).

The process of heating a material to allow molecular or atomic rearrangement is called *annealing* and is important in many types of materials.

CLINICAL SIGNIFICANCE

Ceramics tend to be extremely stable in the biological environment and are therefore perceived as the most biocompatible materials.

Structure of metals and alloys

MICROSTRUCTURE OF METALS

Metals consist of aggregates of atoms regularly arranged in a crystalline structure. Whereas so far we have considered the formation of single crystals, metals will not usually solidify (from what is known as the *melt*) as a single crystal, but instead are formed from a multitude of small crystals.

This happens because there are usually many *nuclei of crystallization* scattered throughout the molten metal. Such nuclei may form when four atoms lose sufficient thermal energy and become able to form a unit cell. These unit cells will grow as more metal atoms reach a low enough energy to join on, and hence crystal formation occurs. This process is known as homogeneous nucleation. It requires highly specialized equipment to grow a single crystal of metal from the entire melt.

More commonly, solidification is initiated by the presence of impurities in the melt. As the temperature drops below the melting point, metal atoms will deposit on these impurities and crystals begin to form. This process is known as heterogeneous nucleation. The crystals (or *grains*, as they are called) will continue to grow until all of the metal has solidified. During their growth, they will begin to impinge on one another, giving rise to boundaries between the crystals where the atoms are irregularly arranged. This boundary is called the *grain boundary*, and is essentially a defect in the crystal structure of the metal.

The process of solidification of a metal is shown schematically in Figure 1.4.1. A fine grain size is usually desirable in a metal because it raises the yield stress, but the reason for this will not be considered now. One way in which to promote a finer grain size is rapid solidification, as used in the casting of dental gold alloys into an investment mould that is held at a temperature well below the melting temperature of the alloy. Alternatively, the presence of many nucleating sites will give rise to a fine grain size. This method is also employed in dental gold alloys by the addition of iridium. The iridium provides many sites for nucleation and acts as a grain-refining ingredient.

It is very useful to be able to study the detailed structure of metals, in terms of the sizes of the crystals, their shape and their composition, because this information can tell us a lot about the properties of the metal and how it was made. Some idea of the structure can be obtained by examining the metal surface under a light-reflecting optical microscope.

Light is reflected from a polished metal surface, but the fraction of the incident light that is reflected from any region will depend on surface irregularities, as irregularities will cause the light to be scattered.

The action of chemicals on a polished surface (known as *etching*) can also reduce the amount of light reflected. A suitably chosen chemical will preferentially attack certain regions of the metal surface. These areas tend to be under high local stress, such as at the grain boundaries, where there is imperfect packing of the atoms. In effect, a groove is produced that will scatter the incident light and therefore show up as a dark line.

This effect is shown schematically in Figure 1.4.2 for a metal which has a very uniform grain structure. All the grains are of roughly the same size and shape; such a grain structure is described as *equiaxed*. An example of the grain structure for a hypo-eutectoid stainless steel, revealed by etching, is shown in Figure 1.4.3. Many other shapes and sizes of grains are possible, and these properties often depend on the methods employed during solidification. For example, if molten metal is poured into a mould with a square or circular cross-section that is held at a temperature well below the melting temperature of the metal, the grains could look something like that depicted in Figure 1.4.4. Crystal growth will have proceeded from the walls of the mould towards the centre.

Many metals are readily deformed, especially in their elemental (i.e. pure) form. This allows them to be shaped by hammering, rolling, pressing or drawing through a die. A large casting, known as an ingot, can thus be turned into any desired shape, be it a wing-panel for a car, the shell of a boat, or a wire.

When deformed in this way, the metal is said to be *wrought*. If we were to examine the microstructure of a wire under the optical microscope, it would be seen to have a structure similar to that shown in Figure 1.4.5. The grains have been elongated in the direction of drawing, and have taken on a laminar structure. Thus, from looking at the microstructure of the metal we can gain a lot of information.

ALLOYS

Elemental metals are not generally of much use because of the severe limitations in their properties. Most metals in common use are a

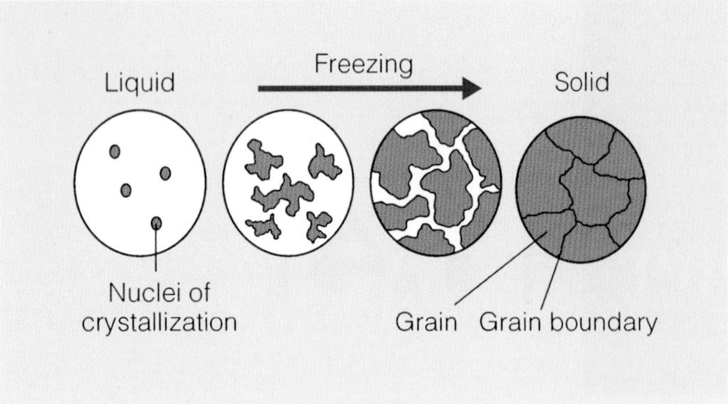

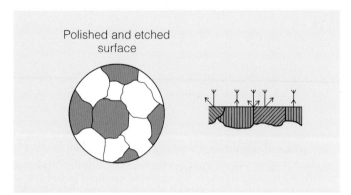

Figure 1.4.1 Solidification of a metal

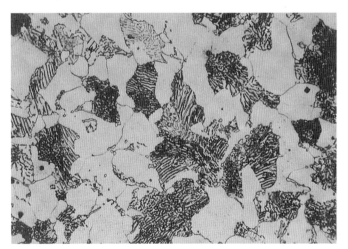

Figure 1.4.2 Reflection of incident light from an etched metal surface

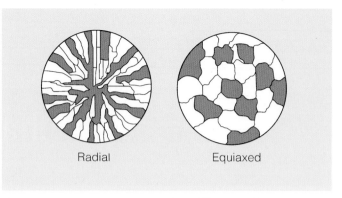

Figure 1.4.4 Grain structures arising from different conditions at solidification

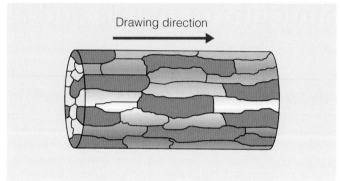

Figure 1.4.5 Elongated grains of a metal drawn into a wire

Figure 1.4.3 Grain structures for hypo-eutectoid stainless steel

mixture of two or more metallic elements, sometimes with non-metallic elements included. They are usually produced by fusion of the elements above their melting temperatures. Such a mixture of two or more metals or metalloids is called an *alloy*. Two elements would constitute a *binary alloy* and a mixture of three is called a *ternary alloy*.

An alloy will often consist of a number of distinct solid phases, where a phase is defined as a structurally homogeneous part of the system that is separated from other parts by a definite physical boundary. Each phase will have its own distinct structure and associated properties.

The commonly cited phases are the gas, liquid and solid phases, as these are markedly different from one another. A substance can exhibit several phases.

For example, water would be considered a single-phase structure, whereas a mixture of water and oil would consist of two phases. Sand would be considered a single-phase system, even though it is made up of lots of individual particles, since each particle of sand is identical.

A phase may have more than one component – as does saline, for instance, which is an aqueous solution of sodium chloride. Similarly, phases in metals can consist of a mixture of metals. Copper can contain up to 40% zinc without destroying its FCC structure. Such a *solid solution*, as it is called, will satisfy some special conditions (see below).

SOLID PHASES

When two different elements are mixed together, the resultant material can be a single-phase alloy or a multi-phase alloy. Which of these is formed depends on the solubility of the one element in the other, and this is governed by the crystalline nature of the elements, and their relative sizes.

There are essentially three different phases which can form in alloys; these are a pure metal, a solid solution or an intermetallic compound. Of these, the solid solution and the intermetallic compound require further description.

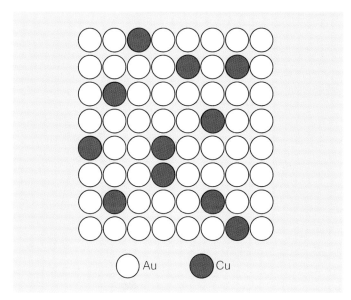

Figure 1.4.6 Substitutional solid solution

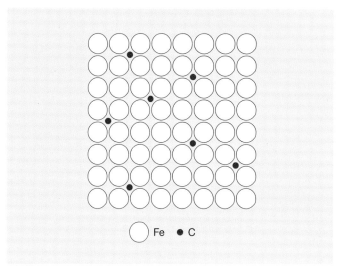

Figure 1.4.7 Interstitial solid solution

Table 1.4.1 Properties of gold and copper

Element	Atomic diameter (Å)	Crystal structure	Valence
Au	2.882	FCC	1 or 3
Cu	2.556	FCC	1 or 2

Solid solutions

A solid solution is a mixture of elements at the atomic level, and is analogous to a mixture of liquids which are soluble in one another. There are two types of solid solutions: substitutional and interstitial.

Substitutional solid solution

If the solute atom can substitute directly for the solvent atom at the normal lattice sites of the crystal, a substitutional solid solution of the two elements will be formed. This will only be possible if:

- the atoms have a similar valency
- the atoms have the same crystal structure (e.g. FCC)
- the atomic sizes are within 15% of each other.

A dentally relevant example of such a system is a mixture of gold and copper (Figure 1.4.6).

Adding any amount of copper will always give a solid solution. Thus, a *substitutional solid solution* can be made to range from 100% gold to 100% copper. This is because these two metals (Table 1.4.1) meet the above conditions.

Other metals that readily form solid solutions with gold are platinum (2.775 Å), palladium (2.750 Å) and silver (2.888 Å), all of which have an FCC crystal structure.

Interstitial solid solution

As the name implies, an interstitial solid solution is achieved when the solute atoms are able to take up the space in between the solvent atoms. For this to occur, the solute atom must, of course, be much smaller than the solvent atom. In practice, the diameter of the solute atom must be less than 60% of the diameter of the solvent atom. This is illustrated for the example of a type of steel that contains a small amount of carbon in iron (Figure 1.4.7).

The interstitial space is usually very limited, and some distortion of the lattice will occur to accommodate the extra atoms. Other elements that readily form interstitial solid solutions are hydrogen, nitrogen and boron.

Intermetallic compounds

An intermetallic compound is formed when two or more metals combine, forming a specific composition or stoichiometric ratio. Examples of metals with specific stoichiometric compositions are some of the phases in the alloy used in the production of a dental amalgam; the alloy may contain regions of an Ag–Sn phase (Ag_3Sn), and a Cu–Sn phase (Cu_6Sn_5).

PHASE DIAGRAMS

Alloys can consist of a wide number of different phases, depending on the composition and temperature, and a means of representing this graphically has been developed, in what is known as a *phase diagram*.

Such a diagram indicates the phases (including the liquid phase) that are present at any given temperature, for any given composition of the alloy.

Solid solutions

The simplest phase diagrams to understand are the binary phase diagrams.

An example of a phase diagram for such a simple system is shown in Figure 1.4.8. This phase diagram is for copper and nickel; the vertical axis represents the temperature and the horizontal axis the composition. Copper and nickel are so close in characteristics that they readily substitute for one another in the crystal lattice, and form an example of a substitutional solid solution. Hence, throughout the compositional range from pure copper to pure nickel, only a single phase occurs.

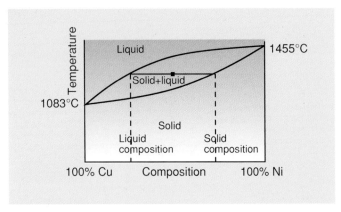

Figure 1.4.8 Equilibrium phase diagram for the Cu–Ni system, where a 50Cu : 50Ni composition at 1300°C produces a mixture of a copper-rich liquid and a nickel-rich solid

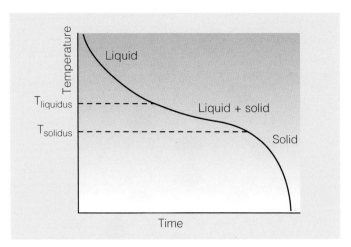

Figure 1.4.10 Cooling curve for an alloy

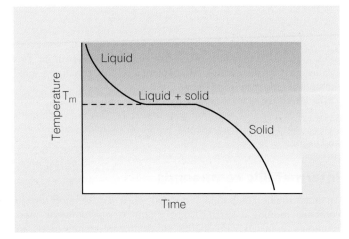

Figure 1.4.9 Cooling curve for a pure metal

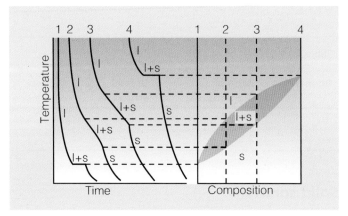

Figure 1.4.11 Construction of a phase diagram

Whereas one might expect the melting temperature of such an alloy to fall somewhere between that of pure copper and pure nickel, it is not immediately obvious why there should be a region where there is a mixture of liquid and solid. The line which defines the transition from pure liquid to a mixture of liquid and solid is called the *liquidus*, and the line which separates the mixture of solid and liquid from the solid is known as the *solidus*.

When a pure metal solidifies, the transformation from a liquid to solid takes place at a well-defined discrete temperature; this is the characteristic melting temperature of the metal. If a temperature–time curve were constructed for such a metal as it cooled, it would look like Figure 1.4.9.

The plateau spans the period during which the metal is solidifying, and the liquidus and solidus are effectively one and the same point. The reason for this plateau is the release of energy (in the form of heat) during the solidification process, which maintains the metal at a constant temperature. This energy is called the *latent heat of fusion*.

When two metals are mixed to form an alloy, the cooling curve looks quite different (Figure 1.4.10), as the alloy solidifies over a range of temperatures. The liquidus and solidus are now separate points on the cooling curve.

The reason for the extended temperature range, covering the transition from liquid to solid for an alloy of copper and nickel, is that the copper and nickel atoms are not identical. As a consequence, in the region between the melting temperatures of the two metals, a copper-rich liquid and a nickel-rich solid are the most stable compounds.

For instance, for a 50:50 composition at 1300°C, solid nickel cannot contain more than 37 w% copper. Any copper atoms above the 37 w% level will therefore appear in the liquid phase, mixed with the remaining nickel. Such a mixture of solid and liquid provides a lower free energy than a single phase alone.

In effect, the solidus and liquidus represent the limits of solubility, and it is these that form the basis of the phase diagram. By creating a series of the cooling curves shown in Figures 1.4.9 and 1.4.10 for a range of compositions, it is possible to build up the phase diagram as shown schematically in Figure 1.4.11.

As the temperature of the 50:50 composition is reduced, so the solubility of copper in nickel increases, until, at approximately 1220°C, all of the available copper can be dissolved in the nickel, and a single solid phase is the most stable configuration.

Partial solid solubility

More usually, the components of materials are not sufficiently soluble to form a complete series of solid solutions. Examples of this are copper and silver, which are sufficiently different in atomic size that their atoms are only partially soluble in one another.

The phase diagram for this system is shown in Figure 1.4.12. For a wide range of compositions, the material will consist of two solid

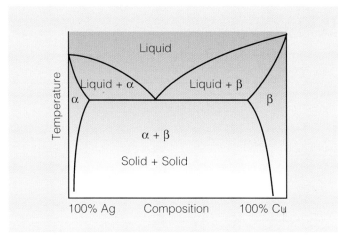

Figure 1.4.12 Equilibrium phase diagram for the Ag–Cu system

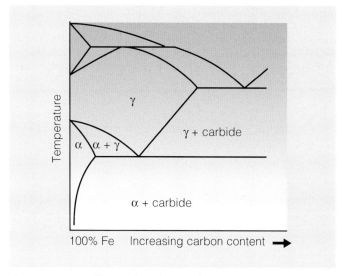

Figure 1.4.13 Equilibrium phase diagram for the Fe–Cu system

phases, one being silver-rich and one being copper-rich; by convention, these are called the α- and the β-phase, respectively. The α-phase consists of predominantly silver, with a small amount of copper dissolved in it, whereas the β-phase consists of copper, with a small amount of silver dissolved in it.

At low concentrations of copper in silver, all of the copper is able to dissolve in the silver, and only a single phase exists. The maximum solubility of copper in silver is 8.8 w%, and this occurs at a temperature of approximately 780°C.

At lower temperatures, the solubility of copper in silver decreases, and the excess copper separates out as the second, β-phase.

Similar behaviour occurs at the other end of the compositional range, where the limited solubility of silver in copper also gives rise to the formation of a two-phase structure.

An interesting and important feature of the phase diagram of the Ag–Cu system is the depression of the temperature of the liquidus at a composition of 72Ag : 28Cu. At a temperature of 780°C, this composition of the alloy can exist as three phases: α, β and liquid. This is called the *eutectic point*, and the temperature at the intersection of the three phases is the *eutectic temperature*. The composition is called the *eutectic composition* of the alloy.

If a eutectic liquid is cooled, it changes directly into two solid phases, without an interposing state as a liquid–solid mixture, something that occurs at all other compositions. This feature of some alloy systems can be utilized to form low melting temperature materials, such as solders.

In the same way that a eutectic involves the formation of two solid phases from a single liquid phase, such a transformation can also occur in solids.

The phase diagram of the Fe–C system, shown partially in Figure 1.4.13, is an example of this. For a composition of 0.8C : 99.2Fe, the solid solution, γ, transforms to a solid solution of carbon in iron, α, and carbide (Fe_3C) at a temperature of 723°C. This is called a *eutectoid reaction*, and differs only from the eutectic in that all three phases are solids.

Such transformations as described (and it should be noted that there are others) are extremely important in determining the microstructure and, consequently, the properties of the alloy.

NON-EQUILIBRIUM CONDITIONS

It must be stressed that the phase diagrams described above are what are known as *equilibrium phase diagrams*. The material would have to

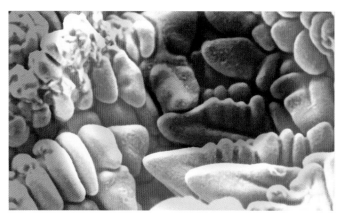

Figure 1.4.14 Scanning electron microscope (SEM) micrograph of the coarse dendritic structure for a CO–Cr alloy

be held at a set temperature for a considerable time to achieve the phase structure shown in such diagrams. In practice, the solidification and cooling rates of alloys do not allow the formation of an equilibrium phase structure.

Above, it was noted that, for a composition of 50Cu : 50Ni at 1300°C, a liquid phase rich in copper and a solid phase consisting of 63Ni : 37Cu coexist. On rapid cooling, it is not possible for these liquid and solid phases to readjust their compositions, and some of the nickel-rich solid will be retained. As the material continues to cool, so a composition richer in nickel will solidify, leaving the remaining liquid, and the subsequently formed solid, richer in copper. The overall effect of this is that the solid will consist of a multitude of crystals with a wide range of compositions, all in the same phase. This formation of a solid with a non-uniform composition is known as *compositional segregation*.

In systems with multiple phases, the phase with the highest melting temperature will always be the first to solidify, followed by the phases with lower melting temperatures. As the first phase solidifies, it tends to form a lattice structure known as *dendrites* (Figure 1.4.14).

Compositional segregation can be eliminated, or reduced, by reheating the alloy to a temperature just below the solidus and holding it at that temperature for some time. This allows the atoms time to diffuse through the system and attain their equilibrium condition.

The process of heat-treating an alloy is known as *annealing,* and if the intention is to achieve a homogeneous composition, it is described as a *homogenization anneal.*

CLINICAL SIGNIFICANCE

In order to obtain the best mechanical properties, alloys rather than pure metals are used in dentistry.

Structure of polymers

INTRODUCTION

Plastics and rubbers, as they are generally called in everyday life, have the common property of being *polymers*. Polymers are long-chain molecules, consisting of many repeating units, as discussed already in Chapter 1.2. Polymers are not a 20th-century invention; they are, in fact, older than human beings themselves, and in one form or another are the basic constituents of every kind of living matter, whether plant or animal.

Examples of naturally occurring polymers are agar, cellulose, DNA, proteins, natural rubber, collagen and silk.

It is only relatively recently that we have begun to understand the structure of polymers and how to make them ourselves. Some examples of synthetic polymers, which are now everyday household names, are PVC (polyvinyl chloride), polyethylene, nylon and polystyrene.

Originally, the synthetic polymers tended to be regarded as substitutes for existing natural polymers, such as rubber and silk. Nowadays, such a wide variety of polymers can be produced that they have entered into every walk of life, satisfying needs that did not previously exist. Pertinent examples are medical applications, such as dialysis and oxygenator membranes, and dental applications such as filling materials.

The starting material for the production of a polymer is the *monomer*. In a material such as polyethylene, the repeating unit is a CH_2 group, with many of these units joined together to form a long chain (Figure 1.5.1a). The monomer from which this polymer is derived is ethylene (Figure 1.5.1b).

A polymer with a similar structure to polyethylene is polypropylene. It is formed by joining molecules of propylene (Figure 1.5.2a). Propylene differs from ethylene in having a methyl group (CH_3) that replaces one of the hydrogen atoms, forming the polymer polypropylene (Figure 1.5.2b).

Polypropylene is slightly more complex than polyethylene, in that the arrangement of the methyl groups can vary so that they:

- are all on one side (*isotactic*)
- alternate from side to side (*syndiotactic*)
- are switched from side to side in a random manner (*atactic*).

A number of polymers based on vinyl monomers are presented in Table 1.5.1.

It should be noted that the chemical routes by which these different polymers are made are quite different, and that it is not a simple matter of modification to form one from the other. Each polymer has its own characteristic repeating unit, or 'fingerprint', and this unit is the basis for the widely differing properties of the polymers.

The most common polymers are those made from the organic compounds of carbon, but polymers can also be made from inorganic compounds, based on silica (SiO_2).

Silicon, being four-valent like carbon, provides the opportunity to form the backbone for the polymer, together with oxygen. An example of a silicone polymer is polydimethylsiloxane (Figure 1.5.3).

When a polymer is formed from a single species of monomer, it is called a *homopolymer*; when different species are included, it is called a *heteropolymer*.

MECHANISMS OF POLYMERIZATION

The monomers shown in Table 1.5.1 all have a double bond in common, which is opened up to allow the monomer to bond to a neighbouring monomer. This process of preparing polymers from monomers is called *polymerization*. There are two ways in which this may be achieved: *addition* and *condensation*.

Addition polymerization

Addition polymerization is defined as occurring when a reaction between two molecules (either the same to form a *homopolymer*, or dissimilar to form a *heteropolymer*) produces a larger molecule without the elimination of a smaller molecule (such as water).

This type of reaction takes place for vinyl compounds, which are reactive inorganic compounds containing carbon–carbon double bonds (see Table 1.5.1). The process of addition polymerization involves four stages to produce these polymers:

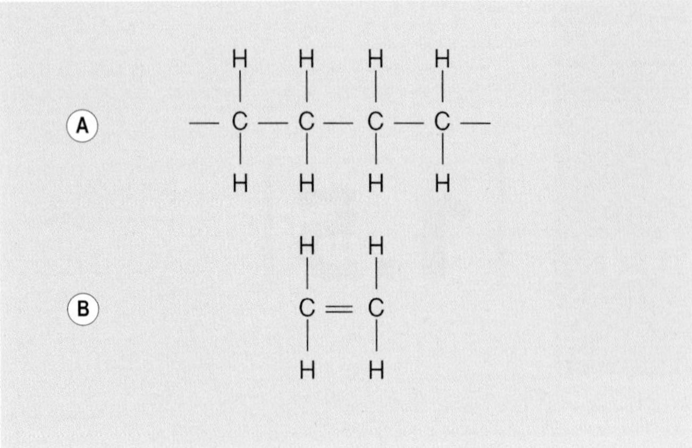

Figure 1.5.1 Polyethylene (a) is derived from ethylene (b)

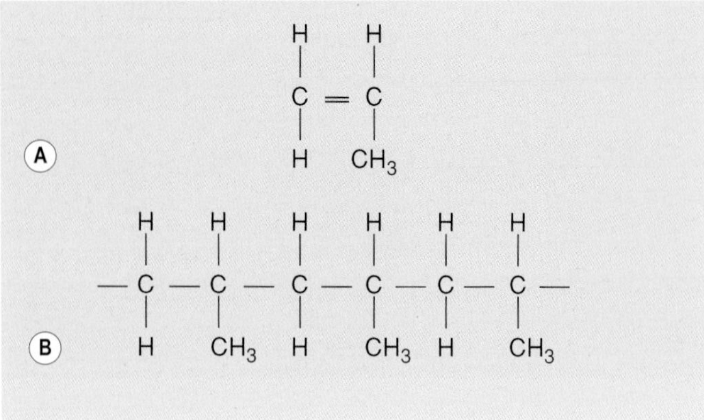

Figure 1.5.2 Propylene (a) polymerizes to give polypropylene (b)

Table 1.5.1 Some monomers and their polymers

Name	Monomer	Polymer
Polyvinyl chloride (PVC)	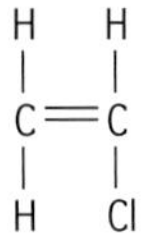	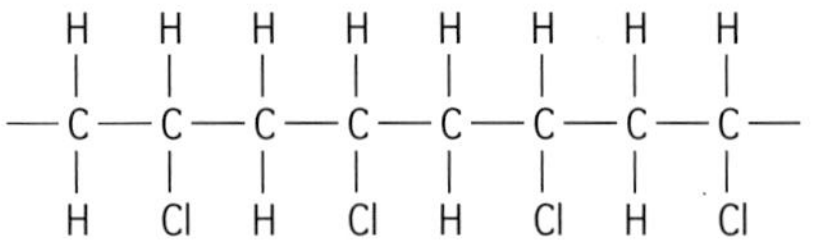
Polytetrafluoroethylene (PTFE)	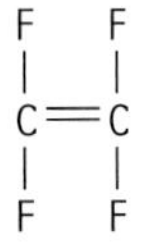	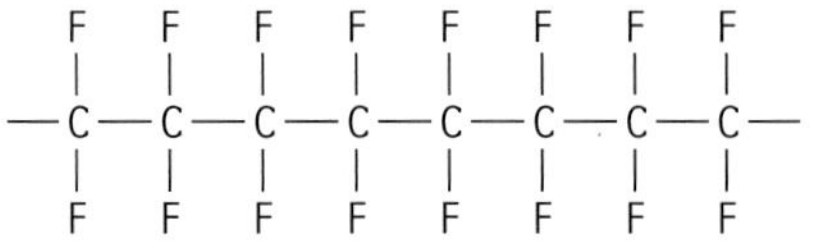
Polypropylene isotactic	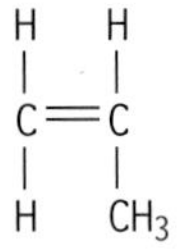	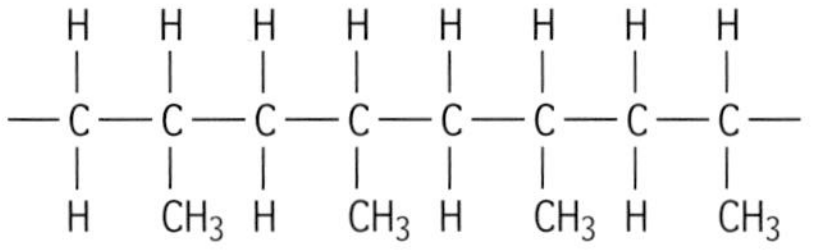
Polyacrylic acid	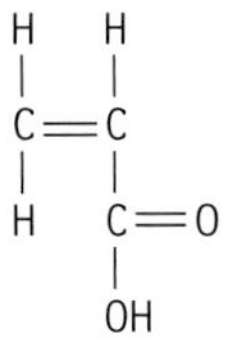	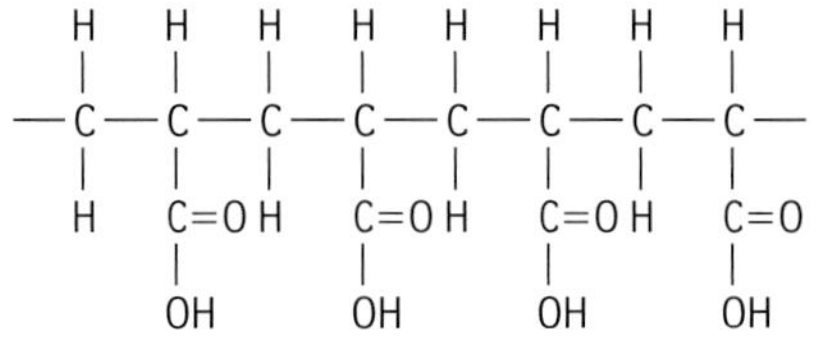
Polymethylmethacrylate	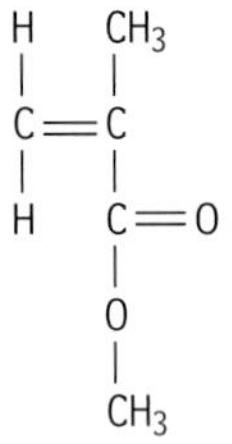	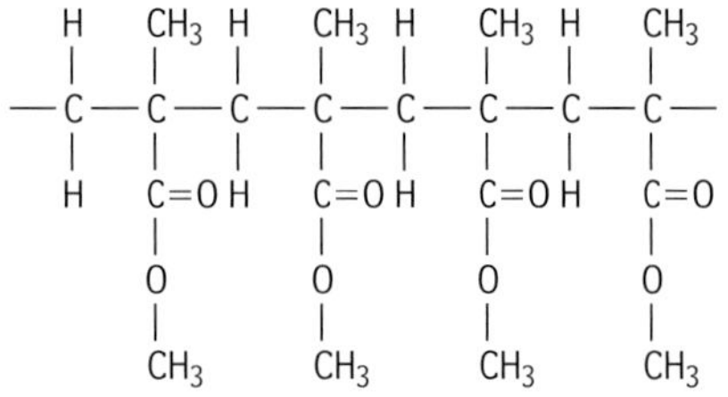

- activation
- initiation
- propagation
- termination.

Activation

The polymerization of a vinyl compound requires the presence of *free radicals* (•). These are very reactive chemical species that have an odd (unpaired) electron. The process of producing free radicals is described as *activation*. Activation occurs, for instance, in the decomposition of a peroxide.

The peroxide commonly used in dental materials is benzoyl peroxide. Under appropriate conditions, a molecule of benzoyl peroxide can yield two free radicals:

$$C_6H_5COO-OOCH_5C_6 \rightarrow 2(C_6H_5COO\bullet)$$

This in turn can decompose to form other free radicals:

$$C_6H_5COO\bullet \rightarrow C_6H_5\bullet + CO_2$$

Such chemical species, known as *initiators,* are able to initiate vinyl polymerization, as described later, and are designated as R•.

Before initiation occurs, however, the benzoyl peroxide needs to be activated. This activation is achieved by the decomposition of the peroxide, due to the use of an *activator,* such as:

- *Heat.* When heated above 65°C, the benzoyl peroxide decomposes, as shown above. This is the method used in the production of acrylic resin denture bases (see Chapter 3.2).
- *Chemical compounds.* The benzoyl peroxide can also be activated when brought into contact with a tertiary amine such as *n,n*-dimethyl-*p*-toluidine (Figure 1.5.4). This method is employed in cold-cured acrylic resins, used, for example, in denture repairs, temporary restorations, orthodontic appliances and special trays (see Chapter 3.2). The same method is also used in chemically cured composite restorative materials, which consist of a base paste containing the tertiary amine activator and a catalyst paste containing the benzoyl peroxide initiator (see Chapter 2.2).

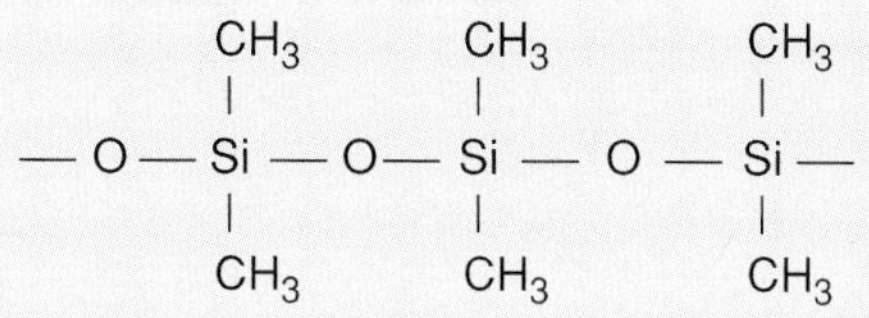

CH₃ ... CH₃ ... CH₃

— O — Si — O — Si — O — Si —

CH₃ ... CH₃ ... CH₃

Figure 1.5.3 The structure of polydimethylsiloxane

- *Light.* Yet another method for the creation of free radicals is employed by light-activated composites; these rely on either ultraviolet light or visible light as the activator of the polymerization reaction. In these instances, other initiators than benzoyl peroxide are employed.

Other forms of free radical production include the use of ultraviolet light in conjunction with a benzoin methyl ether, and visible light with an α-diketone and an amine (see Chapter 2.2).

Initiation

The free radicals can react with a monomer such as ethylene and *initiate* the polymerization process as follows:

$$R\bullet + \underset{\overset{|}{H}}{\overset{\overset{H}{|}}{C}} = \underset{\overset{|}{H}}{\overset{\overset{H}{|}}{C}} \rightarrow R - \underset{\overset{|}{H}}{\overset{\overset{H}{|}}{C}} - \underset{\overset{|}{H}}{\overset{\overset{H}{|}}{C}}\bullet$$

Propagation

The free radical is transferred to the monomer, which can, in turn, react with another monomer:

$$R - \underset{H}{\overset{H}{C}} - \underset{H}{\overset{H}{C}}\bullet + \underset{H}{\overset{H}{C}} = \underset{H}{\overset{H}{C}} \rightarrow R - \underset{H}{\overset{H}{C}} - \underset{H}{\overset{H}{C}} - \underset{H}{\overset{H}{C}} - \underset{H}{\overset{H}{C}}\bullet$$

Repeating this process again and again generates the polymer chain until the growing chains collide or all of the free radicals have reacted.

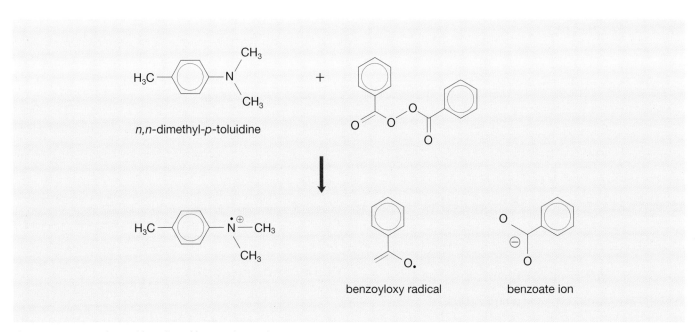

Figure 1.5.4 Benzoyl peroxide activated by a tertiary amine

n,n-dimethyl-*p*-toluidine

benzoyloxy radical

benzoate ion

Termination

Free radicals can react to form a stable molecule:

$$\text{R—C—C}\bullet + \text{R}\bullet \rightarrow \text{R—C—R}$$

Since n will vary from polymer chain to polymer chain, a wide range of long-chain molecules are produced. In most situations, there will also be some unreacted monomer and some *oligomers*, which consist of just a few repeating units.

Condensation polymerization

Condensation polymerization occurs when two molecules (not usually the same) react to form a larger molecule with the elimination of a smaller molecule (often, but not always, water).

In this case, monomer units with a carbon–carbon double bond are not necessary, as shown in the following example of a silicone, which is an inorganic polymer formed by the condensation of silanols:

$$\text{HO—Si—OH} + \text{HO—Si—OH} \rightarrow$$

$$\text{HO—Si—O—Si—OH} + H_2O$$

In this case, R is an organic group, such as a methyl (CH_3), and the by-product is water.

POLYMERIC STRUCTURES

Molecular weight

The molecular weight of a polymer is equal to the number of repeating units (i.e. the *degree of polymerization*) multiplied by the molecular weight of the repeating unit. In both addition and condensation polymerization, the length of the chain is determined by purely random events; not all of the chains will be of the same length and, in general, many different chain lengths will be present. Thus, the molecular weight can only be represented by an average value.

There are a number of ways in which the molecular weight can be determined for a polymer. Two main ones are the *number average molecular weight*, M_n, and the *weight average molecular weight*, M_w.

Number average molecular weight (M_n)

M_n is obtained by counting the number of molecules in a given weight of sample. The general expression would be given by:

$$M_n = \Sigma n_i M_i / X n_i$$

Weight average molecular weight (M_w)

M_w is obtained by measurement of the weight of the molecules in the total sample weight, given by the general expression:

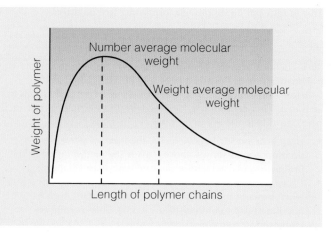

Figure 1.5.5 The molecular weight distribution of a typical polymer

$$M_w = \Sigma w_i M_i / w_i$$

The difference in the definitions for a distribution of molecular weights in a typical polymer is shown in Figure 1.5.5. M_w is particularly sensitive to the presence of high-molecular-weight polymers, while M_n is sensitive to the presence of low-molecular-weight polymers. For example, if equal weights of two polymers of $M_a = 10\,000$ and $M_b = 100\,000$ are mixed, M_w is given by:

$$M_w = (w_a \times M_a + w_b \times M_b)/(w_a + w_b)$$

where w_a and w_b are the weights of M_a and M_b respectively.

In this case, w_a and w_b are equal to $\frac{1}{2}W$, as $M_a = 10\,000$ and $M_b = 100\,000$. Substituting these values in the above expression gives:

$$M_w = (\tfrac{1}{2}W \times 10\,000 + \tfrac{1}{2}W \times 100\,000)/W$$
$$= 55\,000$$

The number average molecular weight is given by:

$$M_n = (n_a \times M_a + m_b \times M_b)/(n_a + m_b)$$

where n_a and m_b are the number of molecules of molecular weight M_a and M_b respectively. In this case, $n_a = 10$ and $m_b = 1$, such that:

$$M_n = (10 \times 10\,000 + 1 \times 100\,000)/11$$
$$= 18\,200$$

The molecular weight of a polymer is of great value in explaining the variations in the physical properties of different polymers. For example, the tensile strength and the elongation required to break the polymer increase steeply for some polymers in the molecular weight range of 50\,000–200\,000.

However, improving the physical properties by increasing the molecular weight is accompanied by a rapid increase in viscosity of the melt, and this raises the glass transition temperature, making it more difficult for the polymer to be processed.

Chain configurations

Polymer chains are held together by weak secondary (or van der Waals) bonds, and by entanglement of the chains if they are sufficiently long. The higher the molecular weight, the more entanglements there will be, giving a stiffer and stronger polymer.

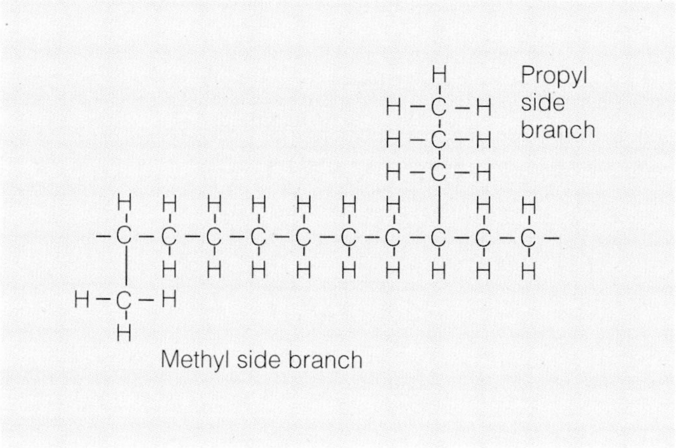

H

H − C − H   Propyl

H − C − H   side

H − C − H   branch

Methyl side branch

Figure 1.5.6 Branched polyethylene

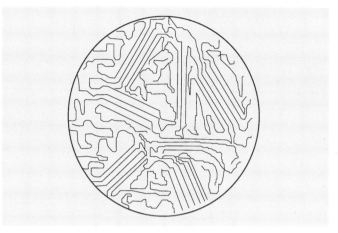

Figure 1.5.7 Partial crystallinity in a polymer

In a polymer such as polyethylene, which has a linear chain configuration, the weak bonds between the chains can easily be broken by increasing the temperature of the polymer. When this happens, the chains can flow past one another so that the polymer softens and readily deforms.

On cooling, the bonds are re-established, and the polymer becomes hard again, retaining the shape it was in at the higher temperature.

The temperature at which a plastic softens such that the molecules can begin to flow is defined as its *glass transition temperature*. These temperatures are similar to those for glasses, except that the temperatures involved are much lower in the case of plastics (see Chapter 1.3).

A polymer that can be softened and subsequently shaped by heating it above its glass transition temperature is known as a *thermoplastic polymer*. Examples of such thermoplastic polymers are polystyrene, polymethyl methacrylate and polyethylene.

For some versions of polyethylene such as low density polyethylene the chains are not linear but are branched (Figure 1.5.6). These branches give the polymer a three-dimensional network structure, which prevents the chains from moving past each other easily, even when heated. Thus, the polymer will retain its properties up to reasonably high temperatures, until chemical breakdown of the polymer structure occurs.

Polymers that decompose on heating without showing a glass transition are known as *thermosetting polymers*.

Crystallinity in polymers

In a polymer the molecules usually twist and turn, coil up and crisscross in a random fashion. Sometimes, however, there will be zones where the molecules are able to lie more or less parallel to each other, as shown in Figure 1.5.7. When this happens, the polymer exhibits a limited degree of crystallinity.

The relative proportions of crystalline and non-crystalline regions in a polymer will depend on the chemical composition, the molecular configuration and the method of processing. These polymers are not wholly crystalline solids, but are composed of a large number of small crystalline regions in close proximity to one another, in an amorphous matrix.

Polyethylene is able to crystallize because of the regularity and simplicity of its polymer chain. As polymer molecules become more complex (whether due to branching or large side groups that restrict the motion of the chain), so it becomes more difficult for them to have crystalline regions.

Cross-linking

When polymer chains are joined together by chemical bonds, the polymer is said to be *cross-linked*. As noted above, cross-linking has a profound effect on the properties of a polymer; it can make the difference between a thermoplastic polymer and a thermosetting polymer. More importantly, it can convert a liquid polymer into a solid polymer, a process used in the setting of many impression materials.

Silicone polymers have a glass transition temperature below room temperature, and therefore are liquids at and above this temperature. When these polymers are cross-linked, the chains are no longer able to slide past each other, and a solid material is obtained. Extensive cross-linking in polymers results in hard, brittle materials.

If the polymer consists of particularly long and flexible molecular chains, there may be cross-linking at several points along their lengths. The molecules can take up a highly coiled configuration when relaxed, and can stretch over long distances (by uncoiling) when stress is applied. When the stress is removed, the chains will again take up their coiled configuration, governed by the cross-links. The amount of extension and the stress that can be borne by such a polymer depends on the lengths of the chains, the degree of cross-linking, and the strength of the bonds.

Materials that show the ability to stretch by large amounts, even to many times their original length, are known as *elastomers*. The characteristic features of an elastomer are that:

- the material is soft and has a low elastic modulus
- very high strains (>100%) are possible
- the strains are reversible
- the material is above its glass transition temperature.

The various polymer chain configurations for polymers are shown in Figure 1.5.8.

COMPOSITION OF REAL POLYMERS

Polymers are very rarely used in their pure form, for the same reasons that pure metals are rarely used in comparison to alloys. Instead, modifications are carried out in order to improve the properties of the polymers.

One such modification that has already been considered is the cross-linking of polymer chains, to form thermosetting polymers from thermoplastic polymers. As thermosetting polymers cannot be

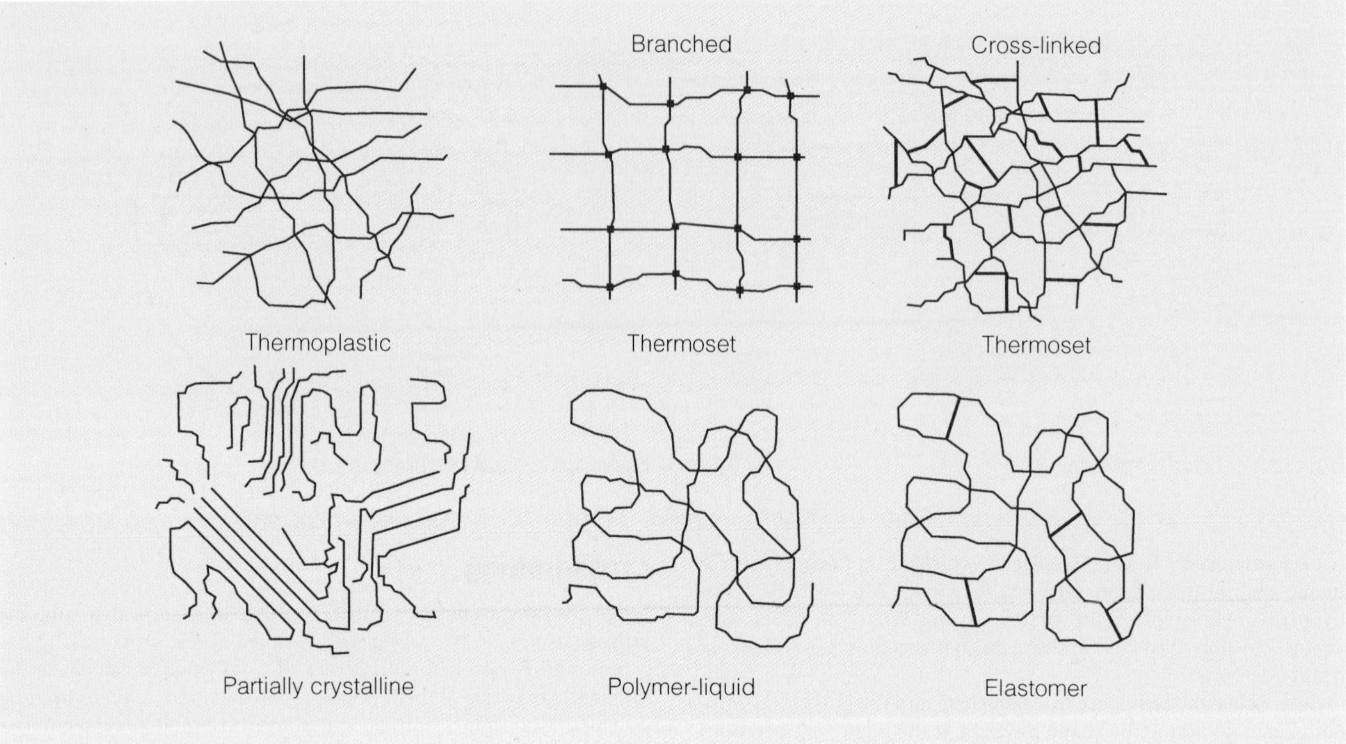

Figure 1.5.8 Polymer chain arrangements

softened and reshaped, the shape of the object has to be created before cross-linking, and this places serious constraints on the means of processing. However, various other processing options are available, such as blending, and the use of copolymers and composites.

Blending

Blending is a process commonly used in the processing of thermoplastic polymers and involves mixing two or more polymers prior to moulding. The properties of the blended polymer will usually lie somewhere between those of the constituent polymers.

As the polymers have to be miscible (i.e. able to mix freely with one another), they tend to be of a similar chemical composition. This places a limit on the changes in properties that are possible by the blending process.

Copolymers

An alternative to blending is the mixing of two polymer-producing systems during the polymerization process; this is *copolymerization*.

For example, if monomer A and monomer B are mixed prior to polymerization they will *copolymerize* to form polymer chains consisting of both A and B monomer units. The sequence of the original monomers in the polymer may be random, producing a *random copolymer*, giving a sequence such as:

$$—A—A—A—A—B—B—A—B—A—B$$
$$—B—B—A—A—B—B—A—B—$$

If the monomers self-polymerize more readily than they copolymerize, what will result is a *block copolymer*, where segments of each homopolymer are linked:

$$—A—A—A—B—B—B—B$$
$$—A—A—A—B—B—B—$$

Such systems can produce polymers with properties that are quite different from the homopolymers. For example, one polymer may be quite rigid, while the other is very flexible. Producing a block copolymer would allow one to control the degree of flexibility of the final material by controlling the length of the blocks and the relative amounts of each polymer.

An example of a block copolymer is ABS (acrylonitrile butadiene styrene), which is formed from a mixture of three polymers. The acrylonitrile and styrene copolymerize to form a glassy block copolymer, while the butadiene forms spherical rubbery regions bonded to the rigid polymer matrix. Although this material has a lower stiffness and creep resistance than polystyrene, it is much tougher, to the extent that it has been considered for the manufacture of car body parts.

Plasticizers

If a low-molecular-weight substance is added to a polymer, it has the effect of lowering the glass transition temperature and the elastic modulus of the material. These plasticizers reduce the forces of attraction between the polymer chains, so the chains become more flexible, and begin to flow past one another at a lower temperature, which accounts for the reduction in T_g.

If enough plasticizer is added, a brittle polymer can be transformed into a soft, flexible and tough polymer.

Plasticizers are usually added to polymers to improve their flow (and hence their processability), and to reduce the brittleness of the product. An example is PVC, which is a very rigid polymer in its pure form, but can be formed into flexible tubing after the addition of plasticizer.

The basic requirement to be met by a plasticizer is that it must be compatible with the polymer, and have a permanent effect. Compatibility means that the plasticizer must be miscible in the polymer, and this implies the need for a similarity in the molecular forces active in the polymer and plasticizer.

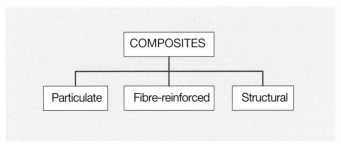

Figure 1.5.9 Classification scheme for composite materials
(Adapted from Callister WD, Materials Science and Engineering: An Introduction. John Wiley & Sons Inc, New York, USA 1994)

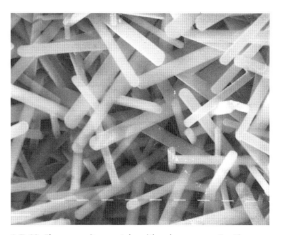

Figure 1.5.10 Fluorcanasite crystals with a large aspect ratio

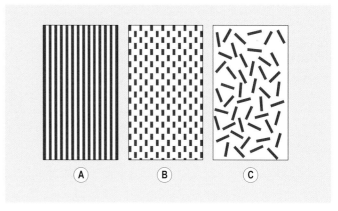

Figure 1.5.11 Schematic representation of fibre-reinforced structures: (a) continuous fibres, (b) short aligned fibres and (c) randomly distributed short fibres

For a plasticizer to be permanent and not easily leached out of the material, it must have a low vapour pressure and a low diffusion rate through the polymer.

A dental example of the use of a plasticizer, is when dibutyl pthalate is mixed with polymethyl or polyethyl methacrylate for the production of soft liners for dentures (see Chapter 3.2).

Composites

A composite may be defined as a combination of materials in which the individual components retain their physical identity. More importantly, a composite material is a multiphase material that exhibits properties of the constituent phases in such a way as to produce a material with a better combination of properties than could be realized by any of the component phases.

In two component composites, it is usual to refer to the *matrix* and the *filler*, the former being the component that binds the filler together. Enamel and dentine are excellent examples of composite structures, being made up of an organic matrix (collagen, proteins, water) and an inorganic filler (hydroxyapatite).

A wide variety of different composite structures can be created, as indicated in the simple classification scheme shown in Figure 1.5.9. In particulate composites, the matrix may be a thermoplastic or a thermosetting polymer. The filler particles may be present simply to reduce the cost, or may be used to perform a specific role, such as to impart colour to an otherwise clear polymer. Their most crucial function, however, is when they are used to improve the mechanical properties of the polymer. For instance, the inclusion of glass in a polymer increases the stiffness, and sometimes increases the strength. The flow properties of elastomeric impression materials are to a large extent controlled by the amount of filler that is included.

The shape and distribution of the filler play an important role in the way the properties are modified. Besides particulate fillers, it is also possible to incorporate fibres or whiskers. The incorporation of fibres in a polymer matrix can have a profound effect on the properties of the resultant composite. Significant improvements in strength and stiffness, while retaining a low weight, can be achieved by the judicious use of fibre reinforcement. Whiskers are very thin crystals that have extremely large length-to-diameter ratios, as is the case with the example of a fluorcanasite structure shown in Figure 1.5.10. Typical tensile strength values for whiskers and fibres are provided in Table 1.5.2. The fibres may be short or long and can be distributed in a number of different ways in the resin matrix, depending on the sorts of properties required (Figure 1.5.11). An example of a structural composite is a material composed of sheets of material stacked one on top of the other, where each sheet may have fibres aligned in a certain direction. This can produce materials that have high strength properties in a multitude of directions (Figure 1.5.12).

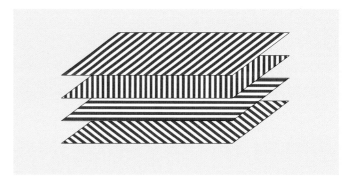

Figure 1.5.12 Laminate structure with sheets of fibre-reinforced resin placed on top of each other in different directions

Table 1.5.2 Tensile strength of fibres and whiskers

Material	Type	Tensile strength (MPa)
Graphite	Whisker	20 000
Silicon carbide	Whisker	20 000
Aluminium oxide	Whisker	14 000–28 000
E-glass	Fibre	3500
Carbon	Fibre	1500–5500
Aramid (Kevlar 49)	Fibre	3500

In dentistry, particulate fillers are most common, with two of their many important applications being in the use of impression materials and resin-based composite restorative materials. The latest developments seek to explore the use of nanotechnology (scale of 1 billionth of a metre), where nanoparticulate fillers are added to resins to improve their properties. There is a growing interest in the dental application of composite materials, not only as a filling material (see Chapter 2.2), but also in the construction of fibre-reinforced resin bridges and endodontic posts (see Chapter 2.7).

CLINICAL SIGNIFICANCE

Polymers are highly versatile materials in that they can be solid or liquid, and brittle or flexible at body temperature, depending on their composition and configuration.

FURTHER READING

Suzuki S (2004) In vitro wear of nano-composite denture teeth. J Prosthodont **13**: 238–243

Xu HH, Eichmiller FC, Smith DT et al (2002) Effect of thermal cycling on whisker-reinforced dental resin composites. J Mater Sci Mater Med **13**: 875–883

Chapter | 1.6 |

Mechanical properties

INTRODUCTION

When one stretches a steel wire or a rubber band, the responses of the materials are quite different. The steel wire will hardly appear to change; although it will become longer, this change is normally so small that it is difficult to perceive. On the other hand, the rubber band will stretch quite readily, and can virtually double in length. Obviously, different materials respond quite differently to the application of a load.

We could make a component and determine its response to an external loading. However, the data collected would be applicable only to that component, and would not allow us to predict the behaviour of a differently shaped component that was made from the same material.

How are we to compare the performances of materials in different applications? Obviously, we need some objective standard of comparison that is independent of the size and shape of the material. Once we have such a standard, it should be possible to compare the properties of different materials, and to predict the behaviour of objects made from them.

The bases for such an objective standard are the quantities called *stress* and *strain*. The description of the mechanical properties of materials is based on these, so we shall now consider them in some detail.

STRESS AND STRAIN

The simplest approach to understanding stress and strain is to consider a rod of material that is held under tension by being subjected to a *tensile force*, or *load*. As shown in Figure 1.6.1, the rod will extend.

Naturally, one would expect the rod to fail (i.e. to snap or to deform irreversibly) under a high enough load. The load at which failure occurs is a measure of the strength of the rod, but it is particular to a rod of those specific dimensions and specific material. The load that the rod could bear without failing would be increased if the diameter of the rod was increased, and would decrease if the diameter were decreased.

The amount of extension of the rod at the time of failure depends on the starting length of the rod, such that the longer the starting length, the greater the extension. Thus, force and extension do not represent the ideal means of defining the mechanical properties of a material.

The way to overcome the dependence on the dimensions of the rod is to introduce the parameters of stress, σ, and strain, e, for the material under test.

The definitions for these parameters are:

- *Stress* is the force per unit cross-sectional area that is acting on a material.
- *Strain* is the fractional change in the dimensions caused by the force.

Thus, if a rod is subjected to a tensile force, F, along its length, the stress, σ, is given by:

$$\sigma = F/A$$

where A is the cross-sectional area of the rod. The units used to measure stress are Newtons per metre squared ($N \bullet m^{-2}$ = Pascal = Pa).

At the same time as when the force is applied, the rod's length changes from its original length L_0, to the extended length L_1. The strain that results, e, is given by:

$$e = L_1 - L_0/L_0$$

This parameter is dimensionless, as it involves the calculation of length divided by a length.

In practice, we can measure the load–extension curve for a material, and then convert this to a stress–strain curve. Once we have this information, it is possible to predict the load–extension curve for a rod of any cross-sectional area and length. We can also compare the response of different materials to the same tensile force.

Stress and strain are not properties in themselves, but allow the definition of a number of mechanical properties that could not be defined otherwise. In the example described above, the stress was generated by a load applied in an axial direction (i.e. along the rod), but in practice, a load could be applied in any direction, and in most situations there will be more than one load involved. These loads give rise to complex stress patterns in the structure.

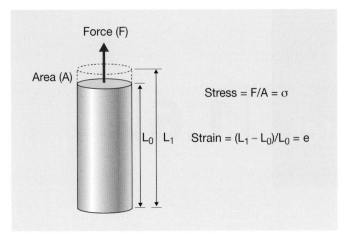

Figure 1.6.1 Rod of material being pulled in a uniaxial direction

The three principal types of stress are tensile stress, compressive stress and shear stress, and these are shown schematically in Figure 1.6.2.

CLINICAL SIGNIFICANCE

When a load is applied to a tooth, this load is transmitted through the material, giving rise to stresses and strains. If these stresses and strains exceed the maximum value the material can withstand, fracture is the most likely outcome.

Definitions of some mechanical properties

A typical stress–strain curve for a metal such as a brass alloy is shown in Figure 1.6.3. It can be used to identify several of a material's properties.

Elastic limit and plastic flow

An important feature of the mechanical behaviour of materials is the relationship between the stress and the strain. Immediately noticeable in Figure 1.6.3 is the fact that this brass alloy does not show a linear relationship between stress and strain along the full length of the curve.

The region where the stress–strain curve is linear is known as the *linear elastic region*, and represents the range where *elastic deformation* occurs. In this region, removal of the stress from the material results in the material returning to its original shape.

Where the curve begins to deviate from its linear path, the material will have exceeded its *elastic limit* and will begin to deform permanently; removal of the stress from the material does not result in the return of the material to its original shape. This is known as *plastic flow*, and is represented by the *region of plastic deformation* on the graph.

Young's modulus

When a material is stressed, it is usually found that the stress is initially proportional to the strain, so their ratio is constant. In other words, the material deforms linearly and elastically. This can be represented by the expression:

$$\sigma / e = E$$

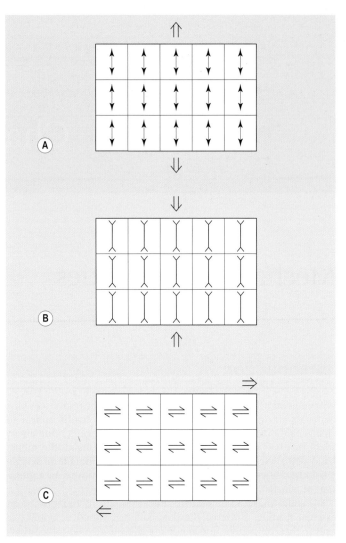

Figure 1.6.2 Three principal types of stress: (a) tensile; (b) compressive; (c) shear

which allows us to define another property of the material: namely, the *Young's modulus*, denoted by E. Young's modulus is the constant that relates the stress and the strain in the linear elastic region, and is a measure of the stiffness of the material.

Note that the stiffness of a rod is dependent on its shape and dimensions, *and* on the Young's modulus of the material from which it is constructed. Once we know the Young's modulus of a material, it is possible to determine the stiffness of any structure made from that material.

Since Young's modulus is obtained by dividing the stress by the strain, the units are the same as those of stress ($N \cdot m^{-2}$). The value of Young's modulus is often very large for real materials. To make the values more manageable, it is usual to express the value of Young's modulus in Gigapascals (GPa), where 1 Pascal is $1 \ N \cdot m^{-2}$, and 1 Gigapascal is $10^{9} \ N \cdot m^{-2}$.

The Young's modulus is often described as simply the *elastic modulus*, or the *modulus of elasticity*.

Fracture strength

It is now possible to define the *fracture strength* of the material, σ_f, since this is simply the stress required to break it.

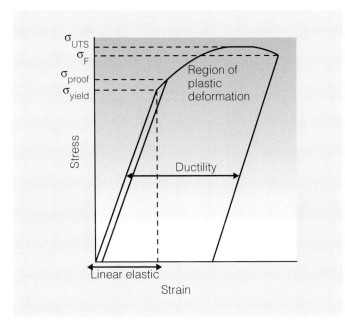

Figure 1.6.3 Stress–strain curve for a ductile metal. UTS: ultimate tensile strength

Table 1.6.1 Fracture toughness data for a variety of materials	
Material	$K_{1c} \cdot$ (MPam$^{1/2}$)
Ductile metals	100–350
High-strength steels	50–154
Aluminium alloys	23–45
Wood	11–13
Nylon	3
Porcelain	1

Yield stress and proof stress

The stress at which plastic deformation begins is defined as the *yield stress*, σ_y. In practice, this point is often difficult to detect since there is a gradual transition rather than a rapid change in the slope of the stress–strain curve.

The quantity known as *proof stress* is used as a measure of the onset of yielding of the material, and is defined as the stress required to produce a certain amount of plastic strain, usually 0.2%.

CLINICAL SIGNIFICANCE

If, at any point in a metal restoration, such as a three-unit bridge, the tensile stress exceeds the yield stress, the restoration will deform permanently.

Ultimate tensile strength

In the tensile response depicted in Figure 1.6.3, there is a maximum stress that the specimen can withstand. This maximum stress is defined as the *ultimate tensile strength* of the material, σ_{UTS}, and is often different from the fracture strength, which, as noted above, is the stress at the point of fracture.

Ductility

The amount of plastic strain produced in the specimen at fracture is called the *ductility* of the material.

Ductility is measured by drawing a line from the point of fracture, which is parallel to the elastic region of the stress–strain curve. Where this line meets the strain axis is the measure of the ductility of the material, and is frequently presented in terms of percentage elongation.

Resilience and toughness

When a wire is bent and then released, it will spring back to its original shape as long as the stress does not exceed the elastic limit.

This is because the energy stored in the wire is recoverable when the stress is released. The amount of energy, which can be absorbed and subsequently released, is an indication of the potential springiness of the material.

The *resilience* is the amount of energy a material can absorb without undergoing any permanent deformation. It is measured from the stress–strain curve as the area under the linear elastic portion of the curve, and is given by:

$$R = \frac{1}{2} \times \frac{P^2}{E}$$

where R is the modulus of resilience, P is the proportional limit and E is the elastic modulus. The units are those of energy per unit volume, $J \cdot m^{-3}$ (1 Joule = 1 N•m).

The total amount of energy that a material can absorb before it fractures is a measure of the *toughness* of the material, and is indicated by the total area under the stress–strain curve. It is also expressed in terms of J•m^{-3}.

Fracture toughness

There are occasions when materials fail suddenly and unexpectedly. This is often as a result of fast fracture, and arises when a crack in the material goes unstable and grows at a very rapid rate. Such failures cause planes to fall out of the sky, ships to break in half and bridges to collapse. This mode of failure is usually associated with materials that have brittle behavioural characteristics, such as glasses and ceramics, although it can also happen for many metals that are not ductile, such as dental amalgam, solders and welds, and for hard brittle resins. The fracture toughness of a material is a measure of the ability of materials to resist propagation of a preformed crack. The method used to measure the fracture toughness of a material is to introduce a crack of known size and shape, and then measure the stress required for this crack to grow and calculate a parameter known as K_{1c}. Typical values for the fracture toughness of a range of materials are presented in Table 1.6.1.

MECHANICAL TESTS

Tensile test

The *tensile test* is a relatively simple test to understand and interpret, and is possibly also the most useful. In this test, a sample of the material is stretched in a uniaxial direction in a tensile tester, as shown in Figure 1.6.4. The test is carried out at a constant strain rate (i.e. a constant rate of extension), and the load is measured from a load cell. The elongation corresponding to the applied load is measured

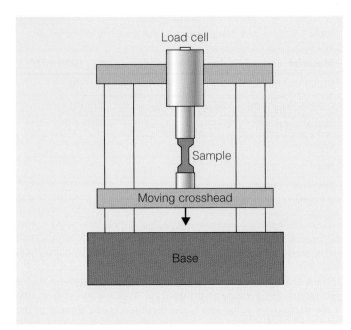

Figure 1.6.4 An arrangement for measuring tensile strength

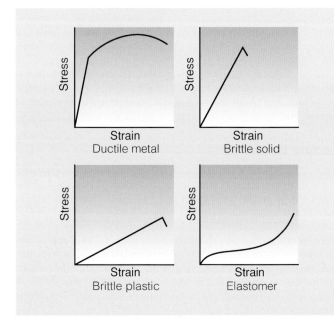

Figure 1.6.5 Stress–strain curves for a range of materials. Note that the stress and strain scales are not meant to be comparable

simultaneously, and can be done in a number of ways, possibly involving measurement of the separation of the moving crosshead, or by attaching strain gauges to the material if the strains are very low. The stress and corresponding strain can then be calculated according to the definitions already described.

A stress–strain curve can be constructed, from which a number of properties can be determined. Some typical examples of stress–strain curves for a range of materials are shown in Figure 1.6.5.

An example of a ductile metal is mild steel, which shows a region of linear elastic behaviour, a well-defined yield point and a considerable degree of ductility. In contrast, a hard brittle solid, such as plaster of Paris, shows only a linear elastic region and then fractures without any evidence of plastic deformation.

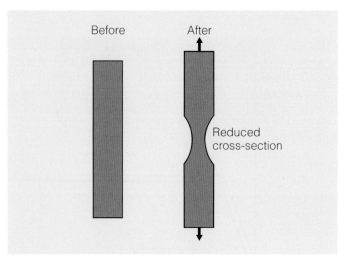

Figure 1.6.6 Necking, exhibited by a ductile material

Many plastics, such as polymethyl methacrylate, are also brittle, although they are less stiff than plaster of Paris. The elastomer, of which silicone impression materials are examples, shows a very different behaviour when compared to the other materials. Firstly, it does not appear to have a linear elastic region, and the region of elastic recovery is very large. The percentage elongation is much higher than that observed with either steel or plaster of Paris, and it is elastic in nature, since the rubber will recover its original dimensions once the stress has been removed. The rubber also has a significantly lower tensile strength.

Necking

During elastic deformation, there is a slight increase in the volume of the material because the atoms which make up the solid are being pulled apart. However, no such change in volume occurs during plastic deformation. During such deformation, an increase in the length of the material must result in a decrease in the cross-sectional area. This tends to occur in a localized region of the material, as shown in Figure 1.6.6, and is known as *necking*. This phenomenon occurs most readily in highly ductile materials.

The results of tensile tests can be very useful when designing structures, because a knowledge of the elastic deformation characteristics of the material is required in order to predict the behaviour of the structure when it is placed under load.

The yield stress determines the maximum stress that the material can safely withstand, and, consequently, the maximum load the structure can withstand, although it is prudent to include some safety factor. The elastic modulus will allow the determination of the stiffness of the structure. For example, a combination of these properties would allow one to determine the resilience or springiness of a metal wire.

If fabrication techniques, such as rolling, wire drawing or pressing, are involved in the manufacture of a product, then it is necessary to know how much plastic deformation the material can withstand. If the material shows high ductility, then it can be shaped, but if it shows no ductility, then shaping by the application of loads will not be possible.

Compression test

For brittle materials in particular, the tensile test is difficult to carry out, and the results usually show a high degree of scatter. An alternative is a *compression test*, which is more easily performed on brittle

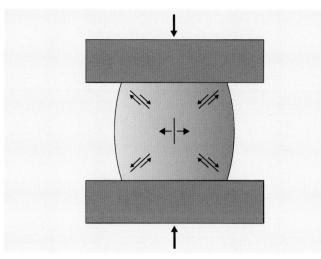

Figure 1.6.7 An arrangement for measuring compressive strength, showing where tensile and shear stresses develop

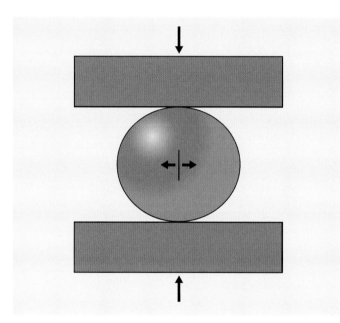

Figure 1.6.8 An arrangement for measuring diametral tensile strength

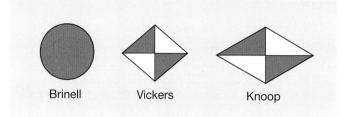

Brinell   Vickers   Knoop

Figure 1.6.9 Surface indenters from different hardness testers

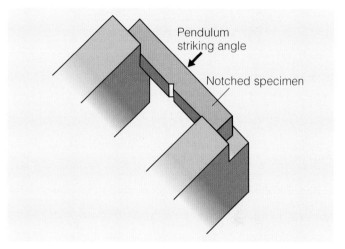

Figure 1.6.10 Specimen arrangement for a Charpy impact test. The pendulum has a hammer head, which is released from a fixed height

materials and has results that show a lower degree of scatter. Another reason why such tests are done on brittle materials is that these materials are only used under conditions of compressive loading.

The configuration for a compression test is shown in Figure 1.6.7. As the sample is constrained by friction at points of contact with the platens of the tester, there is an increase in the cross-sectional area, with the material taking up a barrel shape. This 'barrelling' effect gives rise to a very complex stress pattern in the material (also shown in Figure 1.6.7) that cannot be analysed easily. This makes the interpretation of compression tests very difficult.

A compromise test is the measurement of *diametral tensile strength*, in which a disc of the material is subjected to a compressive load. The load applied to the disc results in a tensile stress in a direction perpendicular to the applied load, shown schematically in Figure 1.6.8. The tensile stress, σ, is calculated as follows:

$$\sigma = 2P\pi/DT$$

where P is the load, D is the diameter of the disc and T is the thickness of the disc. It is a commonly used test for brittle dental materials, because it is simple and provides more reproducible results than a tensile test.

Hardness test

The *hardness test* measures the resistance of a material to an indenter or cutting tool. It provides an indication of the resistance of the material to scratching or abrasion. There is also a reasonable correlation between the hardness of a material and its ultimate tensile strength.

The test involves the use of an indenter, which can be in the shape of a ball (Brinell), a pyramid (Vickers or Knoop) or a cone (Rockwell), which of course must be harder than the material being tested. The indenter is pushed into the surface of the material for a given period of time, leaving behind an impression of the indenter (Figure 1.6.9).

The size of this impression will depend on the hardness of the material. The sizes can be measured, and an empirical hardness number calculated. The choice of hardness tester, to some extent, depends on the nature of material being tested.

Impact test

The *impact test* is designed to test the resistance of a material to the sudden application of a load. A standard notched bar is subjected to an impulse load provided by a heavy pendulum. The arrangement for the test is shown in Figure 1.6.10.

The pendulum is released from a known height, and then strikes and breaks the sample, which is placed across parallel supports. Some of the energy of the pendulum is used up in breaking the sample. From a knowledge of the initial and final height of the pendulum after

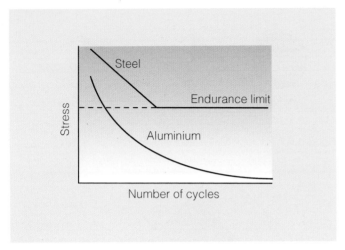

Figure 1.6.11 S–N curves for steel and aluminium

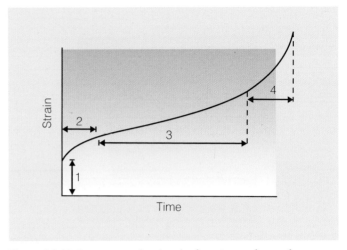

Figure 1.6.12 Creep curve, showing the four stages of creep for long-duration and high-temperature creep conditions

it has fractured the sample, the difference in energy can be calculated. This difference is a measure of the amount of energy that was absorbed by the sample, causing it to fracture. Although the test is empirical, it provides a useful means of comparing the impact resistance of a range of materials. The presence of the notch makes this a very severe test, and provides an indication of the sensitivity of a material to notches in its structure.

Fatigue test

In many practical situations, materials are subjected to fluctuating stresses rather than the static loads that are considered above. The gradual accumulation of minute amounts of plastic strain produced by each cycle of a fluctuating stress is known as fatigue and a clinical situation where such failures may occur is for Ni-Ti files used in endodontics.

Fatigue can lead to failure at stresses well below the yield stress of the material. The test for fatigue strength involves subjecting samples of the material to cyclic loading for a range of loads. The number of cycles required to cause failure is counted in each case.

The stress is plotted as a function of the logarithm of the corresponding number of cycles required to cause failure. This gives an S–N curve, as shown in Figure 1.6.11.

Two forms of behaviour can be observed. For some materials, as the number of cycles of loading is increased, the allowable stress decreases. In other materials, however, there is what is known as an *endurance limit*, which corresponds to a level of stress below which the material can be subjected for an indefinite number of cycles without fracturing.

The fatigue strength is very dependent on the surface characteristics of the material. Improvements in surface finish or surface compressive stresses, which may be induced mechanically or chemically, tend to raise the level of the S–N curve.

The testing environment will also have a profound effect on the S–N curve, with corrosive environments, particularly, lowering the fatigue strength.

CLINICAL SIGNIFICANCE

Whereas a material may be strong enough to withstand the loads placed on it when initially put into use, this does not mean it will always be able to withstand those loads.

Creep test

Under the influence of a constant stress, materials can deform permanently if the load is applied for a long time, even though the stress on the material may well be below its elastic limit. This time-dependent deformation of materials is known as *creep*, and will eventually lead to fracture of the material.

It is particularly important when a material is used at a temperature above about half of its melting temperature or softening point, e.g. some amalgam phases and many plastics. At temperatures 40–50% less than the absolute melting point, creep is negligible.

A typical creep curve is shown in Figure 1.6.12. Four stages of elongation can be identified:

- initial elongation due to the application of the load
- transient or primary creep, which tends to be a large effect
- steady state (secondary) creep
- tertiary creep.

We will not consider the mechanisms that give rise to creep.

CLINICAL SIGNIFICANCE

A wide variety of mechanical properties of materials can be measured. This allows comparisons to be made between dental materials, although their clinical meaning can be a matter of some considerable debate.

Physical properties

INTRODUCTION

The uses to which dental materials are put are not conducive to mass production, as each patient is different from the last, and the material has to be specially moulded each time. As a consequence, most materials used by the dentist and the dental technician require some form of processing before they are hardened.

This processing often involves mixing the materials with others to produce a dough or liquid that can then be placed and shaped to suit the patient's needs. The successful use of dental materials, therefore, requires some understanding of the way in which materials flow when they are mixed, poured or moulded. The study of the flow of materials is known as *rheology*.

When a patient drinks a cup of tea or eats an ice cream, the temperature in the mouth can range from 5 to 60°C. This can result in temperature differences within the tooth that can be quite pronounced. The pulp of the tooth would react severely if it were not protected from these temperatures, which differ greatly from the norm of 37°C. When a filling, crown, bridge or denture is placed, account must be taken of the need to protect the pulp from extremes of temperature. Therefore, the *thermal properties* of the dental materials need to be considered.

The restoration of the human dentition has moved more and more from the purely functional towards the aesthetic. Most patients now demand a level of restoration where it is virtually impossible to detect the fact that the dentist has intervened. Consequently, the *optical properties* of the materials that are selected and used by the dentist have become of great importance.

RHEOLOGICAL PROPERTIES

Rheology is the study of the flow of materials. For liquids, flow is measured by the viscosity, whereas for solids one considers creep and viscoelasticity. Creep has already been described in the previous section and only the viscosity and the viscoelasticity will be considered here.

Viscosity

When a substance flows under the influence of an external force (e.g. gravity), the molecules or atoms come into contact with different neighbours. Thus, bonds must be broken and remade, and this gives rise to a resistance to flow, known as *viscosity*.

For a liquid such as water, the forces binding the molecules together are very weak and easily overcome, so the water flows quite readily and has a low viscosity. For some fluids, the intermolecular attractions are much stronger. This is usually associated with large molecules, such as in the case of treacle. The molecules may even become tangled up in one another, giving rise to very high viscosities. This is what happens with high-molecular-weight polymers.

When we stir a liquid, we are effectively applying a shear stress, and the degree of vigour with which we stir it can be quantified by the shear rate. Such a situation is shown in Figure 1.7.1. The shear stress and the shear rate are defined by:

$$\text{Shear stress} = \eta_s = F/A$$

$$\text{Shear rate} = \grave{e} = V/d$$

A number of methods are available for measuring the shear stress over a range of shear rates for a fluid, and the information collected can be plotted as a *shear stress–shear rate curve*. This relationship is linear for many fluids, and a typical curve for such a fluid is shown in Figure 1.7.2. The slope of the curve is equal to the viscosity, so that the exact scientific definition of viscosity, η, is given by:

$$\eta = \text{shear stress/shear rate}$$

The units of viscosity are Pascal seconds (Pa.s).

The viscous properties of substances that have a linear relationship between shear stress and shear rate are given entirely by this single value of viscosity, and are said to be 'Newtonian' in behaviour.

However, not all materials behave in this simple fashion, and some of the different forms of behaviour are shown in Figure 1.7.3.

Liquids with *plastic* behaviour will not flow until an initial shear stress has been reached. The fluid will then flow in a Newtonian fashion.

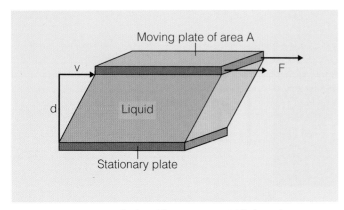

Figure 1.7.1 Shearing of a liquid between two rigid plates that are separated by a distance, d. The upper plate is moving at a velocity, v, relative to the stationary plate, and a force, F, is needed to overcome the resistance from the liquid

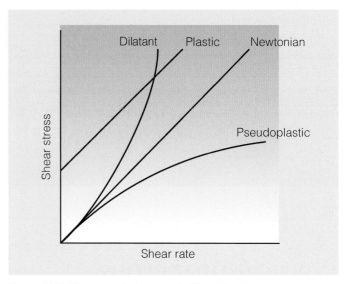

Figure 1.7.3 Rheological behaviour of different liquids

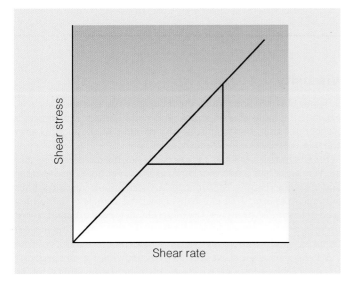

Figure 1.7.2 Shear stress versus shear rate for a Newtonian liquid

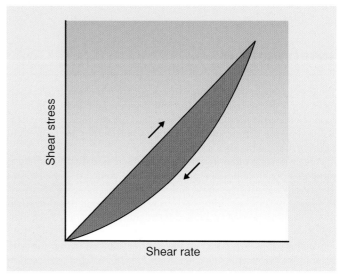

Figure 1.7.4 Thixotropic behaviour

Dilatant liquids show an increase in viscosity as the shear rate goes up. This means that the faster one tries to mix the fluid, the more difficult the liquid becomes to mix. It is not possible to define the flow characteristics of such a liquid by a single viscosity.

For some liquids, an increase in shear rate does not lead to a corresponding increase in shear stress. This means that the liquid becomes easier to mix at higher shear rates than would be the case for a Newtonian or dilatant liquid. This behaviour is described as *pseudoplastic*, and leads to the feature of some liquids that is commonly known as *shear thinning*. A dental example of this type of behaviour is in silicone impression materials, where shear thinning makes the flow of the fluid from a syringe much easier than it would otherwise have been.

Thixotropy

So far, it has been assumed that the viscosity can be determined from a knowledge of the shear stress and shear rate at any one instant in time. For some substances, the viscosity will change at a particular shear rate, and if one plotted the shear stress against the shear rate for such a liquid, one would typically find the response shown in Figure 1.7.4.

In this case, the viscosity for an increasing shear rate is different from the viscosity for a decreasing shear rate, which is an example of *hysteresis*. In such cases, the viscosity of the fluid is dependent on the previous deformations to which the fluid has been subjected.

This type of behaviour occurs when there is some molecular rearrangement caused by the mixing, and a lack of time for the molecules to return to their normal arrangement before mixing again. The effect of this is that the longer the fluid is mixed at a given shear rate, the lower the shear stress and hence the viscosity will be. If the fluid were left for long enough, it would recover and the whole process could be repeated. This type of behaviour is defined as *thixotropic*, and one fluid that exhibits this is non-drip paint.

CLINICAL SIGNIFICANCE

The rheological properties of a material are important, as these have a major influence on the handling characteristics of the material.

Viscoelasticity

A wide range of materials show behaviour that is intermediate between that of a viscous liquid and that of an elastic solid. For an elastic solid, it has been assumed that the relationship between stress and strain is independent of any dynamic factors such as loading rate or strain rate. However, if given sufficient time to do so, some solids show a capacity to rearrange their molecules under the influence of an applied load, and this is reflected in a change in the strain. When the load is then released, the material does not immediately return to its original state. This means that the behaviour of the material is dependent on such factors as the duration and the amount of load applied.

A simple and effective way of visualizing this problem is through the use of models based on a spring and a dashpot, which combine to give a system rather like a shock absorber. The spring represents the elastic element, and the dashpot represents the viscous element. The variation of the strain with time for these models is shown in Figure 1.7.5. For the spring, the application of a load results in an immediate strain that is maintained for as long as the load is applied. Once the load is removed, the spring returns instantaneously to its original state. In contrast, on the application of a load to the dashpot, there is a gradual increase in the strain, which continues to increase for as long as the load is applied. On removal of the load, the strain is not relieved, and the dashpot remains in its new position.

When these two elements are placed in parallel, a simple viscoelastic model is created. The strain response for such a model is shown in Figure 1.7.6. In this model, the dashpot prevents the spring from responding elastically. Now, the dashpot gradually lets the spring approach its desired strained state. On removal of the load, the dashpot prevents the spring contracting to its unstrained state, which it can now only achieve after some time.

A dental example of a group of materials that show viscoelastic behaviour would be that of the elastomeric impression materials. The strain–time curve for such a material, and the corresponding model based on the elastic, viscous and viscoelastic elements are shown in Figure 1.7.7.

In order to avoid excessive permanent deformation of these materials, they should not be loaded for any longer than necessary; this is why elastic impression materials must be removed from the mouth with a short sharp pull. The more rapidly the material is loaded and unloaded, the more elastically the material will respond.

CLINICAL SIGNIFICANCE

Some materials have properties between that of a solid and a liquid, which makes them susceptible to distortion.

THERMAL PROPERTIES

Material can feel warm or cold to the touch. This response of a material to a source of heat, in this case the fingertips, is dependent on the ease with which heat is transferred through the material. A material which readily conducts heat is a *thermal conductor* and a material which resists the conduction of heat is a *thermal insulator*.

Thermal conductivity

One factor which determines the ease with which heat is transferred through a material is its thermal conductivity. The thermal conductivity (K) is defined as the rate of heat flow per unit temperature gradient; its units are $cal \cdot cm^{-1} \cdot s^{-1} \cdot {}^\circ C^{-1}$.

Specific heat

For some materials, the initial 'cold feeling' can rapidly disappear as the material heats up due to the transfer of heat energy from the heat

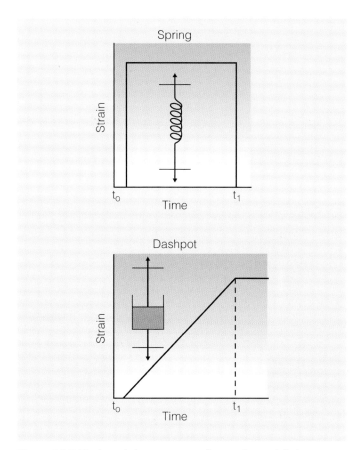

Figure 1.7.5 Elastic and viscous response for a spring and dashpot model

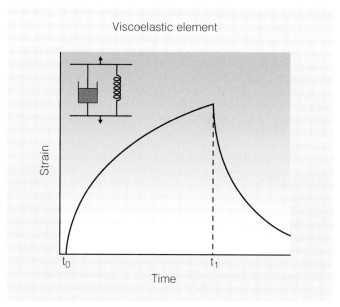

Figure 1.7.6 Viscoelastic behaviour of a spring and dashpot in parallel

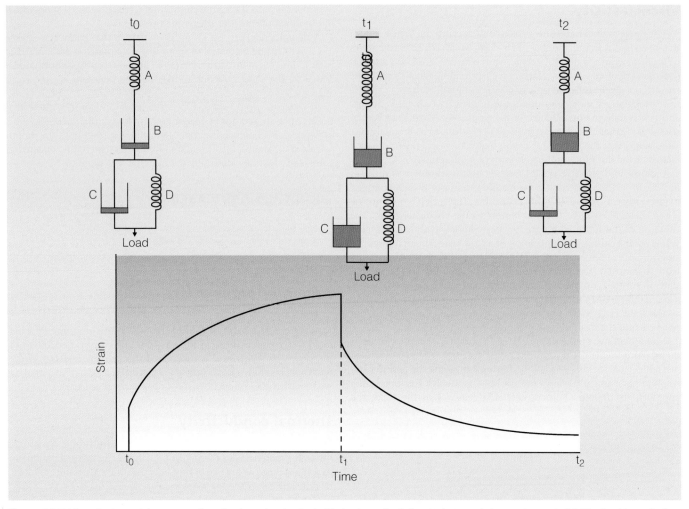

Figure 1.7.7 Viscoelastic model corresponding closely to the rheological behaviour of a fully set elastomeric impression material. The load is applied at time t_0, and spring A extends instantaneously while spring D is prevented from doing so by the dashpot C. With time, dashpots C and B allow further strain to develop. At time t_1, the load is removed, and spring A contracts immediately. Spring D is prevented from doing so by dashpot C. Eventually, at time t_2, spring D has returned to its original length. Some permanent strain remains, since dashpot B will not return to its original state

source to the material. How rapidly the temperature increases depends on the specific heat of the material, which is defined as the heat energy required to raise the temperature of a unit volume by one degree Centigrade. Thus, its units are $cal \cdot g^{-1} \cdot {}^{\circ}C^{-1}$ and the symbol used is C_p.

Thermal diffusivity

The transfer of heat from a hot to a cold source is dependent on both the thermal conductivity and the specific heat, with the former regulating the rate at which the heat enters and passes through the material, and the latter determining the rate at which the temperature will rise as heat enters the material. This is presented by the thermal diffusivity, h, such that:

$$h = K/C_p\rho$$

where ρ is the density of the material. The thermal diffusivity gives a clear indication of the rate of rise of temperature at one point due to a heat source at another point, and may be considered the most relevant in dental applications.

Some typical values of the above properties for a range of materials are presented in Table 1.7.1. An interesting feature is the low diffusivity of water, showing it to be an excellent thermal insulator. For this reason, the Inuit can be quite warm when sheltering in their igloos.

Thermal expansion

When a material is heated, the extra energy absorbed causes the atoms or molecules to vibrate with an increased amplitude. As a consequence, the material expands. The most common way of measuring this expansion is by taking a length of material, heating it to a certain temperature and then measuring the resultant change in length. This change in length, when determined per unit length for a $1 \, {}^{\circ}C$ change in temperature, is called the linear coefficient of expansion, α. This change is so small that it is more usual to express it in terms of parts per million per degree Centigrade (ppm/$^{\circ}C$). Some typical values for α are given in Table 1.7.2.

In an ideal restorative material, the coefficient of expansion would be identical to that of the tooth tissues. If this is not the case, the thermal mismatch can give rise to marginal gap formation and the breakdown of adhesive bonds. Such effects will depend not only on

Table 1.7.1 Physical properties of relevant materials

	ρ (gm·cm^{-2})	C_p (cal·gm^{-1}°C^{-1})	K (cal·cm^{-1}·s^{-1}·°C^{-1})	h (cm^{-2}·s^{-1})
Enamel	2.9	0.18	0.0022	0.0042
Dentine	2.1	0.28	0.0015	0.0026
Silver	10.5	0.056	0.98	1.67
Silica	2.5	0.20	0.003	0.006
Water	1.0	1.00	0.0014	0.0014

Table 1.7.2 Coefficients of thermal expansion

Material	α (ppm/°C)
Enamel	12
Dentine	14
Resin composite	20–55
Fissure sealant	80
Porcelain	12
Glass–ionomer cement	8

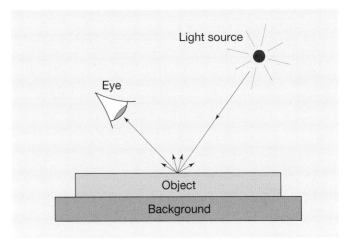

Figure 1.7.8 Perception of an object depends on the light source, the optical properties of the object, and the ability of the eye to discriminate the visible light spectrum landing on the retina

the coefficient of expansion but also on the thermal diffusivity of the material.

Some materials, such as silver, require only a small amount of heat energy to raise their temperature and readily expand or contract. In contrast, composite restorative materials have a low thermal diffusivity. This provides some protection against thermal stimuli, as more heat energy is required to cause a rise in temperature and the corresponding expansion. However, if sufficient heat *is* supplied, the material *will* show a significant expansion/contraction mismatch with tooth tissues.

Fracture of castings can occur due to hot tearing on cooling, when there is a big mismatch between the refractory material and the casting alloy. Dimensional correction of the cooling contraction of alloys is vitally important if crowns and bridges are to fit. Similarly, metal-bonded porcelain relies on a close match of the coefficient of expansion of the metal and the porcelain.

CLINICAL SIGNIFICANCE

The thermal properties of a dental material can influence the sensation of hot and cold food, and can cause mechanical failure due to differential expansion and contraction.

OPTICAL PROPERTIES

In the real world, every object we see is as a result of reflectance of light from that object reaching an extremely sensitive, if somewhat wavelength-limited, photodetector: namely, the eye (Figure 1.7.8). We therefore have a triplet, composed of the light source, the object and the observer. Each of these will influence what we see. Hence, when we place an apple in front of three people and ask them to tell us the colour of the apple, we may well receive three different answers. One

will see it simply as red, another as crimson and yet another as bright red. This is because our colour sensitivity and past experience will be different.

There are three characteristics of the object that govern the nature of this reflected light, namely:

- *Colour.* The colour of an object that our eye detects will be a function of the light source providing the spectrum of light hitting a surface and how the object transforms this spectrum.
- *Translucency.* The amount of light reflected and the spectrum of light reflected from the object and detected by the eye will depend on the ability of the light to travel through the material, where it will change due to absorption and scattering properties of the material and the background against which it is held.
- *Surface texture.* Light can be reflected from a surface, as from a mirror, or scattered in all directions. In the first case, the surface is an ideal reflecting polished surface, while in the second case it is a matte scattering surface.

Colour

The perception of colour is highly subjective, as it is a physiological response to a physical stimulus. For example, the choice of colour of restorative material that we make in order to match a tooth tends to vary slightly from person to person. This happens because the eye is an ill-defined detector of light, followed by interpretation in the brain, of the energy scattered or transmitted by a material. This process will vary from person to person. This can present a real problem for those who suffer from colour blindness, which basically means that their

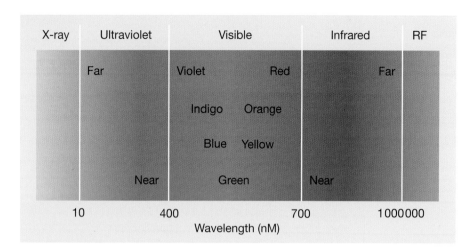

Figure 1.7.9 Spectrum of electromagnetic radiation. RF, radio frequency

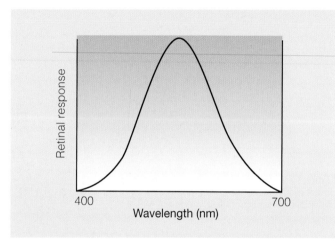

Figure 1.7.10 The relative response of the retina to visible electromagnetic radiation

photo-detector is defective. The *perception* of colour does not therefore lend itself to quantification, but this is not the case for the light itself.

Light is electromagnetic radiation that can be detected by the human eye. Newton (1666) was able to produce a spectrum of different-coloured light by illuminating a glass prism, which split the light into a multicoloured band. This band of light was identical to the colours of the rainbow. He showed that white light is, in fact, the result of combining a broad spectrum of coloured radiation. The spectrum of electromagnetic radiation is shown in Figure 1.7.9. From this, it can be seen that visible electromagnetic radiation occupies only a small part of the total spectrum and is in the range of 380–780 nanometers (1 nanometer (nm) = 10^{-9} m). This spectrum goes from violet (380–450 nm), through blue (450–490 nm), then green (490–560 nm), yellow (560–590 nm) and orange (590–630 nm), and finally to red (630–780 nm).

Light is focused on the retina and triggers nerve impulses that are transmitted to the brain. There are cone-shaped cells in the retina that are responsible for providing sensitivity to different-coloured light, and rod-shaped cells that are sensitive only to the brightness (i.e. the amount of light) that is focused on the retina. The response of the retina to light is indicated in Figure 1.7.10. It shows that the eye is most sensitive to light in the green–yellow range, and is least sensitive at the extremes of the visible spectrum, i.e. the reds and blues.

The cone-shaped cells have a threshold intensity. Exposure to excessive light of a given wavelength can cause these cells to switch off, resulting in eye-strain and a very different perception of colour.

The actual light that we see is not of a single wavelength, but is composed of a mixture of different wavelengths which combine to produce a distinctive colour. The wavelength and intensity spectrum of the light we see depend on the source of the light. The light spectra for daylight and a tungsten filament lamp are quite different, as shown in Figure 1.7.11. This means that the colour of an object will appear different when it is viewed under light from different sources.

In order to allow us to convey colour – for example, to a laboratory being asked to make a crown or a veneer – we need to have some mechanism of describing the colour characteristics of the patient's teeth to which the restoration is to be matched. Various people have attempted to devise a method of quantifying colour and expressing it numerically, with the aim of making colour communication easy and accurate. In 1905, the American artist A. H. Munsell came up with a method for describing colours, which were classified according to their hue, chroma and value:

- *Hue*. This represents the dominant colour (i.e. wavelength) of the spectrum of light from the source. The possible colours are violet, indigo, blue, green, yellow, orange and red. The three primary colours, from which all other colours can be produced, are red, green and blue. This fact is used in TV sets to create a full colour picture from only three distinctly coloured sets of dots.
- *Chroma*. This is the *strength* of hue, in other words how vivid the colour is. On the TV set, this would be represented by the colour adjustment.
- *Value*. This is the brightness or darkness of the object, and ranges from black to white for diffusive or reflective objects, and from black to clear for translucent objects.

Whereas hue and chroma are properties of the object, the value will depend on the incident light, the surface finish of the object and the background if the material transmits light. For this reason, it is important that colour matching should be carried out under a variety of light sources, with bright daylight being by far the best. The basis of the Munsell system is shown in Figure 1.7.12. This three-dimensional representation of colour is not exactly practical, and initially this method of describing colour involved a huge number of paper colour tags, which was later updated to a numerical system. In this system, any given colour is expressed as a letter/number combination as visually evaluated using a Munsell Colour Atlas. However, this system has its limitations in that the colour stability of the atlas is such that it needs to be replaced every 5 years and it has to be viewed under

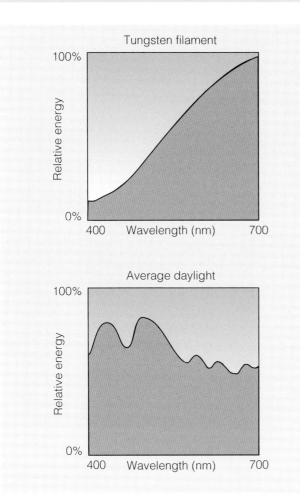

Figure 1.7.11 Light spectra for a tungsten filament lamp and daylight

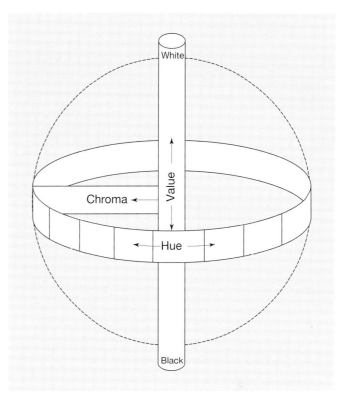

Figure 1.7.12 The three-dimensional Munsell colour scheme for hue, chroma and value

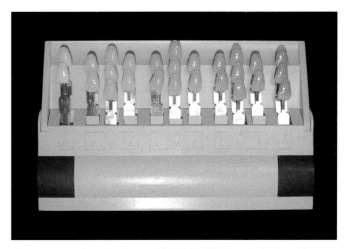

Figure 1.7.13 The VITA Linearguide 3D-MASTER tooth shade guide

standardized lighting conditions. Besides, although it may be adequate for matching the colour of a piece of cloth or a paint, which can be brought close to the atlas, it is not the most convenient method of assessing the colour of a patient's teeth! Also, it has been shown that the range of tooth shades in humans only takes up something of the order of 2% of the Munsell colour space. Hence, for dentistry, a simpler system based on a shade guide has been developed, of which the VITA Linearguide 3D-MASTER is the most recent addition (Figure 1.7.13). The VITA Linearguide 3D-MASTER tooth shade guide is structured on the principle of being able to make a decison in two steps and being able to do so quickly and accurately. A first selection is made with the VITA Valueguide by comparing the shade tabs with the patient's tooth. The Valueguide is numbered from 0 to 5. Once the appropriate value has been selected, the corresponding Chroma/Hueguide is selected and the closest match to the tooth in terms of chroma and hue is chosen. It is important that a shade guide is selected that corresponds with the restorative material being used. Ideally, the shade guide should be manufactured from the same material as that used to produce the restoration.

The fact that objects can change colour under the influence of different light sources is known as *metamerism*. Metamerism occurs when two objects with different light-reflecting properties (spectral graphs) present an identical coloured appearance in specific lighting and observation conditions, and appear different when the lighting or observation conditions are changed. Most shoppers know that trying to match the colour of two garments is best done under daylight rather than under the fluorescent lights of the shop. Ideally, a tooth shade should be determined in daylight conditions, preferably at midday.

Alternatively, it should be done under a daylight-corrected lamp; under no circumstances should conventional lighting be used. The process should be completed in 5–7 seconds, as the eyes tire very quickly.

Another important feature of light is that some objects are able to absorb light of a wavelength near ultraviolet range (300–400 nm), and then release it as light of a longer wavelength (400–450 nm). This is the property of *fluorescence*, and it occurs naturally in tooth enamel. This is the reason why teeth look so white under a fluorescent light and why sometimes crowns, bridges or fillings are more noticeable under a fluorescent light source than under daylight. If the materials used in the construction of the restoration do not have the property of fluorescence, then the restoration will look dark next to the fluorescing natural tooth.

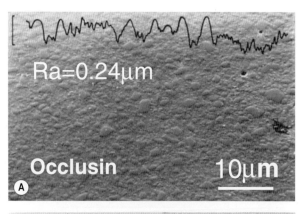

Figure 1.7.14 A simple opacity scale

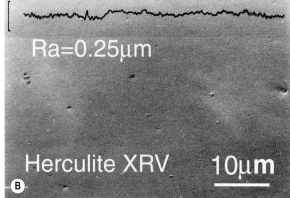

Figure 1.7.15 Surface profiles produced by a profilometer superimposed on scanning electron microscope views of a large particle hybrid composite resin (Occlusin, ICI) and a small particle composite resin (Herculite XRV, Kerr UK Ltd)

Translucency

A *transparent* material such as window glass allows the passage of light in such a way that little distortion takes place, meaning that an object can be seen quite clearly through it. Selective absorption of certain wavelengths may take place, and this forms the basis for optical filters.

A *translucent* material allows some light to pass through it, absorbs some of the remainder, and scatters and reflects the rest from its surface or internal interfaces. An object viewed through such a material would have a distorted appearance.

An *opaque* material is one that does not transmit light, but instead absorbs light and reflects or scatters it from the surface. The colour of the object will depend on which wavelengths of light are reflected and which are absorbed. For example, red glass is red because it allows light with the wavelength of red light to pass through it but absorbs all other wavelengths. Consequently, it would appear opaque if the light source did not contain light with the wavelength of red light, since all the other wavelengths are absorbed.

A simple scale for quantification of the degree of opacity is shown in Figure 1.7.14. In this system, the opacity is presented by a contrast ratio between the daylight reflectance of a specimen of standard thickness (normally 1 mm) when backed by a black standard, and the daylight apparent reflectance when backed by a white standard. The white standard has a reflectance of 70% relative to magnesium oxide ($C_{0.70}$). Restorative materials can be compared easily with enamel and dentine on this scale, to find their relative degrees of opacity.

Surface texture

Whether a material has a shiny or a matte surface texture is a function of how smooth a surface can be. Enamel has a shiny surface because it is extremely smooth and reflects a lot of the light falling on the surface. As a surface gets rougher, the light is scattered and it will begin to appear matte. This is an important consideration with regard to restorative materials, since the appearance of a restored tooth can be spoilt by the restoration having a matte surface finish, making it stand out from the rest of the tooth. The simplest way to assess this is visually, but it can also be assessed numerically using a device known as a profilometer. This device essentially consists of a stylus attached to a long lever arm, which is traced along the surface and records the up-and-down movement of the stylus. An example of such a trace run across the surface of a composite resin restorative material is shown in Figure 1.7.15. It also allows the quantification of the surface roughness by calculating Ra, which is the arithmetic mean deviation of the profile; the higher this value, the rougher the surface.

Chapter | **1.8** |

Chemical properties

INTRODUCTION

The oral environment is an aggressive environment. Materials may dissolve in the water that is present in saliva or release soluble components; they may corrode due to the presence of acids; they may discolour or break down due to absorption of substances from saliva; or they may tarnish and corrode.

All of these possibilities can adversely affect the chemical stability of the materials and limit their durability. The products released may have an adverse effect on the biological environment, both locally and systemically.

Dental ceramics are mostly compounds of oxygen, such as silica (SiO_2) and alumina (Al_2O_3). These are chemically stable under most circumstances and immune from the oxidation process associated with electrochemical (or wet) corrosion. Degradation of ceramics generally involves a process of chemical dissolution. In contrast, metals are not immune to wet corrosion. With the notable exception of some *noble metals*, such as gold and platinum, metals are usually found in nature as compounds (principally oxides or sulphides), from which the metal is extracted. Corrosion of metals is, to all intents and purposes, the reversal of the reactions employed in the extraction process. Frequently, the corrosion product of a metal is very similar to the compound from which the metal was originally extracted. For instance, iron is extracted from naturally occurring iron oxide, and rust is simply hydrated iron oxide. Generally, polymers are not stable either, as many will burn once ignited, showing that the polymer oxidizes readily. However, polymer degradation is generally physio-chemical in nature, such as swelling, dissolution or covalent bond rupture. The latter may be due to heat or radiation and invariably results in a reduction in mechanical properties such as strength and toughness.

CLINICAL SIGNIFICANCE

In general, it could be said that polymers tend to suffer from absorption and loss of soluble components, metals are prone to tarnish and corrosion, and ceramics may be subject to chemical dissolution.

DEGRADATION OF POLYMERS

Water sorption and soluble fraction

Many polymers used in dentistry, such as those used in resin composites, dentures and soft liners, are susceptible to absorption of solvents, particularly water, and the loss of soluble components. The solvent molecule forces the polymer chains apart, causing swelling. As the strength of the bond decreases, the polymer becomes softer, the glass transition temperature is reduced and the strength may be lowered. Nylon is particularly susceptible to water sorption and this is a significant contributing factor to limiting the life of a toothbrush. In the case of resin composites, water sorption is believed to be a contributory factor to the eventual discoloration of the restorations and the hydrolytic degradation of the resin–filler interface. Soft denture liners lose their flexibility due to the loss of water-soluble plasticizers, have an increased propensity to creep, and may even fracture under the osmotic pressure that can build up. Water sorption can have a significant effect on the properties of glass–ionomer cements, as too much or too little water can lead to loss of translucency or surface crazing respectively.

Generally, it is desirable for both the water sorption and soluble fraction of polymers to be as small as possible. This ensures that the polymer retains its characteristic properties, and that no components are leached out which might adversely influence the biocompatibility of the material.

The simplest method of assessing the water sorption and soluble fraction of a polymer is to monitor the weight change of a sample when immersed in water. The detailed analysis of the amount of water sorption by polymeric materials is complicated by the concurrent loss of water-soluble components such as residual monomers or plasticizers, as these two processes take place simultaneously, although at different rates. It is important in the characterization of these factors that the two processes are separated.

Both processes are controlled by the rates of diffusion of water and the water-soluble components through the material, such that the higher the rates of diffusion, the faster water will be absorbed and the faster the soluble fraction will be lost. It is important that any water that the sample has absorbed from the atmosphere has been removed

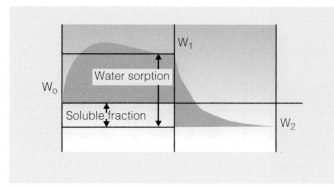

Figure 1.8.1 A schematic representation of the kinetics of water sorption and the dissolution of the soluble fraction

prior to its immersion in water. To this end, samples must be stored in a desiccator until a constant weight is obtained.

The kinetics of a sorption and desorption cycle are shown in Figure 1.8.1. The peak in the weight of the sample in the first cycle is a consequence of the different rates of diffusion of water *into* the sample and diffusion of the soluble fraction *out of* the sample. Water is usually absorbed more rapidly than the soluble components are removed, such that there is an initial rapid weight gain until the sample is nearing saturation. At this point, the loss in weight due to the soluble fraction begins to show, as its release is aided by its dissolution into the absorbed water. The amount of water sorption and the soluble fraction can be calculated from the following:

$$\text{Weight \% water sorption} = (W_1 - W_2)/W_2 \times 100$$

$$\text{Weight \% soluble fraction} = (W_0 - W_2)/W_2 \times 100$$

If the volume, V, at the end of the desorption cycle is calculated, and W_2 replaced by V, then the water sorption and soluble fraction can be expressed in terms of $\mu g/mm^3$, as recommended in the international standard (ISO/DIS 4049).

For most polymers, the amount of water sorption is approximately $30–50 \ \mu g/mm^3$. For resin composites, the value will be lower, due to the presence of the glass fillers, but if this is taken into account, the amount of water sorption into the resin should be in the range given above for polymers. Higher values for water sorption have been recorded for some resin composites, which may be associated with the presence of porosity, free space formed due to removal of the soluble fraction, hydrolytic breakdown of the resin–filler interface, or dissolution of the glass filler.

CLINICAL SIGNIFICANCE

Excessive water sorption can lead to discoloration and degradation of dental restorative materials.

Bond rupture

The degradation of polymers by the breakdown of covalent bonds is known as *scission*. Many polymer properties depend on the molecular weight of the polymer chains. If the polymer chains are broken by chain scission, thus reducing the molecular weight, this can result in a significant loss of mechanical properties. Bond rupture can be due to radiation, heat or chemical attack.

Some forms of radiation, such as ultraviolet (UV) light, can penetrate the polymer and interact with the bonds holding the polymer

together. One possibility is ionization, where the UV radiation removes an electron from a specific atom, converting this atom into an ion. The result is that the bond with that atom is broken and the polymer chain length is reduced. Another possible outcome is that a cross-link may be formed and this can also be utilized to good effect to improve the mechanical properties. An example of this is the γ-radiation of polyethylene to introduce cross-links, which improves its resistance to softening and flow at high temperatures.

If a polymer is subjected to elevated temperatures, this can result in chain scission. This can arise simply due to localized overheating during polishing. The ability of a polymer to resist high temperatures depends on the bond energies between the various constituent parts of the polymer (see Chapter 1.2 for bond energies).

Another factor to consider is the chemical attack of polymers by solvents such as alcohol. The absorption of alcohols causes swelling of the polymer matrix, and the weaker polar interactions between the polymer chains can result in a softer material that is more susceptible to wear. However, there are situations in which the breakdown of the polymer can work to our advantage. An example of this is biodegradable polymers, such as soluble sutures and resorbable implants. In this case, the degradation process converts the polymer to smaller products (carbon dioxide, water, salts etc.), which can be ingested by cells and transported away from the implant site.

TARNISH AND CORROSION OF METALS

Tarnish is a surface discoloration due to the formation of hard and soft deposits, e.g. sulphides and chlorides. Tarnish does not cause a deterioration of the material itself, but can be unsightly, and is easily removed from the surface by polishing the metal. In contrast, corrosion is a chemical reaction between the material and its environment, and is therefore a potentially much more serious problem.

The corrosion process for metals is driven by a decrease in the free energy as the metal reacts with a liquid or a gas. For metallic materials, the corrosion process is normally electrochemical, involving the loss of electrons (e^-) in what is called an oxidation reaction:

$$M \rightarrow M^{n+} + ne^-$$

with the metal becoming a positively charged ion. The site at which the oxidation takes place is called the *anode*. The electrons will transfer or become part of another chemical species in a reduction reaction. For example, in an acid solution containing dissolved oxygen, the reduction takes the form of:

$$O_2 + 4H^- + 4e^- \rightarrow 2H_2O$$

The site of the reduction reaction is known as the *cathode*. All metals are prone to corrosive attack when the environment is sufficiently aggressive. Corrosion is highly undesirable, as it weakens materials and may lead to fracture. Similarly, the corrosion products may react adversely with the biological environment. This latter factor is of major concern in the use of metals in dental applications, such as amalgams, crowns and bridges, rubber dam clamps and orthodontic brackets and archwires.

Dry corrosion

Other than gold and a few other noble metals, all metals will form a surface oxide coating when the surface comes into contact with the oxygen in the air (Figure 1.8.2). Sometimes this thin film of surface oxide can be seen, as is the case of titanium when it can be made to

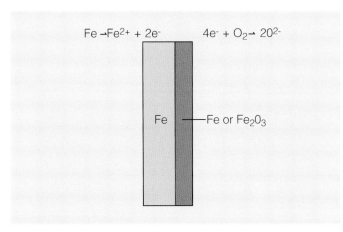

Figure 1.8.2 Oxide formation on the surface of a metal

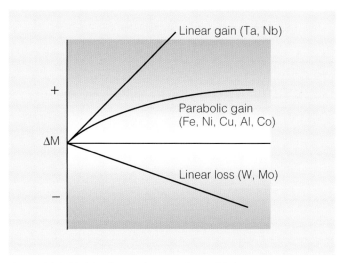

Figure 1.8.3 Weight change due to surface oxidation

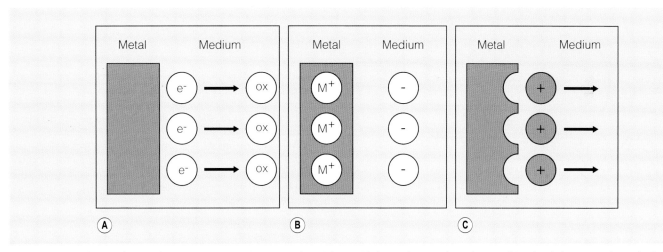

Figure 1.8.4 Oxidation of a metal in an aqueous environment. The oxidator withdraws electrons from the metal in what is known as the cathodic process (a). This causes the metal to become positively charged and the medium negatively charged (b). Due to the positive charge of the metal, metal ions are released, in what is known as the anodic process (c)

produce interference colours that are used to good effect in the production of jewellery.

Since the formation of the surface layer of oxide involves the addition of oxygen atoms to the surface, a material that oxidizes will gain weight. This process can be monitored; the three possible outcomes of such an experiment are shown in Figure 1.8.3. Which of these will actually happen depends on the stability of oxide formed.

If the oxide is very stable, then the corrosion process is self-limiting and there comes a point where the metal ions take so long to diffuse through the thickening oxide layer (whereupon they come into contact with oxygen and react with it) that the oxidation virtually stops. In this case, there is an initial rapid weight gain that gradually tails off; this gives the parabolic weight-gain curve.

Some oxides are not very stable, and as they form on the metal surface, they tend to crack or to separate partially from the surface, exposing the underlying metal and allowing a new oxide coating to form. In this case, there is a gradual build-up of the oxide, causing a continuous gain in weight.

The third possibility, weight loss, is less common and only occurs during the oxidation of certain metals at high temperatures. If the temperature is sufficiently high, the oxide evaporates as soon as it is formed, offering no barrier to further oxidation of the metal. Consequently, weight is lost as the oxide layer evaporates.

These forms of oxidation are described as *dry corrosion*. Most metals are stable under such processes due to the protective first layer of the oxide coating itself. Hence, surplus aircraft are stored in the desert, where it is hot but, more importantly, dry, and cars are less susceptible to rust in hot, dry climates. In the presence of an aqueous environment, different conditions prevail and the material's response is much altered.

Wet corrosion

Wet corrosion can take place in neutral, acid or alkaline environments. When a metal is placed in an aqueous environment, metal ions and electrons are released into the water (Figure 1.8.4).

An oxidator, commonly oxygen dissolved in the water, withdraws electrons from the metal, in what is known as the *cathodic process*. This extraction of electrons produces a current called the *cathodic current*. This loss of electrons from the metal causes the metal to become positively charged, and positive ions are released into the water, producing an *anodic current*.

Table 1.8.1 The galvanic series in seawater

↑	Platinum
	Gold
	Titanium
	Silver
Increasingly inert	Stainless steel
	Copper
	Nickel
Increasingly active	Tin
	Lead
	Cast iron
↓	Aluminium
	Zinc

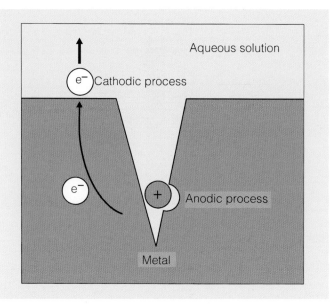

Figure 1.8.6 In crevice corrosion, the oxidation takes place at the surface (cathodic process) and metal ions are released from within the crevice (anodic process)

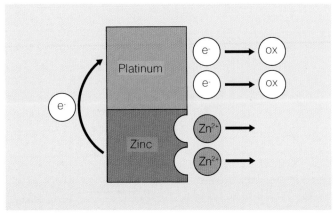

Figure 1.8.5 Galvanic corrosion of zinc in contact with platinum. The noble metal (platinum) is more easily oxidized than the base metal (zinc), such that the anodic process takes place at the zinc surface and zinc ions are released into the aqueous environment

Metals do not oxidize with the same ease and the relative reactivity of metals is presented in what is known as the galvanic series. This is shown in Table 1.8.1 for a series of metals when placed in seawater, where the alloys near the top of this ranking are the least reactive.

If the metal ions are removed from the surface evenly, the process is called *uniform* corrosion. Under suitable conditions, *localized* as opposed to *uniform* corrosion can take place, and this is generally far more dangerous. *Galvanic* and *crevice* corrosion are examples of such localized corrosion.

Galvanic corrosion

Galvanic corrosion occurs when two dissimilar metals are combined, resulting in the corrosion of one of the metals being significantly increased.

A classic example of this is the corrosion of zinc in acid. When zinc is in contact with platinum, as shown in Figure 1.8.5, the platinum reacts very quickly with the hydrogen ions that are supplied by the acid, and releases electrons, producing hydrogen (this is an example of the cathodic process). This generates an electrical imbalance between the zinc and the platinum, such that electrons flow from the zinc to the platinum. This enhances the release of metal ions from the zinc (the anodic process), such that the zinc corrodes faster when it is in contact with the platinum.

To what degree dissimilar metals will be susceptible to this form of corrosion depends primarily on their relative rates of reaction. Platinum is a particularly effective oxidizer. Other noble metals will not have quite the same effect, as they are not quite so effective at oxidation.

A combination of metals behaving in this way is described as a *galvanic cell*, and can occur within alloys due to the presence of different phases with different rates of oxidation. An example is the galvanic cell set up between the γ_1 and γ_2 phases in dental amalgam, where the γ_2 phase corrodes significantly faster than the γ_1 phase.

Crevice corrosion

When there is a sharp crack or fluid-filled space, as shown in Figure 1.8.6, this space is usually depleted of oxygen. The metal ions will still be released into the space and will form corrosion products, whereas the electrons are unable to react because of the lack of oxygen. Thus, the oxidation reaction must take place where there *is* oxygen, which will be at the main surface, such that the electrons will have to travel through the metal, making the base of the crevice anodic and the surface cathodic. Material is therefore lost from the base of the crevice. As the corrosion products are formed, they tend to build up in the crevice such that the supply of oxygen is further restricted. There is nothing to stop this reaction from continuing, which makes this form of corrosion highly insidious. The same process can take place when there is a break in the surface oxide coating, which is known as *pitting* corrosion.

The concentrated attack on one area of the metal is highly undesirable, as it causes the metal to weaken due to the formation and growth of cracks. The damage done is totally out of proportion to the amount of material destroyed by the corrosion process. Thus, localized corrosion is far more dangerous than uniform corrosion.

CLINICAL SIGNIFICANCE

If the conditions are right, corrosion of metals can be a rapid and highly damaging process.

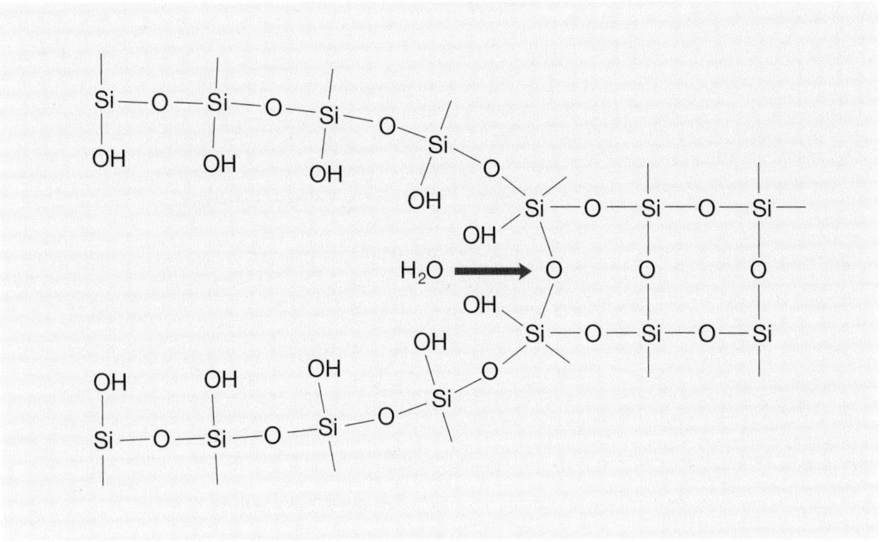

Figure 1.8.7 Crack growth in a ceramic due to local hydration at the tip of the crack

DEGRADATION OF CERAMICS

In contrast to metals, ceramics are in general very resistant to electrochemical corrosion, but are still susceptible to chemical corrosion. For example, a glass made from only SiO_2 and Na_2O will rapidly dissolve in water and CaO is added to reduce its susceptibility to dissolution. On the other hand, the dissolution capabilities of certain acids such as HF are used to great effect to create microscopically roughened surfaces and improve adhesion to resins by the preferential dissolution of certain phases in the ceramic.

Chemical corrosion can also have a profound effect on the strength of ceramics. The failure of ceramics is usually associated with a crack that has become so large that the component can no longer support the stresses applied. This can manifest itself as a sudden disintegration of the ceramic, such as the apparently inexplicable shattering of a drinking glass or car windscreen. These failures are frequently caused by the slow and undetectable growth of a crack until the crack becomes a critical size and progresses spontaneously and catastrophically. Chemical interaction between the ceramic and the environment at the crack tip can have a profound effect on the rate of crack growth. Water or water vapour at a crack tip can react with the Si–O–Si bond at the tip of the crack in a silica-based glass, forming hydroxides (Figure 1.8.7). This process is often referred to as *static fatigue*. When the environmental conditions are combined with high levels of stress in the ceramic, either by the application of an external load or built-in stress, the rate of growth of the crack will be much accelerated. Under such circumstances, the failure may be described as resulting from *stress corrosion cracking*.

CLINICAL SIGNIFICANCE

All materials are susceptible to attack from the oral environment, such that virtually all materials will be degraded in the longer term.

Chapter | 1.9 |

Principles of adhesion

INTRODUCTION

Since the acid-etch technique of bonding to enamel was introduced into dentistry, the use of adhesive procedures has developed to such an extent that it now constitutes a major part of the dental discipline. Many concepts, which have served the profession well for many decades in providing good dental care, have had to be revised in light of these developments and many new techniques and materials have been introduced.

Two examples of new, adhesive restorative procedures that spring to mind readily are resin-bonded bridges and porcelain veneers. These procedures have been possible because of our improved knowledge and understanding of the surface characteristics of enamel and dentine, and of the requirements that need to be satisfied in order to obtain good bonds to them.

These advances in themselves would not have been sufficient, but they laid a foundation for the development of the new materials and techniques that are used in enamel and dentine bonding today. A combination of factors has provided the dentist with a variety of procedures for restoring the dentition. Although these procedures have been available for only a relatively short time, their impact has already been quite considerable.

There are now many materials that we wish to bond to enamel and dentine, and to each other. Consequently, numerous adhesives have been developed to cope with the diversity of the applications; such adhesives include composite resins, glass–ionomer cements and dentine-bonding agents.

New methods of surface preparation, such as etching and silane coupling, have had to be investigated to find ways of using them in conjunction with materials such as the new glass–ceramics and a wide variety of alloys.

It is the variety of applications that has contributed to the growing complexity of adhesive restorative dentistry. In order to appreciate fully and understand the clinical application of adhesive techniques, it is important for the clinician to have a thorough knowledge of the principles of adhesion, the materials employed, the dental adhesive systems and how these are applied in the clinical situation.

WHAT IS ADHESION?

Adhesion can be defined as the force that binds two dissimilar materials together when they are brought into intimate contact. This is distinct from *cohesion*, which is the attraction between similar atoms or molecules within one substance.

Adhesion between solids

At an atomic level, surfaces are rough. This means that, when they are brought into contact, the only places where intimate contact is achieved is at the tips of the *asperities* (Figure 1.9.1). Very high pressures can be generated at these points, such that, in the absence of any contaminants, an effect called *local adhesion* or *cold welding* can result. If an attempt is then made to slide the one surface over the other, a resistance known as *friction* is experienced.

Friction is caused by the need of the local adhesions to be sheared, or broken. In general, the local adhesions are so strong that the shearing process does not take place at the interface but actually within the solids themselves; this explains the general phenomenon of frictional wear.

While frictional forces due to local adhesion can be quite high, adhesion *normal* (i.e. perpendicular) to the surface is usually undetectable. This has been attributed to the build-up of elastic stresses in the normal direction, which are released when the load on the material is removed.

Only very soft metals, such as pure gold, can relieve these elastic stresses by flow and prevent rupture of the junction when a normal load is applied. A dental example of this is the use of cohesive gold.

Adhesion between a solid and a liquid

It is a matter of common observation that a drop of water will cling to the underside of a glass slide. This effect demonstrates the adherence of water to glass that arises by virtue of molecular attraction between the two substances. The attraction is due to secondary (van der Waals) bonds. Even a hard shake of the slide will not remove all

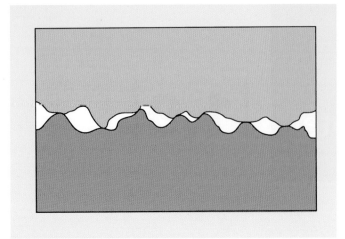

Figure 1.9.1 Point-to-point contact of two solid surfaces at a microscopic level

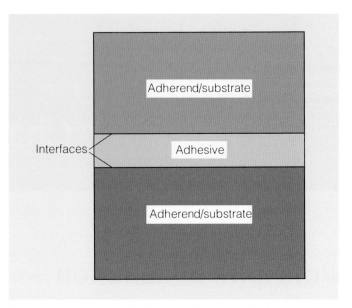

Figure 1.9.2 Terminology for the description of an adhesive joint

of the water and merely drying the glass with a cloth will still leave a very thin residual layer of water. The only way of ensuring that all the water has been removed is by heating the glass in an oven.

This illustrates the good adhesion that may be obtained between a solid and a liquid. Such good adhesion is due to the liquid's ability to make intimate contact with the solid over a large surface area. This is in contrast to the poor adhesion (described above) that usually occurs between two solids, where the contact is at points only.

Thus, one of the fundamental requirements of adhesion is that the two substances to be bonded must be in close contact with each other. The importance of this statement cannot be overemphasized, as a strong bond can be created only in the case of intimate molecular contact. This may seem a simple requirement, but it is not particularly easy to achieve intimate contact at the microscopic level, as noted for solids above.

Given that the distance between the interacting molecules must be less than 0.0007 μm (micrometres; 1 mm = 1000 μm) for adhesion to occur, one appreciates that adhesion is virtually impossible for two solid surfaces. This is a serious obstacle when there is a need for adhesion between two solids, and in order to overcome this, we use a third substance, usually in a fluid or semi-fluid state, to act as an intermediary.

The substance that binds the two materials is defined as the *adhesive*, and the surfaces of the materials are the *adherend* or *substrate*. The point at which the substrate meets the adhesive is described as the *interface* (Figure 1.9.2).

Naturally, what happens at the interface is crucially important to the success or failure of an adhesive bond. This applies equally to industrial and dental adhesives, so it is useful in the first instance to consider the general requirements of an adhesive and then to look more closely at the bonding mechanisms.

CLINICAL SIGNIFICANCE

Before bonding to a surface, one must make sure it is scrupulously clean; otherwise no adhesive bond will form.

CRITERIA FOR ADHESION

When reading the instruction leaflet of any adhesive, one sees that one of the first requirements is invariably that the surfaces to be bonded

are both clean and dry. This is important for a variety of reasons. A clean, dry surface ensures that the adhesive has the best possible chance of creating a proper bond with the solid material. The presence on the surface of anything that could be considered as a contaminant will prevent the formation of a strong bond, since the contaminant itself is weakly bonded to the solid and will prevent the adhesion of the adhesive to the substrate.

The factors that govern the ability of the adhesive to make intimate contact with the substrate are:

- the *wettability* of the substrate by the adhesive
- the *viscosity* of the adhesive
- the *morphology* or *surface roughness* of the substrate.

Wettability

In order for the adhesive to create a bond between two materials, it must make intimate contact with the surfaces of the substrates such that no air voids (which would weaken the bond) are formed. The ability of an adhesive to contact a substrate depends on the *wettability* of the adhesive on that particular substrate. *Good wetting* is the ability to cover the substrate completely, so that the maximum benefit is obtained from whichever adhesive mechanism is activated.

The ability or inability of fluids to wet a surface is frequently encountered in everyday life. An example of a surface that is extremely difficult to wet with water is PTFE (polytetrafluoroethylene), as used in non-stick saucepans. When water is placed on a PTFE surface, it forms globules that will not spread in an even layer across the surface. This is an example of poor wettability. This and the other possible responses are depicted in Figure 1.9.3.

The interaction between the substrate and the adhesive is governed by a driving force that tends to spread the adhesive over the substrate, and resistance to spreading that depends on the viscosity of the adhesive, the surface irregularities and the presence of contaminants. The driving force is provided by the surface energies of the adhesive and the substrate (see below).

Surface energy

In the bulk of a solid or a liquid, the molecules are subjected to attractive forces in all directions, such that the molecule is in dynamic

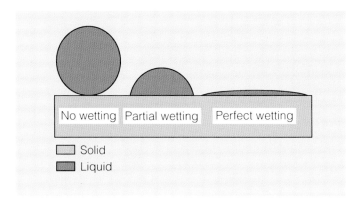

Figure 1.9.3 The possible wetting characteristics for liquids on a solid surface

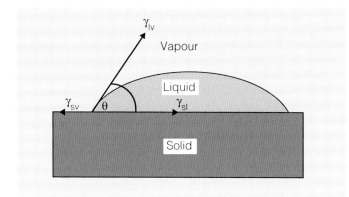

Figure 1.9.4 The contact angle θ between a liquid and a solid, where γ_w is the surface tension between the solid and the vapour, γ_{sl} is the surface tension between the solid and the liquid and γ_{lv} is that between the liquid and the vapour

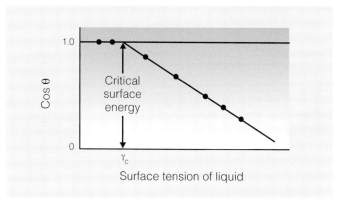

Figure 1.9.5 Zisman plot for the determination of the critical surface energy, γ_c, of a solid

equilibrium with its surrounding molecules. At the surface, however, this delicate balance is destroyed, resulting in a net inward attraction directed towards the large number of molecules in the mass of the material. It is this inward force that gives rise to the *surface energy* of a material. In liquids, the surface energy is known as the *surface tension*.

One of the effects of surface tension is the tendency for liquids to take up a spherical shape in preference to any other. This arises because a sphere has the minimum surface area (and hence the minimum surface energy) for a given volume of liquid, allowing the total energy stored in the liquid to be a minimum.

Whereas the surface tension of a liquid is a real surface stress, in the case of a solid, work is done in stretching and not in forming the surface. The measurement of the surface energy of a solid is not achieved as readily as it is with liquids. An approach that has now gained wide acceptance is one pioneered by Zisman, who introduced the concept of the *critical surface energy*.

Contact angle

When a solid and a liquid make contact, the angle between the liquid surface and the solid surface is known as the *contact angle*, and is dependent on the surface tension of the liquid and the surface energy of the solid (Figure 1.9.4).

By measuring the contact angle between the solid and the liquid, a useful measure of the wettability of the liquid on a particular substrate can be obtained. For perfect wetting, which is the ideal situation for adhesion to occur, this angle should be 0°. In this case, the surface is

completely covered with the adhesive and the maximum bond strength can be achieved. The driving force that gives rise to the tendency, or otherwise, of a fluid to spread on a solid surface depends on the surface tension of the liquid and the surface energy of the solid. At the point where the surface of the liquid meets the surface of the solid, their surface tensions must balance, in order to be in equilibrium:

$$\gamma_{sv} = \gamma_{sl} + \gamma_{lv}\cos\theta$$

This relationship can be rearranged to give the contact angle, θ, and in this form is known as the *Young equation*:

$$\cos\theta = (\gamma_{sv} - \gamma_{sl})/\gamma_{lv}$$

where γ_{sl} is the surface energy at the solid–liquid interface, γ_{sv} is the surface energy at the solid–vapour interface and γ_{lv} is the surface energy at the liquid–vapour interface.

Critical surface energy

If one measures the contact angle of a number of different liquids on the same substrate and plots the cosine of the contact angle against the known surface tension of the liquids, then a linear relationship results.

This relationship is shown in Figure 1.9.5; it shows the linear curve being extrapolated to the point where it crosses the line at which the cosine of the contact angle is equal to 1. This is the situation under which the contact angle will be 0°, representing the condition of perfect wetting.

The value of the surface tension at which the cosine of the contact equals 1 is defined as the *critical surface energy* of the solid. This critical surface energy is equal to the surface tension of a liquid that will *just* spread on the surface of the solid; such a liquid may be real or hypothetical. Any liquid that has a surface tension less than the critical surface energy of the solid will wet the surface of the solid effectively.

Thus, a low surface energy liquid will readily spread over a high surface energy substrate because the surface of the substrate is replaced by a surface with a lower surface energy.

PTFE has a very low surface energy, making it difficult to find liquids with lower surface tensions that could wet it successfully. Another material with a similarly low surface energy is silicone rubber. Again, it is extremely difficult to make anything adhere to this material.

On the other hand, silicone polymers in their liquid form tend to adapt well to most surfaces due to their low surface energies. These polymers are used to great effect in impression materials.

Table 1.9.1 Typical surface energies

Material	Surface energy $\times 10^{-3}$ J m^2
Perfluorolauric acid	6
Methyl chloride	16
Polytetrafluoroethylene (PTFE)	18
Polytrifluoroethylene	22
Ethyl alcohol	24
Polyvinyl chloride (PVC)	39
Water	73
Plate glass	200
Steel	230
Iron oxide	350
Alumina	560
Mercury	488

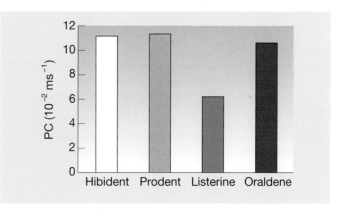

Figure 1.9.6 Penetration coefficients for mouth rinses.
(Adapted from Perdok et al (1990) Physicochemical properties of commercially available mouthrinses. J Dent 1990; 18: 147.)

The penetration coefficient is a measure of the ability of a liquid to penetrate into a capillary space, such as interproximal regions, gingival pockets and pores. An example of the penetration coefficient for mouth rinses is shown in Figure 1.9.6.

Surface roughness

The measurement of contact angles assumes that the surface of the substrate is perfectly smooth. In reality, the surface may be quite rough at a microscopic level. This roughness has the advantage of increasing the potential area for bonding, but can also give rise to the entrapment of air. Such entrapment will significantly reduce the effective bonding area and result in a weak bond. Cracks and crevices constitute surface irregularities and the adhesive must be able to flow into these.

Adhesives with a high viscosity are particularly prone to causing entrapment of air because their stiffness may be such that they bridge the small cracks and crevices in the surface, rather than flowing into them.

In the absence of air, capillary action ensures that the adhesive penetrates the cracks and crevices. For this penetration to occur readily, a high surface tension adhesive is desirable, as this means that the capillary attraction is also high. This effect is demonstrated by the fact that the higher the surface tension of a liquid, the higher the liquid will climb up a capillary placed in it.

The driving force that causes capillary action must work against the pressure of the air that is trapped by the adhesive, and must also overcome the viscous resistance forces. However, the surface tension of the liquid must also be sufficiently low to wet the substrate perfectly. Hence, the ideal adhesive would have a surface tension just below the surface energy of the solid. If this condition is satisfied, then the surface irregularities can be advantageous in improving the bond strength of the adhesive.

An irregular surface has a higher surface area than a smooth surface, so more chemical bonds can be created. If the irregularities are of a particular morphology, such that undercuts are present at the microscopic level, the bond can be enhanced by the process of micro-mechanical interlocking.

MECHANISMS OF ADHESION

First, let us assume that the initial criterion for adhesion is met, in that intimate contact at the molecular level between the adhesive and the substrate is achieved. Let us now look at what happens when the

Examples of the surface energy of a number of substances, expressed in units of J·m^{-2} (N·m^{-1}) for convenience, are provided in Table 1.9.1. In the case of perfluorolauric acid, only condensed inert gases can spread on this surface.

CLINICAL SIGNIFICANCE

An adhesive must be compatible with the surface to be bonded. For example, hydrophobic resins will not stick to hydrophilic surfaces.

Viscosity

For an adhesive to be effective, it must be able not only to make intimate contact with the substrate, but also to spread easily on it, yet not so easily that it is impossible to control. The driving force for the spreading of the liquid is provided by its wettability on the solid surface, and is resisted by the liquid's viscosity. Too high a viscosity is undesirable, as it prevents the fluid from flowing readily over the surface of the solid and penetrating into narrow cracks and crevices.

In general, contact angles are directly proportional to the viscosity of the adhesive, but this can be a misleading statement if the adhesive is a solvent containing additives.

The use of low surface tension solvents with highly viscous solutes will give misleadingly low contact angles. Although a low contact angle is obtained, the resistance to flow offered by the high viscosity of the solute will continue to resist the spreading.

Similarly, a highly filled adhesive, such as a composite resin, can be difficult to spread, which may lead one to think it has a high surface tension and poor wettability. However, the substrate only experiences contact with the low viscosity resin that may readily wet the surface if it has the correct surface tension. Spreading of the composite resin is merely resisted by its own stiffness and not by any reluctance on the part of the resin to wet the underlying surface.

The ability of a liquid to fill cracks and crevices can be quantified by what is described as the penetration coefficient (PC), which is a function of the surface tension (γ) of the liquid and its viscosity (η), according to the equation:

$$PC = \gamma \cos\theta / 2\eta$$

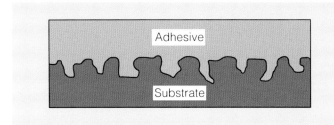

Figure 1.9.7 Microscopic mechanical interlocking between an adhesive and the substrate

materials are in contact, and see how they may interact. An adhesive bond can be mechanical, physical or chemical, and is more usually a combination of all of these.

Mechanical adhesion

The simplest method of adhesion is that of the mechanical interlocking of components. This form of adhesion can result from the presence of surface irregularities, such as pits and fissures that give rise to microscopic undercuts.

A primary condition for this form of adhesion is that the adhesive can penetrate readily into the pits before it begins to set. This condition is determined by the wettability of the adhesive on the substrate, which in turn is governed by the relative surface energies and the resultant contact angle, the ideal situation being that of perfect wetting. To improve the level of contact, any air or vapour in the pits must be able to escape in front of the advancing liquid. If the adhesive is able to penetrate these spaces and subsequently to set solid, it remains locked in by the undercuts (Figure 1.9.7). The degree of penetration will depend both on the pressure used in the application of the adhesive, and on the properties of the adhesive itself.

If the adhesive is to disengage from the substrate, then it must fracture in the process of debonding, as it can not withdraw from the undercut. This is not unlike the concept of retention, used in the placement of restorations, except that it occurs at a microscopic level. However, one important difference is that good wettability is not a prerequisite for macroretention, whereas it is of paramount importance for micromechanical interlocking.

The general view is that undercuts frequently provide important mechanical characteristics, but that they are not usually sufficient to act as the mechanism of adhesion in themselves. There are a number of additional adhesive mechanisms that are due to what can be described as physical and chemical causes. The term *true adhesion*, or *specific adhesion*, is commonly used to distinguish physical and chemical adhesion from mechanical adhesion. However, such terms should be discouraged, as these are inappropriate.

True adhesion implies that there is also false adhesion, but a material is either adhesive or not. Physical adhesion and chemical adhesion are distinguished from mechanical adhesion by virtue of the fact that they involve a molecular attraction between the adhesive and the substrate, whereas mechanical adhesion does not require such interaction at the interface.

Physical adhesion

When two surfaces are in close proximity, secondary forces of attraction arise through dipole interactions between polar molecules (see Chapter 1.2). The attractive forces that are generated can be quite small, even if the molecules have a substantial permanent dipole moment or have a large polarizability.

The magnitude of the interaction energy is dependent on the relative alignment of the dipoles in the two surfaces, but is usually less than 0.2 eV. This is considerably less than primary bonds, such as ionic or covalent, which are typically 2.0–6.0 eV.

This type of bonding is rapid (because no activation energy is needed) and reversible (because the molecules remain chemically intact on the surface). This weak physical *adsorption* is easily overcome by thermal energy, and is not suitable if a permanent bond is desired. Even so, the hydrogen bond in particular can be an important precursor to the formation of a strong chemical bond.

It follows that non-polar liquids will not readily bond to polar solids and vice versa because there is no interaction between the two substances at the molecular level, even if there is good adaptation. Non-polar liquid silicone polymers exhibit such behaviour, and will not form bonds to solids other than themselves; this bonding is only possible because the chemical reaction of cross-linking provides sites for bonding between the solid and the liquid.

Chemical adhesion

If a molecule dissociates after adsorption on to the surface and the constituent components then bond themselves separately by covalent or ionic forces, a strong adhesive bond will result. This form of adhesion is known as *chemisorption*, and can be either covalent or ionic in nature.

The sharing of electrons between the two atoms in the chemical bond distinguishes it from the physical interaction. Adhesives must be strongly attracted chemically to the surface of application in order for strong bonds to form, and require the presence of reactive groups on both surfaces. This is particularly so for the formation of covalent bonds, such as occurs in the bonding of reactive isocyanates to polymeric surfaces containing hydroxyl and amino groups (Figure 1.9.8).

In contrast, a metallic bond is readily created between a solid metal and a liquid metal, which forms the basis for soldering or brazing. The metallic bond is provided by free electrons and is chemically unspecific. However, the bond will only be possible if the metal surfaces are scrupulously clean.

In practice, this means that fluxes need to be used to remove oxide films that would otherwise prevent the metal atoms from meeting.

The mechanical breaking of these chemical bonds becomes the only way of separating the adhesive and the substrate, and there is no reason why these bonds should be broken in preference to any other valence bond. This places a restriction on the strength that can be achieved. If the bond strength exceeds the tensile strength of the adhesive or the substrate, then a cohesive failure of the adhesive or substrate will occur before the bond fails.

Adhesion through molecular entanglement

So far, it has been assumed that there is a distinct interface between the adhesive and the substrate. In effect, the adhesive is adsorbed on to the surface of the substrate and can be considered as being *surface-active*, collecting on the surface but not dissolving in the medium below. In some instances, the adhesive, or a component of the adhesive, is able to penetrate the surface of the substrate and absorb *into* it rather than *on to* it. It should be stressed that the absorption of molecules is a *result* of good wetting and not the cause.

If the absorbing component is a long-chain molecule, or forms a long-chain molecule within the penetrated layer, the resultant entanglement between the adhesive and the substrate is capable of producing very high bond strengths (Figure 1.9.9).

Thus, adhesives must be strongly attracted chemically to the surfaces of application in order to form a strong bond.

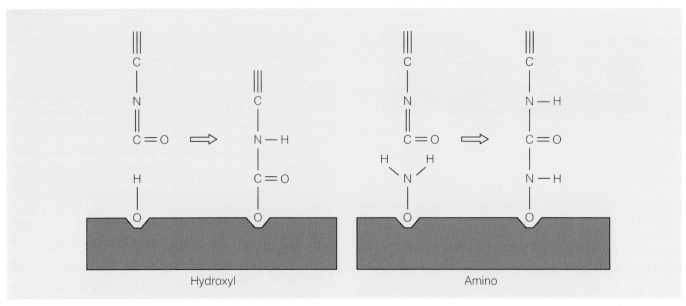

Figure 1.9.8 Covalent bond formation between an isocyanate and a hydroxyl and an amino group on the surface of the substrate

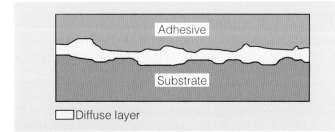

Figure 1.9.9 Diffuse interpenetrating layer arising from molecular entanglement between the adhesive and the substrate

CLINICAL SIGNIFICANCE

It is important to know what type of bond one is trying to achieve so that the bonding steps are understood. This way there is less chance of making an error.

THE STRENGTH OF THE ADHESIVE BOND

A reasonably strong bond can result from the cumulative action of a number of bonding mechanisms that act in concert, such as a large area of intimate contact providing numerous sites for the creation of weak secondary bonds, and the presence of surface undercuts at the microscopic level.

Theoretical strength

It is possible to determine roughly the theoretical strength of an adhesive joint between a liquid and a solid.

If we assume that we have the unit surface area of the solid in contact with the liquid, the energy required to separate these materials will be the difference between the energy of the surfaces when joined and the energies of the individual surfaces when separated (Figure 1.9.10).

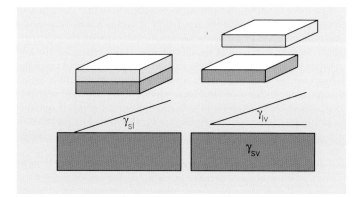

Figure 1.9.10 Separation of a liquid from a solid surface, resulting in the creation of two surfaces

Thus, the work of adhesion per unit surface area can be defined as:

$$W_a = \gamma_{sv} + \gamma_{lv} - \gamma_{sl}$$

This is known as the *Dupré equation*, which states that the work of adhesion is the sum of the surface free energy of the solid and the liquid, less the interfacial energy between the solid and the liquid.

From the Young equation:

$$\gamma_{sv} - \gamma_{sl} = \gamma_{lv} \cos\theta$$

Thus, the work of adhesion can be rewritten as:

$$W_a = \gamma_{lv}(1 + \cos\theta)$$

This adhesion will be a maximum when we have perfect wetting, in which case $\cos\theta = 1$, so:

$$W_a = 2\gamma_{lv}$$

For a hydrocarbon liquid, the surface tension is approximately $30 \text{ mJ} \cdot \text{m}^{-2}$. If it is assumed that the attractive force falls to 0 at a distance of 3×10^{-10} metres, then the force required to pull the liquid

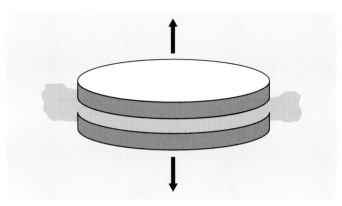

Figure 1.9.11 Two plates held together by a viscous liquid

away from the solid surface is given by the work of adhesion divided by the distance, giving about 200 MPa. This value is, in fact, far in excess of anything found in the real situation. For example, two slides held together by an interposing liquid are difficult to separate by pulling apart but separation is readily achieved by shearing the two slides apart, as the liquid has no resistance to such a shearing action other than its viscosity.

Thus, it is not enough for the fluid adhesive to wet the surface of the substrate and provide a chemical bond. It must also be able to resist tensile and shearing forces, which would cause failure within the adhesive. Increasing the viscosity would make shearing more difficult, and this is the basis on which adhesives, such as single-sided sticky tape, work.

When two plates that are held together by an interposing viscous substance are separated (Figure 1.9.11), the relationship between the force required to do so and the viscosity of the liquid is given by:

$$F = \frac{3}{2}(\pi\eta R^4/h^3)(\delta h/\delta t)$$

where η is the viscosity, R is the radius of the plates, and h the thickness of the adhesive.

We will not concern ourselves with how this expression is derived, but it is based on the need for additional fluid to enter the space between the two plates as they are separated. The expression shows that the force is dependent on the viscosity and the thickness of the adhesive layer. The higher the viscosity of the adhesive and the thinner the adhesive layer, the more force is required to separate the two plates. This expression also shows that the force depends on the rate of separation.

High rates of separation are resisted more strongly than low rates. The adhesive bond is not resistant to long-term low loads, as it would eventually fail by viscous flow in this manner. The best resistance to shear would therefore be offered by a liquid which turns into a solid, as this greatly increases its shear strength.

Real bond strengths

The actual strengths of adhesive joints are found to be at least an order of magnitude smaller than those predicted from theoretical strength calculations. Another common observation is that bond failure does not often take place at the interface between the substrate and the adhesive, but actually somewhere *within* the adhesive, which is essentially a cohesive failure.

Where the failure is genuinely adhesive in nature, it is most probably due to the inability of the adhesive to adapt to the substrate, such that no interaction at the molecular level is possible. Alternatively,

contamination or the entrapment of air or other gases at the interface can prevent a good contact from being established. In this case again, the failure will be at the interface, occurring due to the nucleation and growth of cavities at weak spots along the joint. This highlights the importance of contaminant-free surfaces for bonding.

In practice, the strengths of many adhesive bonds are governed by the presence of stress concentrations in the adhesive or at the interface, rather than being a function of the local forces of attraction at the interface. This is especially the case when the bonded structure is subjected to environmental attack or highly stressed loading conditions. In general, adhesives tend to have poorer mechanical properties (i.e. tensile strength and shear strength) than the substrates being bonded, such that surface and internal defects can play a major role in determining the bond strength of the adhesive joint.

For example, if the exposed surface of the adhesive contains numerous defects, then the probability of finding a defect of a critical size is increased as the exposed surface area of the adhesive is increased. For this reason, it is important that the thickness of the adhesive layer is kept to a minimum. The adhesive must be able to adopt a very thin film thickness, which imposes limits on the addition of fillers that might be incorporated to improve the strength.

There is another reason why the minimal application of adhesives is desirable, and that is because of the shrinkage associated with the setting process of the adhesive. When an adhesive shrinks on setting, the contraction may be away from the surface of the substrate such that debonding of the adhesive occurs immediately after placement. Even if the bond holds out during the initial contraction, the stresses generated may be sufficient to eventually cause breakdown of the bond. The thinner the layer of adhesive, the smaller the shrinkage will be. This is one reason why it is important that indirect restorations such as veneers, crowns and bridges have as good a marginal fit as it is possible to achieve, if the restoration is to be bonded to the tooth structures. The setting shrinkage of resin-based restorative materials such as resin composites, which is a consequence of the polymerization process, can generate very high localized interfacial stresses and contribute to the failure of the bond.

CLINICAL SIGNIFICANCE

More often than not, a bond failure for a compatible adhesive system, such as acid-etched enamel and resin, is usually due to part of the procedure not having been followed properly since, when properly executed, the bond is extremely strong.

ADHESION PROMOTERS

There are many instances in which two materials need to be bonded to each other, but will not do so under normal circumstances because they have no particular affinity for each other and consequently will not wet each other.

A dental example of this would be the desire to obtain a strong and durable bond between the glass filler particles used in a composite resin and the resin itself. To allow these two materials to bond by means other than the physical adsorption of one on to the other (which would be inadequate in itself), it is necessary to modify one or other of the two surfaces to achieve a bond. Sometimes, an intermediary substance can be used that is able to bond to both of the materials in question and such a material is known as a *coupling agent*. Alternatively, it is possible to modify the characteristics of the surface of one of the two materials so that a bond can be created. These materials are known as *primers*.

Coupling agents

The surface of glass, being ionic in nature, readily adsorbs water, forming a well-bonded surface layer which may be many molecules thick. The formation of this water layer cannot be avoided during the commercial processing of glass.

As a consequence of this, when glass is mixed with a resin to produce a composite, be it a fibre composite or a particulate composite, the resin will not wet the surface of the glass and the two are poorly bonded. This has the effect of producing a very weak composite because the glass is not able to take on a load-bearing role and acts merely as a space filler. Some method needs to be devised to dispose of the adsorbed water. One such approach is the use of *coupling agents*. An appropriate coupling agent, applied to the glass, will displace the water on the surface if the bond created between it and the glass is more stable than that between the water and the glass.

The function of the coupling agent is to displace the adsorbed water and provide a strong chemical link between the oxide groups on the glass surface and the polymer molecules of the resin. Silane coupling agents are extensively used for this purpose and have the general formula:

$$R—Si—X_3$$

where R represents an organo-functional group and the X units are hydrolysable groups bonded to the silane. The latter are only present as an intermediate, since they are hydrolysed to form a silanol as follows:

$$R—Si—X_3 + 3H_2O \rightarrow R—Si(OH)_3 + 3HX$$

These trihydroxy-silanols are able to compete with the water on the surface of the glass by forming hydrogen bonds with the hydroxyl groups on the glass surface.

When the silane-coated glass is now dried, the water is removed and a condensation reaction occurs between the silanol and the surface. The two stages involved are shown in Figure 1.9.12. Once this bond is formed, it is no longer susceptible to hydrolysis.

When the resin is now placed in contact with the silane-treated glass, the organo-functional group, R, reacts with the resin, and forms a strong bond to it. For this process to succeed, it is important that the organo-functional group is so chosen so as to be compatible with the particular resin system employed.

This approach produces a strong, water-resistant bond. Without the coupling agent, the bond would deteriorate rapidly as water diffuses through the resin and re-adsorbs on to the glass surface, displacing the resin.

The bond, as depicted in Figure 1.9.12, will be very rigid, as the organo-functional groups are very short. Strains generated by shrinkage during setting, or possibly by differential thermal shrinkage, could be sufficient to cause the bond to fail. This problem can be overcome by making sure that the organo-functional groups consist of reasonably long molecules, providing the necessary degree of flexibility. In a sense, the interface created by the use of coupling agents should be treated as two interfaces: namely, the glass–silanol interface and the resin–organo-functional group interface.

Two commonly used silane coupling agents are γ-methacryloxypropyltriethoxysilane and γ-mercaptopropyltrimethoxysilane.

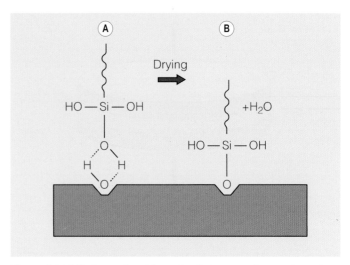

Figure 1.9.12 Hydrogen bond formation between a silane and a surface hydroxyl group (a), which, after drying, forms into a covalent bond with the release of water (b)

Primers

Primers, like the coupling agents, are another group of substances that seek to make the surface of the substrate more amenable to accepting a bond. Primers are usually applied in conjunction with an adhesive.

A typical example of a primer is one that is used to seal the surface of wood prior to applying the adhesive. If a primer were not applied, the adhesive would be soaked up by the porosity of the wood, such that none remained at the interface.

There are many dental examples of primers, such as phosphoric acid, which is used for preparing the enamel surface, and the wide variety of dentine conditioners, which are used in conjunction with dentine-bonding agents. Unfortunately, in the dental literature, the distinction between primers and coupling agents is lost, and the two terms are used interchangeably.

SUMMARY

Adhesion is not a simple phenomenon; nor is it comprehensible with a single model. The formation of an adhesive bond depends on a multitude of factors and rarely involves a single adhesive mechanism.

CLINICAL SIGNIFICANCE

Adhesion has become one of the major cornerstones of dentistry. In operative dentistry it has created the opportunity to produce a marginal seal around restorations. In prosthetic dentistry it has provided the opportunity to explore new materials and techniques. There is no aspect of dentistry that has not been touched in some way by our improved understanding of the molecular interactions between materials at their interfaces.

Section | 2 |

Clinical dental materials

A wide variety of materials are used in the dental surgery by the dentist, the dental surgery assistant and, more recently, the dental therapist. It is important that the manner in which these materials are to be handled and for which clinical applications they are appropriate are well understood.

A significant contributory factor to the failure of restorations is the inappropriate use and abuse of dental materials. This problem can be minimized by ensuring a thorough understanding of the composition and chemistry of dental materials and an appreciation of their physical and mechanical properties.

Chapter | 2.1 |

Dental amalgams

INTRODUCTION

Dental amalgam had a fairly inauspicious beginning, early in the 19th century, when it was used as a restorative material, being made by mixing Spanish or Mexican silver coins with mercury. Dental amalgams have come a long way since then, and are still a part of everyday dental practice.

The development of dental amalgams is due, in no small way, to one of the most famous dentists ever, G.V. Black, who recognized the need to determine the properties of dental amalgams with some accuracy, if their performance was ever going to be predictable. At the beginning of the 20th century, because of his research work, amalgams could be produced with reasonably predictable handling characteristics.

Over the years, our understanding of these materials has advanced considerably, but up until the late 1960s, there was little change in this field and the composition was very much as it had been for the preceding 50 years.

During the last 50 years, it seems as though the developers of dental amalgams have tried to make up for this lack of activity, with new formulations appearing at frequent intervals. There has been an onslaught on the traditional applications of this material by new materials, such as the resin composites and the glass–ionomer cements. While this has led to some exciting new developments in dental amalgams, it has made the dentist's job more difficult, as the selection of the best available product at the best possible price becomes more and more complicated.

In this section, the development of the amalgams from the late 1960s to their current status is charted, highlighting the important advances made.

THE STRUCTURE OF TRADITIONAL DENTAL AMALGAMS

Composition

An amalgam is formed when mercury is mixed with another metal or metals. Mercury is liquid at room temperature (solidifying at $-39\,°C$),

and it reacts readily with metals such as silver, tin and copper, to produce solid materials. When the dentist selects a certain dental amalgam, it is effectively a selection of the alloy with which the mercury will be mixed and react.

Strictly speaking, the term *dental amalgam* cannot be used until one is referring to the material produced as a consequence of the reaction between the mercury and the alloy. This alloy can vary either in composition or in form, and dental amalgam manufacturers use this variability to produce a wide range of products.

Alloy

The alloy used in the traditional dental amalgams consists of a mixture of silver, tin, copper and sometimes zinc and/or mercury. A typical composition may be as shown in Table 2.1.1.

Silver is the main constituent, present in combination with tin as the intermetallic compound Ag_3Sn, known commonly as the *γ phase*. The phase diagram for the Ag–Sn system is shown in Figure 2.1.1, and shows that the Ag_3Sn phase is the third pure phase in the system, hence the Greek symbol γ.

This γ phase reacts readily with mercury to form the dental amalgam. Copper is present to increase the strength and hardness of the amalgam, and a more pronounced effect is produced when the copper content is increased beyond 6%, but this will be dealt with later. Zinc may be present as a result of the initial production of the alloy, and is not considered to serve any useful purpose in the amalgamation process. Mercury is sometimes added to provide a more rapid reaction, in what is referred to as *pre-amalgamation*.

The alloy is used in the form of a powder, and the size and shape of the particles in this powder are critical to the handling characteristics and the final properties of the restoration. The alloy powder is available as either *lathe-cut* particles or spherical particles, as shown in Figure 2.1.2.

Lathe-cut

The lathe-cut particles are produced by machining a solid ingot of the alloy on a lathe. The chippings that are produced are graded, and only those in the right size range are used in the powder to be amalgamated with mercury.

Table 2.1.1 Constituents of a typical dental amalgam alloy

Constituent	% of total
Ag	67–74
Sn	25–28
Cu	0–6
Zn	0–2
Hg	0–3

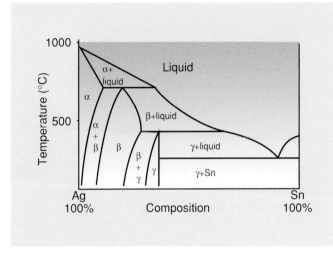

Figure 2.1.1 Phase diagram for the Ag–Sn system

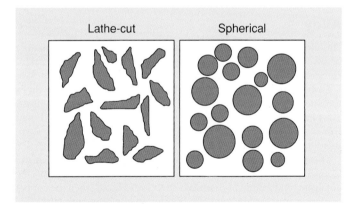

Figure 2.1.2 Schematic representation of the lathe-cut and spherical shapes of alloy particles used in amalgams

The alloy is available as coarse-, medium- or fine-grained powder, and each will handle slightly differently. The individual chippings will have become highly stressed during the machining, and this makes their surfaces very reactive to mercury. A consequence of this is that the setting reaction is far too rapid unless heat treatment (which relieves the internal stresses) is applied. The heat treatment is usually carried out by placing the powder in boiling water.

Spherical particles

The production of the spherical particles is by a quite different route. The various ingredients of the alloy are melted together and then sprayed into an inert atmosphere, where the droplets solidify as small,

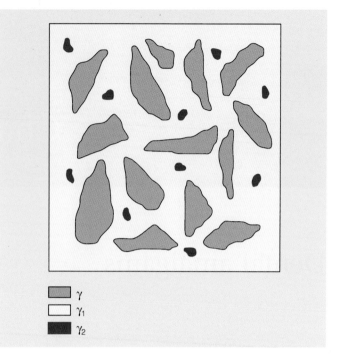

Figure 2.1.3 Schematic representation of the microstructure of a lathe-cut alloy-based amalgam

spherical pellets of various sizes. This method of manufacture has the advantages that no further machining processes are required, and that the composition of the alloy can be readily altered. What is important to the manufacturer is that the yield of particles of the correct size is as high as possible, since this minimizes the cost of production. The particles that are rejected because they are either too big or too small are simply recycled.

Mercury

The mercury used in the preparation of an amalgam needs to be very pure; otherwise a surface layer of contaminants is formed that interferes with the setting reaction. For this reason, the mercury is triple-distilled. The purity can easily be checked by visual examination. If a dull surface is observed, as opposed to the usual highly reflective surface, the mercury is contaminated.

Setting reaction

The setting reaction between the Ag–Sn alloy and the mercury is initiated by a vigorous mixing of the two ingredients. This mixing causes the outer layer of the alloy particles to dissolve into the mercury, forming two new phases, which are solid at room temperature. The reaction is as follows:

$$Ag_3Sn + Hg \rightarrow Ag_3Sn + Ag_2Hg_3 + Sn_7Hg$$
$$\gamma + mercury \rightarrow \gamma + \gamma_1 + \gamma_2$$

| powder | liquid | unreacted alloy | amalgam | matrix |

As can be seen from the reaction, not all of the alloy particles dissolve in the mercury. On the contrary, a considerable amount remains, so that the final structure is one of a core of γ held together by a matrix of predominantly γ_1, which is interspersed with γ_2. The structure of the set material is shown in Figure 2.1.3.

The copper in the lathe-cut alloy is present in the form of discrete areas of Cu₃Sn, and remains mainly within the original alloy in its unreacted form.

In the case of the spherical particles, the copper is uniformly distributed, and the alloy could be more accurately regarded as a ternary alloy of silver, tin and copper. Hence, in the final structure of the spherical alloy amalgam, the copper is not present as a discrete phase but is widely distributed throughout the material. Although some voids will inevitably be present, in a well-condensed amalgam there will be very little porosity.

PROPERTIES OF TRADITIONAL AMALGAMS

It is not the intention here to cover all aspects of the properties of dental amalgams, and only those properties of some importance to clinical use and development of new alloys will be considered.

Strength

The strength of an amalgam is extremely important, since the restoration has to be able to withstand the considerable loads generated during mastication, and any lack of strength is likely to lead to marginal ditching of the restoration or even gross fracture.

Although most attention has been paid to the final compressive strength of the set material, it is perhaps more important to consider the tensile strength and the rate at which the final strength is acquired.

As might be imagined, the final strength of the amalgam will be a function of the properties of the individual phases. It is not easy to determine the properties of the three main phases of an amalgam, but micro-hardness measurements suggest that the γ phase and the γ_1 phase have a similar hardness, while the γ_2 phase is considerably softer. The tensile strength of the γ_2 phase has also been measured to be only a fraction of that of the original γ phase, with the γ_1 phase falling in between (Table 2.1.2).

This means that the weak link within the amalgam structure is the γ_2 phase, and if its proportion in the final composition could be minimized, a stronger amalgam would result. The amount of γ_1 and γ_2 formed is strongly dependent on the amount of mercury in the final composition. The higher the mercury content, the weaker the material will be, because larger amounts of the weaker phases will be produced.

The final mercury content of the amalgam is dependent on the quality of the condensation technique more than anything else, with a properly condensed amalgam having a mercury content of just less than 50%. Besides the condensation technique, the size and shape of the alloy particles will also affect the final mercury content. The initial ratio of alloy to mercury is lower in amalgam made with spherical alloy particles than with lathe-cut alloy particles because the

material is more easily condensed. With spherical alloy particles, a final mercury content of about 45% is readily achievable.

The particle size is also important. For a given amount of alloy that is to be amalgamated with mercury, choosing smaller alloy particles results in more of the alloy surface being exposed to the mercury. This means that more of the alloy will dissolve in the mercury, producing more of the mercury-containing phases. Consequently, too small a particle size is contraindicated.

Whatever the form of the alloy used, the conscientious removal of excess mercury during the placement of a restoration is vitally important.

Flow and creep

It has been postulated that the excessive flow of an amalgam, resulting from repeated occlusal loading, can cause flattening of contact points, overhanging margins, and protrusion of the restoration from the tooth surface at the margin. The latter has been implicated as a major source of marginal breakdown. Although flow is measured for amalgam in laboratory tests, the measurement is usually carried out over a short period very soon after mixing and is therefore of limited clinical relevance. A more appropriate measurement would be that of creep. This is the flow caused by loads acting over long periods. Creep is dependent on both the yield strength of the material and the temperature of the environment, and only becomes a serious problem when the environmental temperature is greater than half the melting temperature of the material.

Since the amalgam phases have very low melting temperatures (about 80°C) and the restorations are subjected to repeated loadings, there is the possibility of creep occurring. The phases most prone to creep will be the mercury-based γ_1 and γ_2 phases. Consequently, the lower the proportion of these phases present (as may be achieved by proper condensation), the less susceptible the amalgam will be to creep.

Corrosion

It is well recognized that amalgams corrode in the oral environment. Indeed, corrosion is often cited as an advantage, in that the corrosion products help to produce a good marginal seal. However, crevice corrosion, caused by the formation of an oxidation cell in the marginal gap, can cause a rapid deterioration in the properties of the amalgam. The corrosion process is especially associated with the γ_2 phase.

The γ_2 phase is considerably more electronegative than the γ and γ_1 phases. This means that, in the presence of an electrolytic solution, the γ_2 phase will act as the anode of the oxidation cell and will gradually dissolve. The reaction is as follows:

tin-mercury phase + oral fluids → tin salts + free mercury
Sn_7Hg + oxygen → oxides & chlorides + Hg

Normally, the formation of oxides would help to slow down the corrosion process by forming a protective surface coating. However, in the gap between the amalgam and the tooth tissues, a surface oxide is not formed, as the reaction products from the corrosion process precipitate out. The process is also very insidious, since the production of free mercury allows further reaction with γ, and the formation of more γ_1 and γ_2. This process will severely weaken the amalgam structure, and is often cited as a cause of marginal breakdown.

Table 2.1.2 Tensile strengths of phases of amalgam

Phase	Tensile strength (MPa)
γ	170
γ_1	30
γ_2	20
Amalgam	60

CLINICAL SIGNIFICANCE

Traditional dental amalgams suffer from a lack of strength and excessive creep and corrosion.

HIGH-COPPER-CONTENT DENTAL AMALGAMS

From the above discussion of the properties of the traditional dental amalgams, it can be deduced that an improvement in their performance may be possible if their strength could be increased. This strengthening is possible by reducing the amount of γ_1 and γ_2, or better still if the weak and corrosion-susceptible γ_2 phase could be eliminated from the structure entirely, with the added benefit that creep could be reduced.

Dispersed phase amalgams

In the early 1960s, attempts were made to increase the strength of dental amalgams by increasing the copper content of the alloy.

The idea was that the copper would act as a dispersion-strengthening agent. A spherical alloy (basically silver and copper) with a high copper content was added to the conventional lathe-cut alloy. The choice of the spherical particles was made essentially because it was easier to alter the composition of spherical particles than lathe-cut particles on an experimental basis. The potential advantages, in terms of easier condensation, were also recognized at that time.

As it turned out, the increase in the copper content of the alloy resulted in a modification of the setting reaction, which proved to be highly beneficial.

The first reaction is the same as for the traditional alloys, but this is followed by a second reaction:

$$\gamma_2 + Ag\text{—}Cu \rightarrow Cu_6Sn_5 + \gamma_1$$

Thus, the final amalgam contains little or no γ_2. The structure of this amalgam is shown in Figure 2.1.4.

Initially, it was thought that all of the γ_2 was eliminated by this reaction, but it has since been recognized that some γ_2 will remain, although it is only a small and probably insignificant amount.

The modification in the setting reaction has resulted in a number of interesting and important changes in the properties of the amalgam, namely:

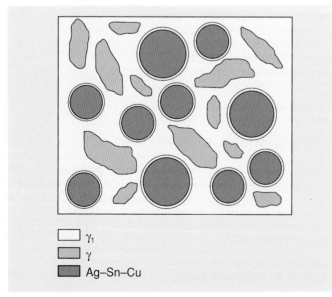

- γ_1
- γ
- Ag–Sn–Cu

Figure 2.1.4 Schematic representation of the microstructure of a dispersed-phase amalgam. The halo around the spherical particles is a Cu–Sn phase

- a higher compressive strength
- a more rapid set to full strength
- a reduction in creep
- a reduced susceptibility to corrosion.

Other high-copper-content formulations

With these sorts of improvements, it was not long before the idea of the *all-spherical high-copper amalgams* came into being. These combine all of the advantages of easier condensation with those mentioned above, and a number of such products are now available.

The powder in these cases is a ternary spherical alloy of silver, tin and copper and has a setting reaction as follows:

$$Ag\text{—}Sn\text{—}Cu + Hg \rightarrow Ag\text{—}Sn\text{—}Cu + \gamma_1 + Cu_6Sn_5$$

The reluctance of many dentists to convert from a lathe-cut alloy to a spherical alloy has led to the introduction of *high-copper-content all-lathe-cut alloy* formulations. The composition of these alloys is essentially the same as for all of the spherical alloys, except that there are wide differences in the total copper content, which can vary from 12 to 30%. As yet, it is not known what the optimum percentage of copper is.

For those dentists who prefer the dispersed-phase type of alloy, there are now a number available that have a mixture of spherical and lathe-cut particles, where both particle types have the same composition of ternary Ag–Sn–Cu alloy.

SELECTION AND USE OF DENTAL AMALGAMS

In the selection of the appropriate dental amalgam, there are two major factors that need to be considered:

- variables under the control of the manufacturer
- variables under the control of the operator.

Both of these will have a profound effect on the properties of the dental amalgams, such as their handling characteristics and their clinical performance.

The clinical performance of an amalgam restoration is dependent as much on the correct choice of the alloy as it is on the use of a good operative procedure. The need for a good procedure involves all of the stages of amalgam placement, from the proportioning stage to the final polishing.

Manufacturer's variables

The variables under the control of the manufacturer are the composition and the particle size and shape of the alloy.

Composition

The most obvious differences in composition relate to the copper content of the alloy, and the first question that might be asked is *'Should I use a traditional or a copper-enriched amalgam alloy?'*

The evidence obtained from controlled clinical trials indicates very strongly that the performance of the high-copper amalgams is superior to that of the traditional amalgams. The rate of marginal breakdown is most certainly lower than that of the traditional low-copper-content alloy systems, although this by itself does not necessarily mean that the longevity of these two systems will be very different.

Table 2.1.3 Selected properties of some dental amalgams

Material	Manufacturer	Type	% Cu content	% Creep	Compressive strength (MPa)	
					1 hour	24 hours
Amalcap-F	Ivoclar	Lathe-cut	6	2.5	94	410
Dispersalloy	J&J	Admix	12	0.25	226	440
Sybralloy	Kerr	Spherical	30	0.05	315	500

It should be remembered that the traditional amalgams have provided excellent service for many years, and that a lifetime in excess of 10 years is by no means uncommon for these restorations, showing the potential of this amalgam. More often than not, the premature failure of an amalgam restoration is related to inadequate operative technique. Nevertheless, in the hands of experienced operators, and under highly controlled conditions, high-copper amalgams have been shown to perform better.

Why the high-copper amalgams should give better clinical performance is not as yet clear. The resistance to creep has improved significantly, but so has the resistance to corrosion. Both of these have been implicated as causes in the reduction in marginal breakdown, but it is not clear whether the reduced corrosion or the reduced creep is responsible for the improved properties. Perhaps it is as well to be pragmatic and just accept that there is an improvement in performance, whatever the cause.

A feature of the high-copper amalgams is their increased compressive strength, when compared to the traditional alloys. Just 1 hour after placement, the high-copper-content amalgams can be twice as strong as the traditional amalgams, and this must contribute to a reduced incidence of gross fractures. It should be noted, though, that the final compressive strength may not be that different (Table 2.1.3).

Another feature of the high-copper amalgams is that they do not contain any zinc. Since zinc is understood to be the source of delayed expansion when an amalgam becomes contaminated with saliva, this is an additional advantage.

One disadvantage that has been noted with some of the high-copper amalgams is that their surfaces are more prone to tarnish.

Particle size and shape

The particles' size and shape need to be considered seriously because they not only determine the handling characteristics of the alloy, but also affect the final composition.

There is a tendency to opt for the alloys that have a very fine particle size because they are easily carved to give a very nice surface finish. However, the small particle size of the powder means that more mercury will react with the alloy, giving a higher final mercury content, and hence higher proportions of γ_1 and γ_2. In addition, the early compressive strength of these amalgams is much lower than those of amalgams made with larger-sized alloy particles.

Some studies have shown that the use of a very fine alloy powder gives rise to a higher rate of marginal breakdown, and that its use is contraindicated.

In contrast, the coarse-grained alloys are difficult to carve because particles are easily dislodged from the surface during the initial set. Medium or fine particles appear to be the best compromise in this respect.

The concern over particle shape is a choice between lathe-cut and spherical alloy or, perhaps, a mixture of the two. This is very much a matter of personal preference, but it is said that the spherical-alloy systems condense more readily than the lathe-cut alloy compositions.

In the end, this is something that only the dentist can decide, by being prepared to try different types of amalgams.

CLINICAL SIGNIFICANCE

Clinical evidence is now sufficient to be able to say that high-copper-content amalgams are the amalgams of choice and the balance has most certainly swung in their favour.

Operator variables

The variables that are under the control of the dentist and which may affect the final quality of the restoration are:

- proportioning of the alloy and mercury
- trituration
- condensation
- carving and polishing.

Proportioning

Proportioning is most commonly carried out using volumetric dispensers or preproportioned capsules. The advantages of the latter are that the dentist does not have to worry about getting the right ratio of alloy to mercury (as this is prefixed by the manufacturer), and that there is less danger of mercury spillage during the handling stages of amalgam placement. Unfortunately, the capsules are more expensive than buying the alloy powder in bulk.

Thus, the volumetric dispenser is a more attractive proposition to some dentists, but it does limit the choice of alloy to the fine-grained variety, since the medium- or coarse-grained alloys tend to produce erratic mixes. On the other hand, the volumetric dispenser allows more freedom in the alloy-to-mercury ratio, which is a feature that appeals particularly to those dentists who like to start from a fairly wet mix. The high initial mercury content should present no problem as long as a good condensation technique is employed. It is important that a sufficiently plastic mix is obtained to allow proper amalgamation and handling; a dry mix should be avoided at all costs. Generally, a 1:1 ratio of alloy to mercury will suffice for the lathe-cut alloys, but for the spherical alloys a higher ratio of alloy to mercury is allowed because of the lower total surface area of the spherical particles.

The lower mercury content in this case does not mean that this reduces the need for the removal of excess mercury. It is important that the final mercury content is as low as possible, and a good condensation technique is still required.

Trituration

Trituration is one of the most important of the operator variables. Adequate trituration is essential to ensure a plastic mix and thorough amalgamation. The trituration time that is needed is dependent on both the type of alloy being used, and the dispensing and mixing system.

The spherical alloys tend to mix more readily and in general require a shorter trituration time. This is because the particles are more easily wetted than the lathe-cut particles.

The exact trituration time depends on the mixing system. For a system running at a speed of 4000 rpm and a throw of some 50 mm, amalgamation times can be as short as 5 seconds. For a slower system, with a speed of 2600 rpm, the trituration time can be 20 seconds or more.

The general recommendation is that it is better to err on the side of over-trituration than under-trituration. If it is found that the amalgam comes out looking crumbly or dry, which might give the appearance of having set already, in fact the trituration time must be *increased* and not decreased, as is often thought; the extra trituration will provide a more plastic mix with a longer working time. However, if the trituration time is set too long, this will reduce the setting time because the material heats up during the vigorous mixing action.

Trituration times also affect the dimensional changes that occur when amalgams set. Ideally, the material should expand slightly on setting, as this aids marginal adaptation and will reduce the potential for marginal leakage.

Prior to the introduction of capsules and amalgamators, the traditional amalgams contained large alloy particles which were hand-triturated; these formulations showed a slight expansion once fully set. The dimensional change with time is shown in Figure 2.1.5.

There is an initial contraction as the mercury diffuses into the alloy. This is followed by an expansion as the γ_1 phase forms, due to the γ_1 crystals impinging on one another and producing an outward pressure which opposes the contraction. This occurs only if sufficient mercury is present to produce a plastic mix.

The introduction of high-speed mechanical amalgamators, low mercury : alloy ratios, small alloy particle sizes and high condensation pressures reduces the amount of mercury in the mix and favours a contraction of the amalgam, such that modern amalgams show a net contraction on setting.

Condensation

The most important demands on the condensation technique are that as much excess mercury is removed as is possible, that the final restoration will be non-porous and that optimum marginal adaptation is achieved so as to prevent postoperative sensitivity.

For the lathe-cut alloys, a final mercury content of 45% can be achieved. Although reductions below 50% mercury have little effect on the compressive strength after 24 hours, a much higher early compressive strength is achieved and the susceptibility to creep is much reduced. A high early strength reduces the likelihood of gross amalgam fracture during the first few hours after placement. This applies equally well to the spherical alloy systems, except that in these cases the final mercury content should be approximately 40%.

The important components in condensation are the use of maximum force, the use of suitably sized condensers in relation to cavity size, the use of multiple and rapid thrusts, and the placement of small increments.

Although condensation pressures of 30–40 N are generally recommended, this does not mean that lower condensation pressures will result in a poorer result, as low condensation pressures can be compensated for by the placement of small increments. The placement of large increments will not only lead to the formation of large amounts of γ_1 and γ_2, but will also produce a high level of porosity.

The condensation of the spherical alloy amalgams requires a different approach from the lathe-cut systems. As the mix flows more readily under even light pressures, small loads need to be applied by larger condensers, if possible. However, close marginal adaptation appears to be more difficult with the spherical alloy amalgams, which is due to the coarser grain structure of the spherical alloys.

Carving and polishing

The ability to carve an amalgam is a function of the size and shape of the alloy particles. In general, the spherical alloys produce a better initial surface finish than the lathe-cut alloys.

The need for polishing an amalgam at a second visit is a matter of some debate. Some would argue that polishing is necessary for no other reason than that it improves the aesthetics, while others would point to the high level of residual mercury in the surface layer and feel that this needs to be removed.

It may be true that a thin surface layer will have a preponderance of the γ_1 and γ_2 phases, but this layer is likely to be so thin that it would soon be worn away. Similarly, a controversy exists concerning the need, or not, for burnishing. It used to be said that the burnishing of amalgams will give rise to a mercury-rich surface layer, which would increase the possibility of corrosion or fracture. However, more recent studies would indicate that the overall effect of burnishing is to increase surface hardness, reduce porosity and decrease corrosion, while also improving the marginal adaptation of the amalgam.

An as-carved surface finish for an amalgam is decidedly rough, and some form of additional finishing is necessary. The option is either to recall the patient the next day in order to polish the restoration or, alternatively, to burnish the restoration at the time of placement. Burnishing may be an effective substitute for conventional polishing of lathe-cut amalgams and, so long as either is used, a better marginal integrity is attained.

LIMITATIONS OF DENTAL AMALGAMS

The use of dental amalgams has been the subject of considerable discussion since the introduction of the new resin composites and glass–ionomer cements. Some have even suggested that the use of amalgams should be discontinued. Given that amalgams have given excellent service for some 100 years, this would seem a rather extreme viewpoint. Nevertheless, dental amalgams have a number of shortcomings.

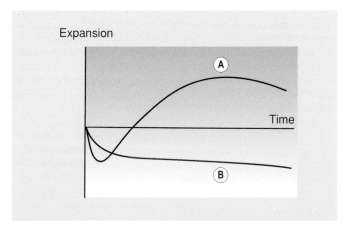

Figure 2.1.5 Dimensional change for a traditional hand-mixed amalgam (a) and a modern mechanically mixed amalgam (b)

Poor aesthetics

Being metallic restorations, amalgams are not the most visually attractive of options, although if they are polished more regularly than is the current practice, they *can* look quite presentable.

The polished finish is lost with time, due to tarnishing. Although there is an increasing demand from patients for more aesthetic restorations, in the case of posterior restorations, durability is the most important consideration.

Mercury toxicity

It cannot be denied that mercury is a highly toxic substance and its use demands the greatest of care. The main sources of mercury exposure arise from:

- accidental spills
- poor mercury hygiene
- direct contact with mercury
- amalgamators
- placement of new and removal of old restorations.

The most serious potential hazard is from mercury vapour, and the most significant source of this vapour is spillage of mercury in the surgery. The use of amalgam capsules should minimize this risk.

Dental surgery staff are most at risk from mercury contamination, since the material is dealt with on a daily basis. If any spillage should occur, it is in the interests of everybody, particularly the dental staff, that it is dealt with immediately and thoroughly. Any mercury left lying around will gradually vaporize and thence be inhaled. The threshold for air/mercury exposure hazard for the general population is $50\ \mu g/m^3$ of air. It is known from the experience of workers in factories dealing with mercury, e.g. thermometer workshops, that if this threshold is exceeded, signs of mercury poisoning will appear. These include leg cramps, itching, rashes, excessive perspiration, rapid heartbeat, intermittent low-grade fevers, irritability, marked personality change, insomnia, headaches, hypertension, chronic fatigue and nerve dysfunction.

Appropriate mercury hygiene procedures must be used, and these include:

- the use of a no-touch technique
- the use of mechanical amalgamators with good seals
- the storage of mercury and old amalgams under water in unbreakable, tightly sealed containers
- the cleaning up of spilled mercury immediately.

Patients are perceived to be less at risk from mercury inhalation than dental staff. Certainly, there is some ingestion by inhalation of mercury vapour during the placement of a freshly mixed amalgam, but this is believed to be well below the $50\ \mu g/m^3$ threshold. However, there have been a number of occasions when patients have reacted very badly to the presence of amalgams in their mouth, due to a delayed hypersensitivity reaction to mercury. Rare as these allergic reactions are, the symptoms can be quite severe, and the dentist should be aware of such a possibility. There have also been reports of local lichenoid-type reactions associated with amalgam fillings, and removal of the amalgam restoration is recommended when there is clear contact between the restoration and the lesion.

Besides mercury vapour inhalation, wear and corrosion will contribute to the overall body burden of mercury. On average, the mercury intake into the body from dental amalgam fillings is believed to be well below the threshold level of $30\ \mu g/day$ recommended by the World Health Organization. However, it should be appreciated that this is only an average and it is possible that some patients, possibly due to excessive chewing or bruxism, can have a mercury level in their body well above the average. It has also been shown in vitro that carbamide-based bleaching agents can increase the release of mercury from amalgam restorations. Thus, patients claiming to have symptoms of mercury toxicity should be treated with care and consideration.

The continued use of dental amalgams has become a controversial issue in a number of countries in Europe. In the primary dentition, the use of dental amalgam has been much reduced with the advent of compomers and resin-modified glass–ionomer cements, such that in only a few countries is amalgam the material of first choice. Mercury from fillings contaminates the environment and adds to the overall mercury burden in the community. In some countries where there are careful controls on the use of mercury, this can mean that dental amalgam can be a significant contributor to the overall mercury burden. In such circumstances, a strong case can be made for discontinuing the use of dental amalgams as long as it is recognized that the cost of dental treatment will go up as a consequence of such a decision. Although the use of mercury in dentistry accounts for only 3% of the total amount used worldwide, all dentists should be encouraged to use stringent mercury hygiene in dental practice and implement waste-management procedures that prevent mercury from entering the environment.

CLINICAL SIGNIFICANCE

It is important to emphasize the safe handling of dental amalgam to the whole of the dental team at every opportunity.

Nevertheless, concerns about the biocompatibility of mercury amalgams are sufficient for serious consideration to be given to alternative alloys.

One approach is to replace mercury with gallium, which has the second lowest melting temperature after mercury. When alloyed with tin and indium, a liquid is produced at room temperature. Alloy powders with a composition close to that of the alloys used in mercury amalgams are mixed with this liquid, which produces a workable mix that can be condensed into the cavity. Although the resulting alloy has physical and mechanical properties similar to those of mercury amalgam, excessive setting expansion and poor handling properties need to be overcome before these materials can be considered as a viable substitute.

In another approach, the use of liquid metal is eliminated altogether by relying on the cold welding of pre-alloyed silver-coated particles. Cold welding takes place where there is silver-to-silver contact between the particles. This process is promoted by exposure of the particles to a mild acid so as to remove any surface contaminants, which would interfere with the cold welding. One problem with this material is the high compaction pressure needed to consolidate the silver particles. Although a promising material, it is still at the developmental stage and not yet available commercially.

High thermal conductivity

As one would expect from a metallic material, the thermal conductivity of dental amalgams is very high. Problems presented by this, such as pulpal sensitivity due to the hydrodynamic effect of pumping fluid through the marginal gap and up and down the dentinal tubules, are readily dealt with by suitable cavity preparation techniques, involving the use of varnishes or liners (see Chapter 2.4).

Galvanic effects

When two metallic restorations consisting of metals with different degrees of electronegativity are placed in close proximity to one another in an electrically conducting medium (in the dental case, this medium is saliva), it is possible that a galvanic cell will be set up.

The resultant currents can cause patients discomfort or leave a strong metallic taste in the mouth, and can accelerate the corrosive breakdown of the more electronegative metal. Consequently, although the problem rarely arises, the use of different metals in the mouth is not recommended.

Lack of adhesion

The need for the use of retentive cavity designs with dental amalgams imposes a severe constraint. Often, large amounts of perfectly sound enamel or dentine are removed, under the banner of 'extension for prevention'. This principle is questionable, as amalgam can never be a substitute for healthy tooth tissues. New ideas in cavity preparation have been developed, with the aim of minimizing the loss of healthy tooth tissue, but these can never be as conservative as the approach of using adhesive restorative materials. In order to overcome this criticism of dental amalgams, it has been suggested that bonding of amalgam to teeth can be carried out, as this would have the benefits of reinforcing the tooth, aiding retention and preserving tooth structure. Generally speaking, adhesion is achieved by the combination of a dentine-bonding agent and a luting resin, which are placed prior to the placement of the dental amalgam, although other options, such as self-adhesive resins, have also been advocated. The benefits accruing from this approach are debatable, except, perhaps, in situations where retention is seriously compromised.

Lack of strength and toughness

As noted previously, dental amalgams are very brittle, low-tensile strength-restorative materials. The way to deal with this is to use the material in bulk, as this reduces the degree to which the restoration will bend and flex, which in turn reduces tensile stresses. Hence cavity preparations are designed such that thin sections of the amalgam filling are avoided. This means that boxes have to be cut deep and margin angles need to be as near to 90° as possible. The consequence of this is that dental amalgams inherently do not conserve tooth structure. Hence, in situations of small primary caries lesions, the use of dental amalgam may well be contraindicated as being too destructive of tooth tissue, and an alternative material, such as a composite resin, would be preferable.

Limited lifespan of dental amalgam restorations

Hundreds of thousands of amalgams are placed each year and, on average, half of these are replacements of existing restorations. The longevity of amalgam restorations has been the subject of a number of clinical studies, with some suggesting that half need replacement within 4–5 years.

On average, the survival time of amalgam restorations is inversely proportional to their size. To compound this problem, every time an amalgam restoration is replaced, the cavity outline is increased by at least 0.5 mm, leading to a larger restoration. In general, then, the smaller the restoration, the longer it will survive.

Of all the disadvantages mentioned above, the lack of longevity and the destructive nature of the procedure are matters of the greatest concern. Ways of making restorations last longer will be considered in the next section.

IMPROVING THE LONGEVITY OF AMALGAM RESTORATIONS

Several workers over the last few decades have cast a critical eye over established amalgam techniques. The reasons for replacement of amalgam restorations are usually associated with:

- tooth fracture
- recurrent caries
- gross amalgam fracture
- marginal breakdown.

The latter may arise from fracture of either the amalgam margins or the enamel margins. Of the factors cited, the most common reason for replacing an amalgam restoration (accounting for some 70% or replacements) is considered to be recurrent caries.

Some of the failures are unavoidable, being related to inadequacies in the properties of the amalgams, but others *can* be avoided by considering the amalgams' limitations and by adopting appropriate techniques by avoiding faults in cavity design and poor clinical technique.

Tooth fracture

Weakened tooth structure

The more tooth tissue that is removed, the weaker the tooth becomes. A dental amalgam acts as an effective space filler, but since it has no adhesive qualities, it does not help in strengthening the underlying tooth structure. Thus, techniques involving the minimal removal of tooth tissue should always be employed.

By cutting enamel along the plane parallel to the prism direction, it is possible to keep outline form to a minimum. This practice also ensures that cavo-surface angles will be close to 90°, which is optimal for the amalgam, with acute cavo-surface angles encouraging marginal breakdown of the amalgam.

There are now a number of adhesives available that allow bonding of the amalgam to the tooth tissues. The bond will provide additional support to both the restoration and the cusps, which should help to strengthen the restored tooth crown. As the durability of the bond is as yet unknown, the design of the cavity should still be such as to avoid potential sites for fracture. With severely weakened cusps, alternative techniques, such as gold onlays or resin-bonded ceramics, might have to be considered.

Undermined enamel

The principle of providing flat walls and floors to a cavity can give rise to undermined enamel, as shown in Figure 2.1.6 for a box in a proximal restoration. The unsupported enamel will break free and leave a gap, which can lead to recurrent caries.

Residual caries

It is of paramount importance that any residual caries is removed. If not, the caries will spread and undermine the cusp, eventually causing it to fracture. The leakage of bacterial toxins will also cause pulpal inflammation.

Recurrent caries

Contamination

Contamination of the cavity with blood or saliva will result in poor adaptation of the restoration to the cavity margins.

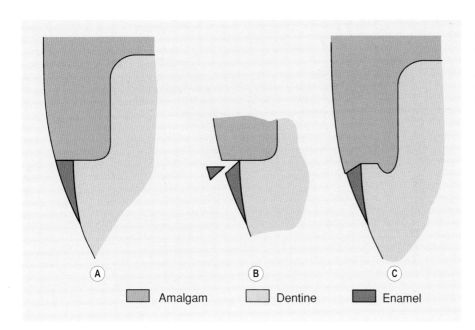

Figure 2.1.6 If the gingival floor of the proximal box is finished (a), then unsupported enamel will break away (b) and lead to recurrent caries. Bevelling the enamel (c) prevents this occurring but it is necessary to place a groove in the gingival floor of the dentine to resist the displacement of the restoration proximally

Amalgam   Dentine   Enamel

Poor matrix techniques

A poorly adapted matrix band can be the cause of proximal overhangs, or of poor contact points with the adjacent teeth. Overhangs are particularly prone to plaque accumulation, and may initiate recurrent caries. If the overhang is subgingival, it may cause soft tissue irritation and can eventually lead to bone loss and pocketing. Overtightening of the matrix band can cause the fracture of tooth cusps that have been weakened by the removal of large amounts of tooth tissue.

Poor condensation

As already noted, poor condensation results in porosity of the amalgam and the presence of excess mercury, both of which reduce the strength of the amalgam. Marginal adaptation will also be poor, increasing the potential for marginal leakage, recurrent caries and corrosion. For good condensation, it is important that the amalgam is well mixed, and that the appropriate trituration time is selected. Under-trituration, in particular, should be avoided, as this will result in a dry amalgam mix that will not condense properly.

Gross amalgam fracture

Shallow preparations

Dental amalgams have a very low tensile strength. When placed in thin sections they are subjected to bending forces and will break. Shallow preparations are only acceptable in very small restorations, where the surface area is small compared to the depth. For large mesial occlusal distal restorations, there must be sufficient depth to the cavity on the occlusal floor to provide enough bulk to resist the bending forces. This may require the removal of large amounts of sound tooth tissue.

Non-retentive proximal boxes

A frequently observed failure of mesial occlusal, distal occlusal or mesial occlusal distal restorations is the fracture of the proximal boxes from the occlusal section of the filling. To some extent, this is due to the low tensile strength of the amalgam restoration, as an occlusal load can force the amalgam to splay outwards. However, sharp

internal line angles aggravate the situation, which ultimately leads to the fracture and loss of the box. The risk of this happening can be reduced by cutting retention grooves in the lateral walls and gingival floor of the boxes. This technique ensures that the box is self-retentive and opposes the splaying action from an occlusal load by resisting the displacement of the restoration in a proximal direction. An added advantage is that an occlusal lock is not required for retention of the restoration. Thus, the additional preparation of occlusal fissures is not required when a primary lesion is confined to the proximal surface only; this type of preparation is generally described as a 'wedge' preparation.

Sharp internal line angles

The presence of sharp internal line angles concentrates stress at these sites, which increases the risk of fracture of both the tooth and the filling, as shown in Figure 2.1.7. Such sharp angles are avoidable, and rounded internal surfaces should be the aim. For example, proximal boxes should be pear-shaped, to conform to the extent of the underlying lesion, and should not be cut with sharp line angles in their corners.

Marginal breakdown

Incorrect cavo-surface angles

The primary cause of marginal breakdown of a restored tooth is the presence of an incorrect cavo-surface angle, leading to marginal fracture of the enamel or the amalgam. Marginal breakdown of the amalgam occurs more readily when the amalgam has an acute margin angle. Amalgam is extremely brittle and has a very low tensile strength (60–70 MPa) so any resultant thin wedges will fracture very easily as they bend under the application of an external load. This contrasts with gold alloy inlays, which do not show symptoms of marginal breakdown of the alloy because this material is tough and ductile. Consequently, marginal breakdown is less likely to occur with margin angles greater than 70°, as this avoids thin wedges of the amalgam.

The practice of cutting perpendicular cavity walls on the occlusal aspect of the cavity is conducive to producing an acute margin angle for the amalgam (Figure 2.1.8a). Changing the angle for the whole of the cavity wall is not possible, as this may cause the cavity outline to

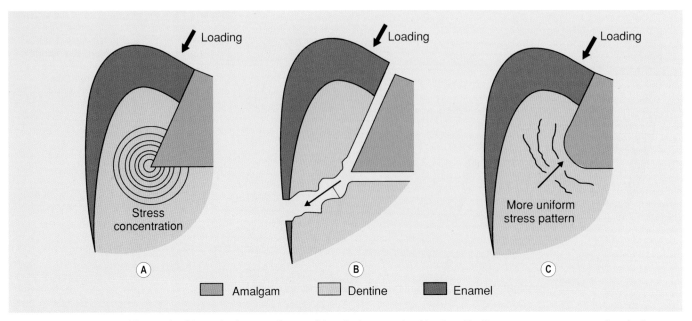

Figure 2.1.7 Sharp internal line angles (a) may lead to cusp fracture (b) under heavy occlusal loading. Tensile stresses are concentrated at the line angle, and can be considerably reduced by creating rounded line angles (c)

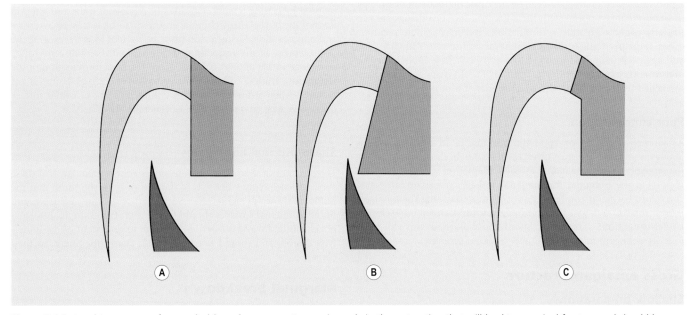

Figure 2.1.8 An obtuse cavo-surface angle (a) produces an acute margin angle in the restoration that will lead to marginal fracture and should be corrected. In (b), the cavo-surface angle is now closer to the ideal but may give rise to a pulpal exposure. An acceptable method is shown in (c), where adjustment is confined to the enamel without increasing the outline form

come close to the pulp horn or to perforate it (Figure 2.1.8b). An acceptable method of overcoming this problem is to confine the sharp angulation to the enamel only, as depicted in Figure 2.1.8c.

For occlusal cavities of minimal width it is not necessary to prepare 90° cavo-surface angles in the enamel because the amalgam may be carved flat without interference with the opposing dentition. The amalgam margin angle will then be obtuse, which will give the margin added strength due to the support of the underlying bulk of the restorative material.

Great care should be employed in the preparation of cavity margins, so as to avoid undermined enamel or acute margin angles in the amalgam.

Delayed expansion

In the case of zinc-containing alloys, the entrapment of saliva in the material as it is being placed can result in a phenomenon known as delayed expansion. The water reacts with the zinc as follows:

$$H_2O + Zn \rightarrow ZnO + H_2$$

Bubbles of hydrogen gas are formed within the amalgam. The pressure rises over time, as more and more hydrogen is produced and stored in the bubbles. Eventually, the pressure is so great that the bubbles expand, causing an expansion of the restoration. This expansion occurs during the early stages of slow-setting amalgams, as they are unable to resist this pressure until they are fully set. The expansion can give rise to a downward pressure on the pulp, or cause the restoration to sit proud of the surface. The former will cause pulpal pain and the latter will lead to marginal breakdown. In badly broken-down teeth, the expansion could also cause cuspal fracture. This hazard can be minimized by using proper isolation and the selection of an amalgam with a rapid set.

Overfilling, underfilling and overcarving

If a cavity is overfilled and is not then carved back sufficiently to provide a smooth transition from the tooth surface to the restoration surface, a ledge will result. This ledge will eventually fracture, and give the appearance of marginal breakdown of the restoration. This would encourage the dentist to replace the restoration, when, perhaps, all that is needed is to trim it back so that it is flush with the tooth surface. Such unnecessary treatment can be avoided by ensuring that the surface has been properly carved in the first place. Equally, underfilling or overcarving can result in an acute amalgam margin angle that will give rise to marginal breakdown.

Creep and corrosion of the amalgam

The problems associated with amalgam as a filling material have already been covered in detail, both in terms of the limitations imposed by their mechanical and physical properties and their handling. Most short-term failures are avoidable if the above factors are addressed and if careful attention is paid to the detail of cavity preparation and the handling of the materials. In the longer term, amalgams will eventually fail. When such failures are specifically material-related, they are usually associated with creep or corrosion that has caused marginal breakdown.

CLINICAL SIGNIFICANCE

Ideally, the amalgam alloy of choice should show little or no creep, and should have a high corrosion resistance. The laboratory and clinical evidence indicates that an admixed zinc-containing, high-copper-content amalgam is the preferred choice.

SUMMARY

Dental amalgams will continue to be the restorative material of choice for many clinical situations. If careful attention is paid to material selection and handling, and there is an appreciation of their limitations, amalgams should provide the patient with restorations that will give satisfactory function for many years.

CLINICAL SIGNIFICANCE

Since all the aesthetic alternatives to dental amalgam are more time-consuming to place and involve more complex procedures, while dental amalgams have a proven track record of good clinical performance, this material will continue to be one of the most convenient restorative materials for posterior use. Nevertheless, aesthetic demands from patients and a desire on the part of the dentist to preserve tooth structure will drive down the use of dental amalgams.

FURTHER READING

Baratieri LN, Machado A, Van Noort R et al (2002) Effect of pulp protection technique on the clinical performance of amalgam restorations: three-year results. Oper Dent 27(4): 319–324

Buerkle V, Kuehnisch J, Guelmann M et al (2005) Restoration materials for primary molars – results from a European survey. J Dent 33: 275

Elderton RJ (1984) New approaches to cavity design. Brit Dent J 157: 421

Letzel H, van 't Hof MA, Marshall GW et al (1997) The influence of the amalgam alloy on the survival of amalgam restorations: a secondary analysis of multiple controlled clinical trials. J Dent Res 76: 1787

Mahler DB (1997) The high-copper dental amalgam alloy. J Dent Res 76: 537

Mjor IA (1985) Frequency of secondary caries at various anatomical locations. Oper Dent 10: 88

Qvist V, Poulsen A, Teglers PT, Mjör IA (2010) The longevity of different restorations in primary teeth. Int J Paediatr Dent 20(1): 1–7

Ritchie KA, Burke FJ, Gilmour WH et al (2004) Mercury vapour levels in dental practices and body mercury levels of dentists and controls. Brit Dent J 197: 625

Roulet J-F (1997) Benefits and disadvantages of tooth-coloured alternatives to amalgam. J Dent 25: 459

Sarkar NK (1978) Creep, corrosion and marginal fracture of amalgam fillings. J Oral Rehab 5: 413

Setcos JC, Staninec M, Wilson NH (2000) Bonding of amalgam restorations: existing knowledge and future prospects. Oper Dent 25: 121

Shaini FJ, Fleming GJ, Shortall AC et al (2001) A comparison of the mechanical properties of a gallium-based alloy with a spherical high-copper amalgam. Dent Mater 17: 142

Staninec M, Hold M (1988) Bonding of amalgam to tooth structure: tensile adhesion and microleakage tests. J Prosthet Dent 59: 397

Summitt JB, Burgess JO, Berry TG et al (2004) Six-year clinical evaluation of bonded and pin-retained complex amalgam restorations. Oper Dent 29: 261

Xu HH, Eichmiller FC, Giuseppetti AA et al (1999) Three-body wear of a hand-consolidated alternative to amalgam. J Dent Res 78: 1560

Resin composites and polyacid-modified resin composites

INTRODUCTION

A composite, as the name implies, consists of a mixture of two or more materials. Each of these materials contributes to the overall properties of the composite, and is present in its discrete form (see Chapter 1.5). Resin-based composites are possibly the most ubiquitous materials available in dentistry as they are used in a huge variety of clinical applications, ranging from filling materials, luting agents, indirect restorations and metal facings to endodontic posts and cores.

A further addition to this already extensive range of resin-based dental materials is the polyacid-modified resin composite, or compomer for short. In this chapter we will first consider the resin composites and then explore how the compomers differ from the resin composites.

COMPOSITION AND STRUCTURE

The resin-based composite restorative materials ('composites' in brief) that are used in dentistry have three major components:

- an organic resin matrix
- an inorganic filler
- a coupling agent.

The resin forms the matrix of the composite material, binding the individual filler particles together through the coupling agent (Figure 2.2.1).

Resin matrix

The resin is the chemically active component of the composite. It is initially a fluid monomer but is converted into a rigid polymer by a radical addition reaction. It is this ability to convert from a plastic mass into a rigid solid that allows this material to be used for the restoration of dentition.

The most commonly used monomer for both anterior and posterior resins is Bis-GMA, which is derived from the reaction of bisphenol-A and glycidylmethacrylate. This resin is commonly referred to as Bowen's resin, after its inventor. It has a higher molecular weight than methyl methacrylate (MMA), which helps to reduce the polymerization shrinkage (Figure 2.2.2). The polymerization shrinkage value for MMA resins is 22 vol. %, whereas for a Bis-GMA resin it is 7.5 vol. %. There are also a number of composites that use a urethane dimethacrylate resin (UDMA) rather than Bis-GMA.

Bis-GMA and urethane dimethacrylate monomers are highly viscous fluids because of their high molecular weights; the addition of even a small amount of filler would produce a composite with a stiffness that is excessive for clinical use. To overcome this problem, low-viscosity monomers known as *viscosity controllers* are added, such as MMA, ethylene glycol dimethacrylate (EDMA) and triethylene glycol dimethacrylate (TEGDMA); the latter of these is most commonly used. The chemical structures of some of these monomers are presented in Figure 2.2.3.

To ensure an adequately long shelf life for the composite, it is essential that premature polymerization is prevented. To this end an *inhibitor*, such as hydroquinone, is included, usually in amounts of 0.1%, or less.

The resin matrix also contains the activator/initiator systems for achieving the cure. These components depend on the type of reaction employed, which may be either chemical curing or visible-light-activated curing.

Filler

A wide variety of fillers have been employed in composites to improve the properties. This practice began in the late 1950s, when fillers such as quartz were introduced into MMA-based filling materials. The inclusion of fillers offers five potentially major benefits:

1. The polymerization of MMA monomer is subject to a high polymerization shrinkage (21 vol. %), even when used as a powder–liquid system (7 vol. %). By incorporating large amounts of glass fillers, the shrinkage is much reduced because the amount of resin used is reduced and the filler does not take part in the polymerization process. However, shrinkage is not totally eliminated and will depend on the monomers used and the amount of filler incorporated.

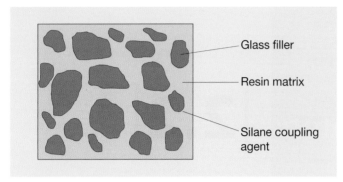

Figure 2.2.1 The structure of a composite restorative material

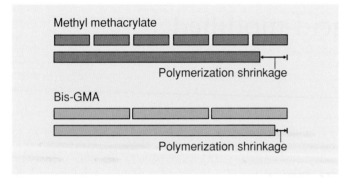

Figure 2.2.2 Polymerization shrinkage of a small and large monomer-based system. GMA, glycidylmethacrylate

2. Methacrylate monomers have a high coefficient of thermal expansion (~80 ppm/°C). This coefficient is reduced by the addition of ceramic fillers, which have a coefficient of expansion similar to that of tooth tissues (8–10 ppm/°C).
3. The fillers can improve mechanical properties such as hardness and compressive strength.
4. The use of heavy metals, such as barium and strontium incorporated in the glass, provides radiopacity.
5. The fillers provide the ideal means of controlling various aesthetic features such as colour, translucency and fluorescence.

The developments in filler technology lie at the root of many of the improvements that have led to the composites that are used today.

Coupling agent

In order for a composite to have acceptable mechanical properties, it is of the utmost importance that the filler and the resin are strongly bonded to each other. If there is a breakdown of this interface, the stresses developed under load will not be effectively distributed throughout the material; the interface will act as a primary source for fracture, leading to the subsequent disintegration of the composite.

The bond is achieved by the use of coupling agents that are incorporated into the resin. These coupling agents are silanes and the one most commonly used in glass-filled resin composites is γ-methacryloxy-propyltriethoxysilane, or γ-MPTS for short, shown in Figure 2.2.4 (see also Chapter 1.9).

It is extremely important that there is a strong and durable bond between the resin and the filler particles. First, if there is no bond, then stress transfer between the resin and glass will be inefficient and, as a consequence, most of the stress will have to be carried by the resin matrix. This will result in excessive creep and eventually fracture and

wear of the restoration. Second, the lack of bonding between the resin and the glass filler particles will create crack initiation sites. Since the resins do not have a high resistance to the propagation of cracks, this makes the composite susceptible to fatigue failure (Figure 2.2.5).

The fundamental problem is that resins are hydrophobic, whereas silica-based glasses are hydrophilic due to a surface layer of hydroxyl groups bound to the silica. Hence, the resin does not have a natural affinity to bond to the glass surface (Figure 2.2.6). The solution to the problem lies in the use of a suitable coupling agent. The silane coupling agent has been so chosen as to have hydroxyl groups on one end, which are attracted to the hydroxyl groups on the glass surface. The other end consists of a methacrylate group that is able to bond to the resin via the carbon double bond (Figure 2.2.7). A condensation reaction at the interface between the glass and the silane coupling agent ensures that the silane is covalently bonded to the glass surface (Figure 2.2.8). Improvements in the quality of the bond between the resin and the glass filler have contributed significantly to the development of wear-resistant composite restorative materials that can be used for both anterior and posterior teeth.

DEVELOPMENTS IN COMPOSITES

A look at the changes in composites over the last couple of decades readily identifies two important areas of development:

- new resin technology
- new filler technology.

Resin technology

Polymerization techniques

The process by which the composite paste turns into a hard material is the *polymerization* of the monomeric resin matrix.

With the early composites, this was achieved by supplying two pastes, a mixture of which would contain the necessary ingredients for polymerization. There would be an activator, such as a tertiary amine, in one paste, and an initiator, usually benzoyl peroxide, in the other (see Chapter 1.5 for details of this curing system).

In the early 1970s, ultraviolet (UV)-light-activated composites became available. In these materials, UV light was used to create free radicals to start the polymerization process. The energy of the UV light is sufficient to break the central bond of benzoin methyl ether to create two free radicals. Thus only a single paste was necessary, which would not set until exposed to UV light. However, there were some serious drawbacks with the use of the UV-light-cured systems. UV light can cause soft-tissue burns and can also cause damage to the eye. Hence protection needed to be used and generally great care needed to be exercised in the use of these light-curing units. The UV light source is a mercury discharge lamp, which is expensive, suffers from the problem that the intensity of the light output gradually reduces as the lamp gets older, and has a limited depth of cure due to the high degree of light absorption taking place as it travels through the composite.

Nevertheless, the practice of having a single paste, which would set hard on demand, was readily adopted by the dental profession and opened the way for the introduction of the visible-light-activated (VLA) composites. VLA composites use camphoroquinone as the source of free radicals. The energy for excitation is lower than that of benzoin methyl ether such that light with a wavelength in the blue range (~460–480 nm) is very effective. This has the advantage that a cheaper quartz halogen light source can be used and is potentially less damaging and that the light is more readily transmitted through

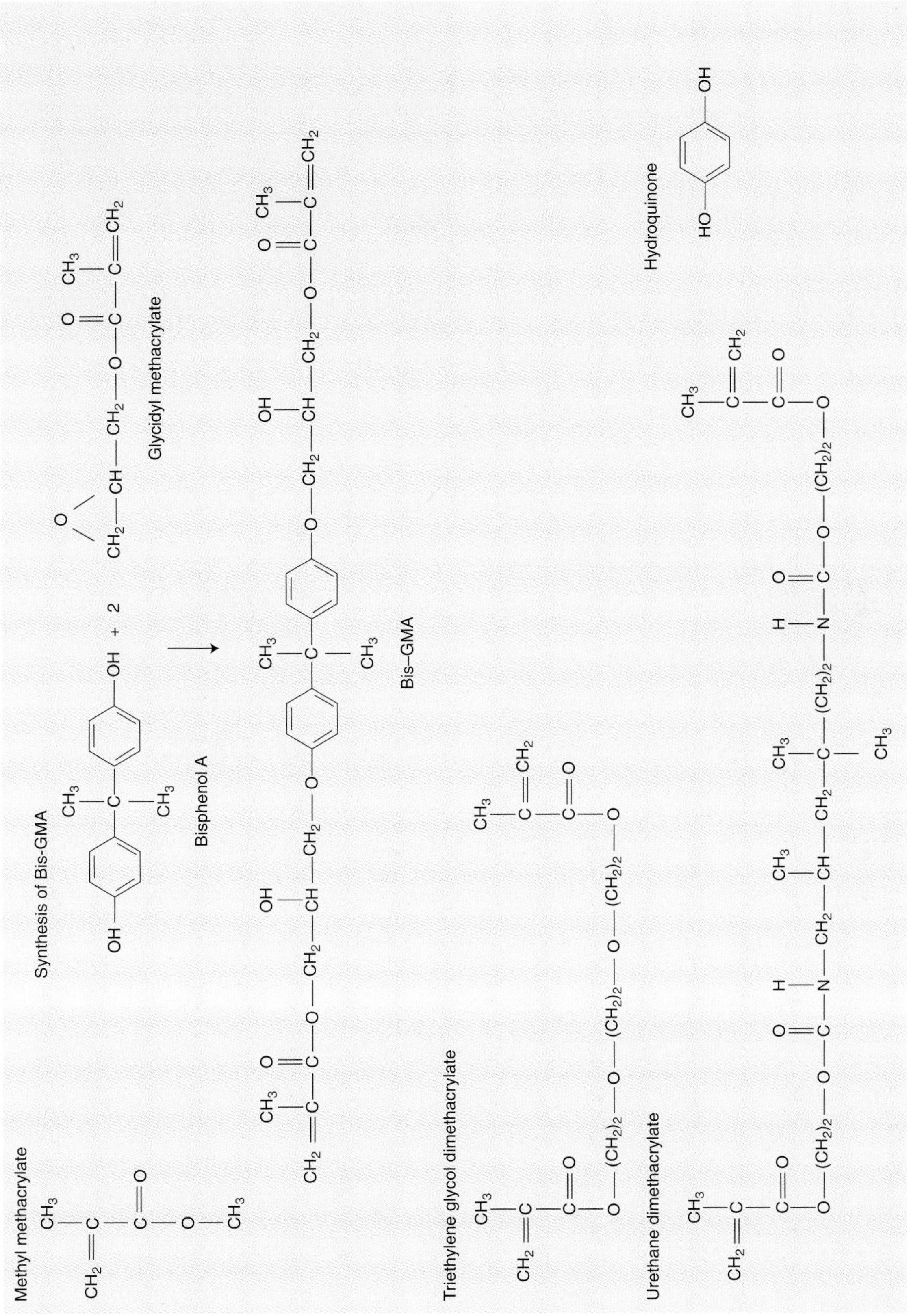

Figure 2.2.3 The chemical structure of some monomers

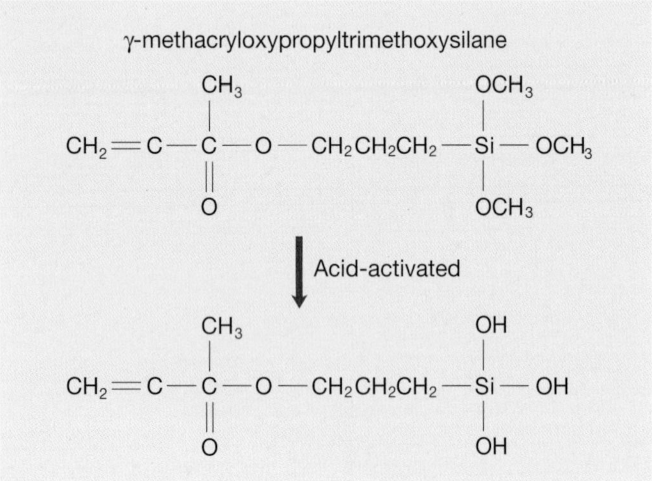

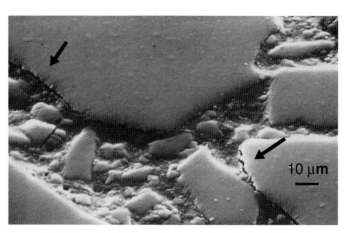

Figure 2.2.4 Structure of silane coupling agent before and after acid activation

Figure 2.2.5 Scanning electron microscope view of a lack of bonding between the resin matrix and the glass filler

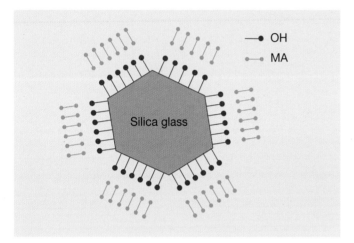

Figure 2.2.6 Schematic of resin monomer molecules being repelled by the glass surface due to the presence of hydroxyl groups on the glass

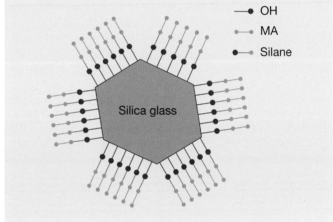

Figure 2.2.7 Schematic of silane coupling agent acting as a link between the methacrylate resin and the hydroxylated glass surface

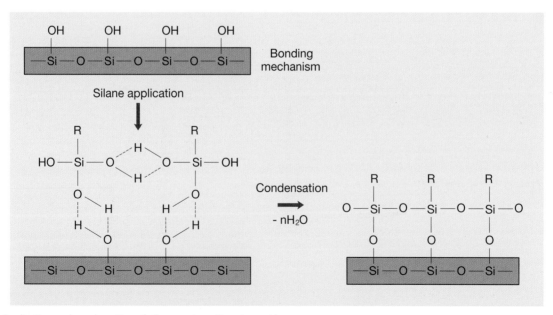

Figure 2.2.8 Application and condensation of silane on to a silica glass surface

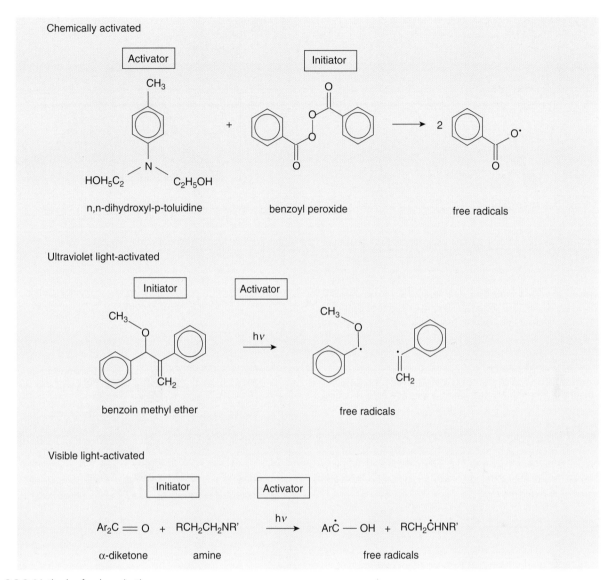

Figure 2.2.9 Methods of polymerization

the composite, providing greater depth of cure. Special filters are used to remove UV and infrared light for the output, so as to avoid soft-tissue burns and any excessive temperature rise respectively.

The curing methods are summarized in Figure 2.2.9.

Safety

Concern has been expressed about the safety aspects of the use of high-intensity UV light, and avoidance of these problems has been facilitated by the new VLA systems. The use of the phrase 'visible light' instils a feeling of safety, since it is something that we are exposed to all the time. Nevertheless, it is advisable not to expose oneself unnecessarily to the light from the visible-light production units, as high-intensity blue light can cause eye damage. The use of high-intensity light itself can have a harmful effect on the retina, and there is also the potential of damaging the retina due to the 'blue-light hazard'. Little is known about the blue-light hazard and how serious a problem it might be. These potential problems are readily resolved by using suitable eye protection, and it is better to err on the side of caution in these matters.

Colour perception

Another difficulty that the discerning dentist needs to be aware of is that caused by a long period of exposure to high-intensity light. Such exposure can upset one's colour perception, meaning that the selection of suitable shades of composites then becomes a real problem, especially when performing multiple restorations or when applying composite veneers.

Oxygen inhibition

Where there is an air interface with the resin, the resin will not cure and a sticky surface is readily discernible. This is of benefit when carrying out an incremental placement procedure, as it ensures that the layers of composite will be well bonded to one another. However, it can be a problem when the last increment has been placed. When it is possible to use a matrix strip, this is usually sufficient to exclude the oxygen and the resin will be fully cured up to the surface. For most resin systems, this oxygen-inhibited surface layer is very thin and extends no more than a few micrometres below the surface. Thus it

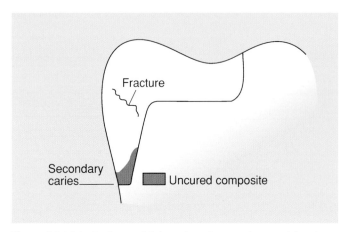

Figure 2.2.10 Lack of cure of light-activated composite material at the base of a proximal box

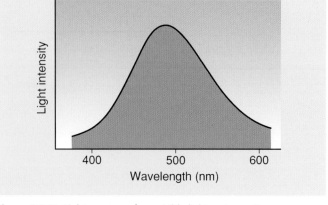

Figure 2.2.11 Light spectrum for a visible-light curing unit

is easily wiped off with a cotton pledget, e.g. when fissure sealing. However, there are some resin systems where the oxygen inhibition is considerable and a special gel needs to be used to avoid contact with oxygen in the air.

Limited depth of cure

Another reason why the VLA composites have replaced the UV systems is that the depth of cure that can be achieved with UV light is considerably less than that obtained with visible light.

In particular, there is a danger of incomplete curing with the UV systems when it is used for deep restorations, which would be a serious drawback in posterior applications. For the UV-cured composites, the maximum depth of cure is little more than 2.0 mm, while for the VLA composites a depth of cure of 3–4 mm is possible with a *good light source* and *good technique*.

Nevertheless, the depth of cure is limited for both systems, and there is always the danger that deeper parts of the restoration will not be fully cured. This is especially problematic with the proximal boxes of posterior composites (Figure 2.2.10). All can appear perfectly satisfactory on the surface, but the bases of the boxes of composite may not be fully cured, particularly when metal matrix bands are being used. A high degree of conversion of the C=C double bond in the resins is highly desirable to achieve the optimum mechanical properties and this relates to the curing time and the power of the light curing unit.

Any lack of cure provides a poor foundation for the restoration and may lead to fracture. This is due to a lack of support at the cervical margins, caused by washout of the uncured restorative material and the development of recurrent caries.

There are a number of points that need to be emphasized. The light source used with VLA composites is more accurately described as *blue light* rather than *visible light of extremely high intensity*. The typical output from a good-quality, visible-light source would produce a spectrum as shown in Figure 2.2.11. The selectivity is necessary to ensure optimal degree and depth of cure.

For all light-activated composites, the conversion from a paste to a solid material relies on the ability of the light to access and initiate the curing in all parts of the restoration. The degree to which the light can penetrate the composite is limited, so the depth to which the material can be cured is limited. A number of factors affect the depth of cure:

- *The type of composite.* As light hits the composite, it is reflected, scattered and absorbed as shown in Figure 2.2.12, and this limits the amount of penetration that is achieved. This is a particular concern for the darker shades of composite, and

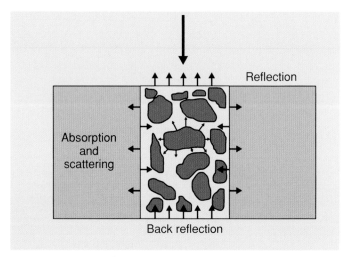

Figure 2.2.12 Reflection, scattering and absorption of light as it enters the composite

special care should be taken that these are cured to the full depth of the restoration, using an incremental technique and long exposure times.

- *The quality of the light source.* The cure of the resin in VLA composites is most effectively initiated by light in the wavelength range 450–500 nm. The light source should be designed so as to produce its maximum light output at approximately 460–480 nm, where the maximum of the camphoroquinone absorption coefficient is located (see Figure 2.2.11). Thus, it is not enough simply to have a high light output, but it must also be of the correct wavelength. Deterioration of the light source also occurs, and it is important that the quality of the output is checked at regular intervals. A variety of inexpensive light meters are now available for this purpose.
- *The method used.* The tip of the light guide should be placed as close as possible to the surface of the restoration, as the curing efficiency drops off dramatically when the tip is moved away from the surface. In fact, the light intensity on unit surface area drops off with the inverse square of the distance between the light source and the resin, as shown in Figure 2.2.13. Every effort must be made to ensure that the light tip does not become contaminated with composite, as this will reduce the curing efficiency on subsequent use. The material should be

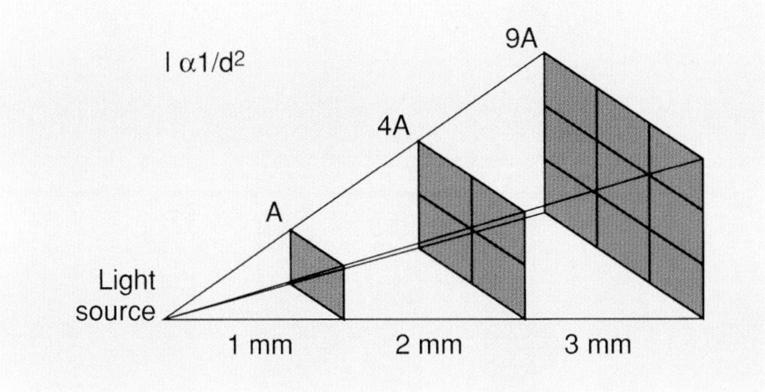

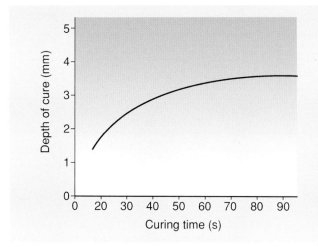

Figure 2.2.13 Relationship between intensity (I) of the light and the distance (d) from the light source to the surface

Figure 2.2.14 Depth of cure as a function of curing time

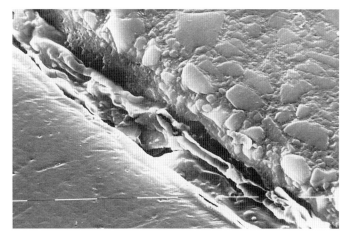

Figure 2.2.15 Scanning electron microscope view of the marginal gap formed due to polymerization shrinkage of the composite

curing to a depth of greater than 2 mm should be avoided, and exposure to the light source should be for at least 40 seconds. If the cavity to be filled is deeper than 2 mm, an incremental packing technique must be employed.

Light curing units

Besides the quartz halogen light curing unit described above, there are a number of other lamps on the market. These include the blue-light-emitting diode (blue-LED), argon laser and plasma (xenon) arc lamps.

The blue-LED light curing unit has the advantage that it only emits light within a very narrow wavelength range around 460–480 nm. It is therefore ultra-energy efficient and can be operated with a small rechargeable battery, making it very mobile. However, the bandwidth of the light may be so narrow that, for some composites using a visible light curing method not incorporating camphoroquinone, its optimum light curing condition may lie outside this bandwidth. Should this be the case, then the composite will not cure or, worse still, will only cure partially, giving the impression that it has cured.

The argon laser has the advantage that it provides a very high-intensity light source, which can be optimized for the initiation of polymerization. The argon laser produces a greater depth and degree of cure in a shorter time than the halogen light curing units. This may seem very attractive at first sight, as it can significantly reduce the time of light curing by reducing the exposure times and the number of increments used in a build-up. However, the rapid cure may compromise the integrity of the resin–tooth interface, as it does not allow any stress relaxation during the curing process. It is possible that using a pulsed rather than a continuous laser can reduce this problem. One serious drawback with these curing lights is the cost, being an order of magnitude more expensive than the quartz halogen and blue-LED light curing units.

The plasma arc light curing units can deliver approximately the same high light intensity as the argon laser but at a lower cost. However, as with the argon laser, the rapid conversion of the resin can produce high shrinkage stresses and the narrow bandwidth of the light can mean that some composites will not cure.

Polymerization shrinkage

As previously noted, a long-recognized and serious drawback with composites is polymerization shrinkage. In a sense, the whole field of adhesive restorative dentistry grew from this limitation of composites, because there would invariably be a marginal gap as the composite shrinks away from the cavity wall on setting (Figure 2.2.15).

exposed to the light for no less than the recommended time, so that there is no danger of undercuring. For large restorations, the light tip may not be large enough to cover the whole of the restoration and there may be a tendency to fan the surface. This should not be done, as it is impossible to tell how long any particular area of the surface has been exposed. If fanning is carried out, it must be followed up with further curing, one spot at a time. For large surfaces, it is important to ensure that the spots overlap.

There is a tendency on the part of some manufacturers to recommend curing times of as little as 20 seconds, as this obviously reduces the time it takes to complete a particular procedure. This may be sufficient for applications where only a very thin layer of the composite is to be applied, but will be insufficient when adopted for extensive restorations. Curing times should be at least 40–60 seconds.

In situations where light access presents a problem, such as distal boxes of a mesial occlusal distal restoration in a posterior composite, aids to curing, such as light-conducting wedges and transparent matrices, must be considered. Curing for excessively long times is, however, not a means of getting greater depths of cure. The depth of cure for a particular composite used in conjunction with a particular light source reaches a limit, which cannot be exceeded (Figure 2.2.14). Thus, curing times of more than 60 seconds tend to be inefficient.

The interpretation of the values for the depths of cure that are quoted in the literature is fraught with difficulty. As yet, there is no recommended definition of depth of cure, and since it is highly technique-dependent, comparison of data from different sources is virtually impossible. The general rule that should be followed is that

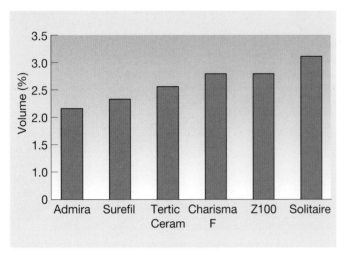

Figure 2.2.16 Volumetric polymerization shrinkage comparison of a range of commercially available composite filling materials. Data were obtained from technical literature provided by Voco GmbH, Cuxhaven, Germany

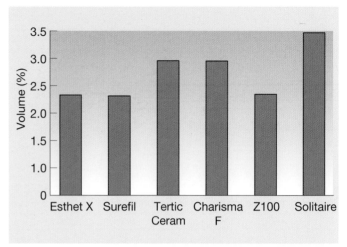

Figure 2.2.17 Volumetric polymerization shrinkage comparison of a range of commercially available composite filling materials. Data were obtained from technical literature provided by Dentsply Detrey GmbH, Konstanz, Germany

Composites do not have any intrinsic defence mechanisms against caries attack, unlike glass–ionomer cements (GICs) and amalgams. Hence, once a gap is formed, micro-leakage will occur, which can quickly lead to the spread of recurrent caries.

It should be noted that, while the development in light curing units has been focused on maximizing the degree of conversion of the monomer, this also maximizes the amount of polymerization shrinkage.

The polymerization shrinkage of a composite is dependent on the type of resin employed and the amount of resin present in its unpolymerized form. Most dental composites use resins with comparable polymerization shrinkage values. In general, a higher proportion of glass filler results in a lower final shrinkage. Such highly glass-filled composites do not necessarily have lower shrinkage values than the microfilled resins, as the latter use prepolymerized particles which may themselves be as highly filled as the glass particle systems.

Ideally, the polymerization shrinkage of the composite should be as low as possible, since this enhances marginal adaptation, reduces the possibility of breakdown of the bond to the tooth tissues, and inhibits the development of recurrent caries. The traditional amalgams minimize this problem because they show a slight expansion on setting, and, in due course, the gap fills with corrosion products. For high-copper-content amalgams, the shrinkage on setting is of the order of 0.1 vol. %, as compared with 2–3 vol. % for a composite. Typical values for polymerization shrinkage are shown in Figure 2.2.16. However, a note of caution is needed when examining such data, since it is difficult to find a reliable method of quantifying polymerization shrinkage and, as Figure 2.2.17 shows, a different manufacturer will tend to rank composites in a different way. Nevertheless, it is apparent that, with current resin technology, the lower limit of polymerization shrinkage is around 2.0 vol. %.

Despite major advances in the field of adhesive dental materials (see Chapter 2.5), polymerization shrinkage has been implicated as a primary source of interfacial breakdown, resulting in visible white lines or invisible cracks in the enamel and resin at the margins. The latter are only visible clinically when using transillumination and magnification. During the setting process, shrinkage stresses develop because the material is constrained by the adhesion to the cavity walls. These stresses can be sufficient to cause breakdown of the interfacial bond, whereby the advantage of the adhesive procedure is lost. This is particularly so for the bond to dentine, which is less strong than

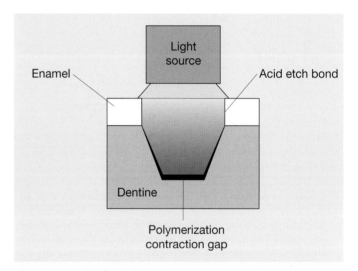

Figure 2.2.18 Gap formation as a consequence of polymerization shrinkage

that achieved to acid-etched enamel, and, as a consequence, the shrinkage tends to occur towards the acid-etched enamel-bonded interface if the bond to the dentine breaks down (Figure 2.2.18). The gap that forms between the restoration and the dentine will give rise to postoperative sensitivity due to the hydrodynamic effect. If any of the margins are in dentine, then the breakdown of the bond will also give rise to marginal leakage. This is especially a problem when composites are placed subgingivally in proximal boxes.

CLINICAL SIGNIFICANCE

The recommendation for the use of composites is that these should only be used when all the margins are in enamel.

Various options to overcome these problems have been proposed, which include using chemically cured composites in the base of boxes, as it is believed that the shrinkage tends to be towards the cavity walls.

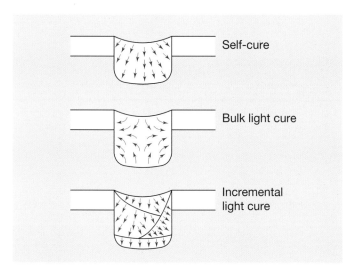

Figure 2.2.19 Various proposed options for filling a proximal box and minimizing the effects of polymerization shrinkage. The direction of the polymerization shrinkage stresses is indicated by the arrows

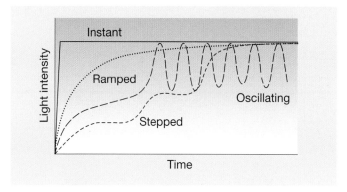

Figure 2.2.20 Light intensity profiles for slow start visible light curing units

The use of incremental placement techniques, combined with through-the-tooth curing, is another approach that is believed will encourage polymerization shrinkage towards rather than away from the cavity walls (Figure 2.2.19).

Another potential problem is that the shrinkage will cause the cusps of the tooth to be pulled inwards so that they become highly stressed. This effect has been suggested as a source of pulpal sensitivity following the placement of posterior composites. This effect can be exacerbated if a rigid, tightly bound matrix band is used during placement of a posterior composite.

It is obvious that the elimination or at least a significant reduction in the polymerization shrinkage of the resin matrix would represent a major leap forward. The steps taken to avoid or minimize the consequences of polymerization shrinkage are by far the most time-consuming aspects of the procedure for the placement of composite fillings and do not really resolve the problem satisfactorily. Ways of possibly improving the marginal integrity of composite restorations include:

- the development of improved dentine-bonding agents and bonding procedures to better resist the polymerization shrinkage stresses
- the use of a low modulus lining material to act as a stress absorber
- slowing down the rate of reaction by using a so-called 'soft-start' light curing unit.

Development in dentine-bonding agents continues, but there is a limit as to how much a high bond strength can compensate for polymerization shrinkage stresses and it is possible that this limit has already been reached. The idea of using a low elastic modulus liner carries with it the penalty that stresses generated by occlusal loads cannot easily be transferred across the interface between the tooth and the restoration, and may cause high stresses elsewhere in the tooth structure. The third approach is based on the idea that a reduction in the rate of reaction would allow more time for the polymerization shrinkage stresses to be dissipated by a process of flow from the free surface and stress relaxation. This has led to the introduction of a variety of soft-start blue-light curing units, using ramped, stepped and oscillating light-curing profiles (Figure 2.2.20). The clinical effectiveness of all these approaches is a matter of considerable debate in the dental research literature.

New resin technologies

Since the incorporation of glass fillers as a means of reducing polymerization shrinkage has probably gone as far as it can go (see below), the solution will most likely have to be found in the development of new resins that show little or no shrinkage on curing. A variety of different resin systems are presently being explored that include modifications of existing methacrylates such as ormocers and stress-decreasing resins and alternative chemistries such as siloranes.

Ormocers

Whereas methacrylate-based resin matrices consist of purely organic material, an alternative type of inorganic-organic copolymer resin was developed for the polymer industry more than 20 years ago and the concept adapted for use in dental resin composite restoratives. This developed into the ORMOCER®, which stands for ORganically MOdified CERamic and is a registered trademark of Fraunhofer Gesellschaft, Germany. It consists of organic reactive species with carbon double bonds for polymerization, which is bound to an inorganic Si–O–Si network (Figure 2.2.21). This inorganic-organic network exhibits a similar viscosity to Bis-GMA and thus the matrix will also contain some viscosity controllers such as TEGDMA. Admira (Voco, Cuxhaven, Germany) is a currently available ORMOCER dental restorative product.

Stress-decreasing resins

A new technology has been developed in the form of what is described as a stress-decreasing resin; it is based on the incorporation of a molecular chain that acts as a means of absorbing polymerization shrinkage stress by acting as a spring/polymerization modulator (Figure 2.2.22). Based on the scientific evidence gathered to date, the 'polymerization modulator' reduces stress build-up on polymerization without a reduction in the polymerization rate or conversion. It is claimed that, by use of the polymerization modulator, the resin forms a more relaxed network and provides a significantly reduced polymerization stress. A commercially available example of this new technology is a 'Smart Dentin Replacement' known as SDR™ from Dentsply. It should be noted that this material is primarily designed to act as a dentine substitute such that the cavity is filled up to the dentino-enamel junction with this material and then a resin composite veneer is placed over the top.

Siloranes

Unlike acrylic resins, which set by a free-radical addition polymerization, epoxy-based resins set via a quite different curing mechanism.

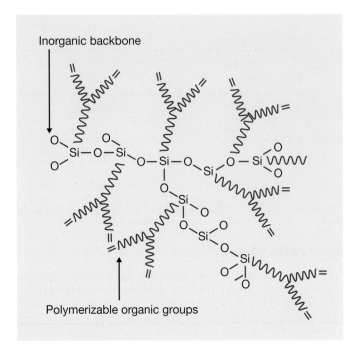

Figure 2.2.21 Ormocer chemistry

Epoxy resin formulations harden by cationic polymerization. The term 'epoxy' refers to an oxygen-containing ring molecule that contains a three-membered 'oxirane' ring. The curing process involves ring-opening, which results in a lower net shrinkage, and the delayed consumption of reactive species can provide stress relaxation throughout polymerization, which may reduce polymerization shrinkage stress. An example of this approach that has found application in dentistry is the silorane (Figure 2.2.23), which has comparable mechanical properties to existing methacrylate composites, with reduced water sorption, improved reactivity and lower polymerization stress rates throughout curing. These novel resins also eliminate the oxygen-inhibited layer and exhibit increased ambient light stability. The material is available in a commercial form as Filtek Silorane from 3M/ESPE.

Despite the apparent reduction in polymerization shrinkage achieved in the new resin systems, it must not be assumed that this will result in a concomitant reduction in shrinkage stress. A range of other factors such as the filler loading, elastic modulus of the resin composite, shrinkage rate and gel-point have a contribution to make. Consequently, this continues to be a matter of considerable debate in the dental materials research community.

New filler technology

Criticisms of the early composites were that they had rough surface finishes and a disappointing resistance to wear. Both of these are directly affected by the choice of filler used in the composite. The factors of interest in the selection of the filler are:

- composition
- particle size.

Composition

The filler most used until quite recently was quartz, but today most composites employ one or other of a variety of silica-based glass fillers, including colloidal silica, lithium-aluminium silicate glass and silica glasses containing barium or strontium.

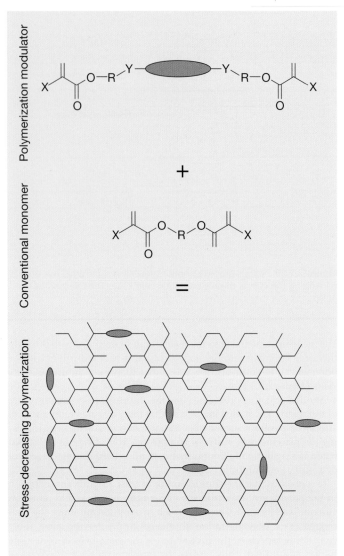

Figure 2.2.22 Stress-decreasing resin system

The glass formulation is critical because it has a major effect on the colouring of the composite. Its refractive index must closely match that of the resin to avoid excessive scattering of incoming light occurring, which would result in poor aesthetics and poor depth of cure.

The inclusion of barium or strontium provides radiopaque versions of the composites, and this aids the detection of recurrent caries. Quartz is by far the hardest material used as a filler, but composites formed in this way are not radiopaque. The silica glasses are considerably softer, which some argue improves the surface finish of the composite.

Average particle size and distribution

The average particle size and particle size distribution of the filler are important as they determine the amount of filler that can be added to the resin, without the necessary handling characteristics being lost. Particle size also has a pronounced effect on the final surface finish of the composite restoration, in that the smaller the filler particle size, the smoother the composite will be. (It should be said that the hardness of the filler, relative to the matrix, is another factor that should be considered when considering the quality of the finish.)

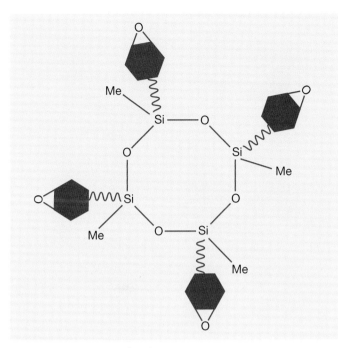

Figure 2.2.23 Structure of a silorane monomer

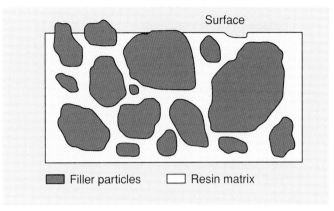

Filler particles   Resin matrix

Figure 2.2.24 Filler particles protruding from the surface due to preferential removal of the resin matrix

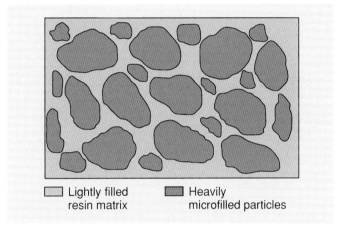

Lightly filled resin matrix   Heavily microfilled particles

Figure 2.2.25 A heterogeneous microfilled resin, using prepolymerized particles that are added to the resin containing a small amount of colloidal silica

The earliest filler used in composites was quartz, which had an average particle size of up to 70 μm. Changing to softer glasses has allowed a reduction in the size of the filler particles and, by choosing a suitable combination of sizes, it has been possible to increase the filler loading of the resins considerably. A filler loading as high as 74% by volume has been claimed for some of the posterior composites, which is well above the usual 55–60% volume obtained for many anterior composites. Of course, such a high filler loading may not be desirable with the anterior composites, as the quality of the aesthetics could be compromised; this is clearly not of the same importance for the posterior composites.

CLASSIFICATION OF COMPOSITES

It is possible to categorize dental composites into five main groups, according to the nature and the particle size of the filler.

Traditional composites

"Traditional" composites contained glass filler particles with a mean particle size of 10–20 μm and a largest particle size of 40 μm. These composites had the disadvantage that the surface finish was very poor, with the surface having a dull appearance due to filler particles protruding from the surface as the resin was preferentially removed around them, as shown in Figure 2.2.24.

Microfilled resins

The first microfilled resins were introduced in the late 1970s, and contain colloidal silica with an average particle size of 0.02 μm and a range of 0.01–0.05 μm. The small size of the filler particles means that the composite can be polished to a very smooth surface finish. The very small particle size of the filler means that it provides a very large surface area of filler in contact with the resin. This high surface area (compared to that of the filler used in the traditional composites)

means that it is very difficult to obtain a high filler loading, as a large amount of resin is required to wet the surfaces of these filler particles. If the filler is added directly to the resin and a reasonably fluid consistency is to be maintained, then the maximum filler loading that can be achieved is only of the order of 20 vol. %.

To ensure an adequate filler loading, a two-stage procedure for the incorporation of the filler has been developed. A very high-filler-loaded material is first produced by one of a variety of techniques. This material is then polymerized and ground into particles of 10–40 μm in size, which is subsequently used as a filler for more resin. Thus, what is finally obtained is a composite containing composite filler particles (Figure 2.2.25). Although the filler loading of the prepolymerized particles can be as high as that of the large particle composites, the overall glass content is still considerably less (~50 vol. %).

Hybrid or blended composites

Hybrid composites contain large filler particles of an average size of 15–20 μm and also a small amount of colloidal silica, which has a particle size of 0.01–0.05 μm (Figure 2.2.26). It should be noted that virtually all composites now contain small amounts of colloidal silica, but their behaviour is very much determined by the size of the larger filler particles.

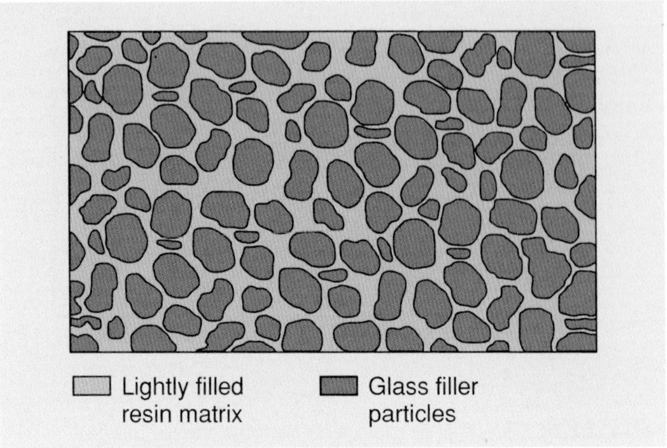

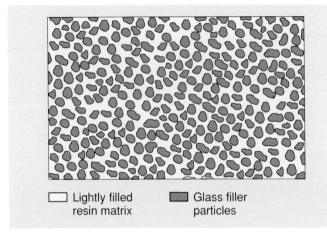

Figure 2.2.26 Structure of a hybrid composite, consisting of large filler particles in a resin matrix containing colloidal silica

Lightly filled resin matrix   Glass filler particles

Figure 2.2.27 A small particle-filled composite

Lightly filled resin matrix   Glass filler particles

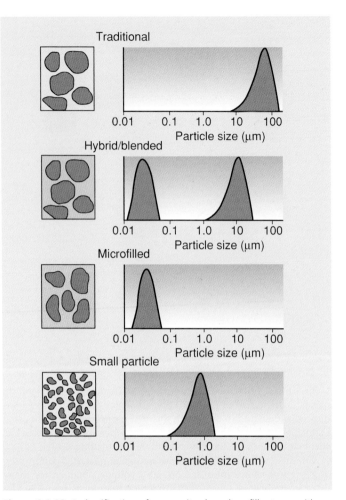

Figure 2.2.28 A classification of composites based on filler type, with the horizontal axis as the logarithmic scale of the particle size

Small-particle hybrid composites

Improved methods have allowed the grinding of glasses to particle sizes smaller than had previously been possible. This has led to the introduction of composites having filler particles with an average particle size of less than 1 μm, and a typical range of particle sizes of 0.1–6.0 μm, usually combined with colloidal silica (Figure 2.2.27). The smaller-sized filler particles allow these composites to be polished to a smoother surface finish than those with larger particles. These composites can achieve a highly polished surface finish because any surface irregularities arising from the filler particles must be much smaller than the filler particles and therefore will be below the resolution of the wavelength of light (0.38–0.78 μm).

Nanocomposites

Since the early 2000s there has been a vogue for the branding of materials and other products as 'nano', and there are now a number of dental composites on the market that are described by the manufacturers as 'nanocomposites'. Nanotechnology has had, and continues to have, a profound effect on many fields, including materials science, medicine and the food and cosmetics industries. There can be no doubt that some of the developments made possible by embracing nanotechnology have allowed academic and industrial scientists to make significant leaps forward in many areas. It is, however, important for the modern dentist not to be seduced simply by the 'nano' badge on a dental material, but to consider the evidence carefully.

Nanomaterials are defined as materials that include components with at least one dimension of the order of less than 100 nm. Practically speaking, composite filler particles are usually approximately equiaxed and thus nanocomposites contain filler particles with a diameter of 100 nm or smaller. Of course, many composites that have been around for some 20 years or more contain filler particles of this scale and so, in one sense, the new wave of nanocomposites could be viewed as simply a rebranding of old materials.

Although a degree of scepticism might, therefore, rightly be applied to dental composites with a 'nano' label, it appears that active research in this area may yet lead to some useful advances, particularly as regards the aesthetic properties of this class of material. It has been shown, for instance, that some modern composites with fillers of ~75 nm displayed superior gloss retention and reduced opacity without seriously compromising mechanical properties.

Summary

The classification proposed above is shown schematically in Figure 2.2.28 in terms of the particle size distributions. In order to increase the filler loading to its maximum, it is possible to select fillers with two or more complementary particle size distributions. The filler with the smaller particle size distribution fills in the spaces left between the larger filler particles (Figure 2.2.29). This has meant that the packing density of composite restorative materials has been increased, while the size of the filler has been reduced.

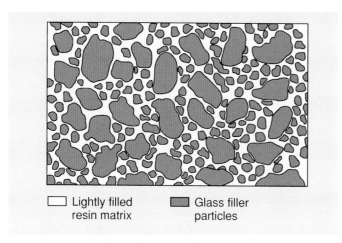

Lightly filled resin matrix   Glass filler particles

Figure 2.2.29 Bimodal particle size distribution

By ensuring that the aesthetics are not compromised, composites can be used for both anterior and posterior applications.

PROPERTIES

Handling characteristics

Despite the introduction of VLA, the placement of composite resins is demanding and technique sensitive. Composite resins are not intrinsically adhesive to enamel and dentine, and, therefore, acid etching with phosphoric acid and the application of a dentine-bonding agent is required. When combined with the need for incremental placement and careful attention to light-curing procedures, this means that the placement of a composite restoration can be expected to take up to three times as long as that for an amalgam of comparable size. The proper placement of a composite restoration and careful oral hygiene maintenance by the patient are all the more important because, should recurrent caries occur, the caries tends to progress more rapidly than with other filling materials.

There have been a number of developments relating to the rheology of composite resins. Ideally, the viscosity of a composite should be such that it can be condensed into large cavities and, at the same time, is able to flow into inaccessible spaces. The material should not flow under its own weight so that it can be sculpted but will flow readily when being pushed. Compared with dental amalgams, composites can have a tendency to stick to the instruments and this can create problems in achieving good marginal adaptation. In an effort to improve the marginal adaptation of composite restorations, so-called 'flowable' composites were introduced in the late 1990s. At the same time, 'packable' composites appeared on the market, which sought to have handling characteristics similar to that of dental amalgams by having an increased viscosity.

In order to produce flowable composites, the manufacturers have reduced the filler loading and, so as not to have to reduce it too much, the particle size of the glass filler may also have been increased. Flowable composites can be difficult to control due to their low viscosity. Hence these materials are ideally suited for small preparations such as abrasion preparations, margin repairs and preventive resin restorations. With the reduced filler loading and larger filler particle size, these materials are not recommended for situations involving high levels of stress or wear.

The production of packable composites can be achieved by a slight increase in filler loading of 1–2 vol. % and a change in the rheology

of the resin matrix. This is not as easy as it sounds since the filler loading of most composites has already been maximized and simply adding more filler will make the composite crumbly and cause cracking. The increased viscosity can be accomplished in a number of different ways:

- by increasing the filler particle size range, which improves the packing density, such as a trimodal particle size distribution
- by modification of the filler particle shape such that particles have a tendency to interlock, making it more difficult for them to flow past each other
- by modification of the resin matrix such that stronger intermolecular attractions are created (e.g. replacing the hydroxyl groups on the Bis-GMA with hydrogen for hydrogen bonding) and thus raising the viscosity
- by the addition of dispersants (rheological control additive), which lower the viscosity and allow an increase in the filler loading.

As with most things, there is a price to pay for the increased filler loading. These materials tend to be more opaque and have an inferior surface finish; despite the increased filler loading, the mechanical properties appear to be no different from those of the universal composites such as the small-particle hybrids. Since the aesthetics are compromised, the manufacturers provide only a limited range of shades. These materials therefore have a limited range of applications and are most suited for posterior applications, such as small to moderately sized class II preparations. Due to the high viscosity, adaptation can be a problem and there is an increased potential for trapping air, resulting in voids at the margins or in the bulk of the restoration. For this reason, it has been suggested that a thin layer of flowable composite is first placed in the base of the proximal box before the packable composite is placed.

It should be appreciated that both the flowable and the packable composites have been developed as a response by manufacturers to requests from dental practitioners to produce composites with special handing properties. Hence these composites do not represent a major advance in the context of their physical and mechanical properties. In fact, the flowable composites have inferior mechanical properties and the packable composites have inferior aesthetics compared with the universal composites.

Biocompatibility

Composite resins are complex structures, and various components and breakdown products are released from these materials. These include uncured resins and diluents and additives, such as UV stabilizers, plasticizers and initiators. Weight losses of up to 2% have been reported, although this is highly variable, as it depends largely on the degree of cure that has been achieved. Some of the materials eluted from composites have been shown to be cytotoxic and delayed hypersensitivity associated with composite resins can occur. However, this should not be interpreted as being an indication that these materials present an unacceptable risk to the patient's health as the amounts released are very low and delayed hypersensitivity reactions associated with composite resins are rare.

Some concerns have been expressed regarding the use of bisphenol-A and bisphenol-A-based monomers in composite restorative materials, as these materials have been shown to be capable of inducing changes in oestrogen-sensitive organs and cells. However, studies of leached components tend to show that it is the low-molecular-weight monomers, such as MMA and TEGDMA, that leach out, rather than such high-molecular-weight monomers as Bis-GMA and UDMA. Hence it becomes an issue not unlike that associated with amalgams: namely, whether or not the low dose of leached components with oestrogenic activity from composite resins presents an unacceptable risk to the patient. For the present, it is believed that the safety of composite resins should not be of concern to the general public.

Water sorption and solubility

Water sorption should be minimized for composites because excessive water sorption has a detrimental effect on the colour stability and the wear resistance. If the composite can absorb water, then it is also able to absorb other fluids from the oral cavity, which results in its discoloration.

Water sorption occurs mainly as direct absorption by the resin. The glass filler will not *absorb* water into the bulk of the material, but can *adsorb* water on to its surface. Thus, the amount of water sorption is dependent on the resin content of the composite and the quality of the bond between the resin and the filler. As such, it would perhaps make more sense to relate the value for the water sorption to the resin content of the composite. This would show whether or not the amount of water sorption is that predicted from a knowledge of the water sorption characteristics of the resin alone or if it is unduly high.

Data shown in Table 2.2.1 indicate that, when the filler content of the restorative material is taken into account, marked differences between the water sorption values for a range of composites become apparent.

The intrinsic water sorption for the resin appears to be around 40–45 $\mu g \cdot mm^{-3}$, but for two of the composites in the table, the water sorption is 2–3 times what might have been expected. The question is, 'Where does this extra water go?'

A high water sorption value for a composite (when corrected for the amount of filler present) may indicate a number of possibilities. It is possible that the material has a high soluble fraction, which dissolves and leaves a space into which the water can flow (this is possibly due to incomplete cure of the resin). In addition, the resin may contain air voids, introduced during mixing or placement. Another possibility is that hydrolytic breakdown of the bond between the filler and the resin has occurred, allowing adsorption on to the surface of the filler particles. This has two important consequences. First, as the bond between the filler particles and the resin is lost, the filler will lose its effectiveness as a reinforcing agent, resulting in a rapid deterioration of the restoration. Second, the filler particles lose their surface cohesion, resulting in a high rate of wear. Thus, a worrying combination of features for a composite would be a high filler loading combined with a high value for water sorption.

It is often suggested that the water sorption may, to some extent, compensate for the polymerization shrinkage, but water sorption is a gradual process taking many months to complete. This can readily be shown from a knowledge of the diffusion coefficient, D, of water in a composite, which is typically of the order of 1.25×10^{-9} $cm^2 \cdot s^{-1}$. For a sample of 2 mm thickness, the material would require 166 days to reach equilibrium, and if the sample is 5 mm thick, the time taken to reach equilibrium is in excess of 3 years. Thus, water sorption cannot prevent interfacial debonding, since it cannot counteract the instantaneous shrinkage that occurs on setting. In due course, the slight swelling may well improve the marginal adaptation of the restoration, but the chances are that, by then, it will be too late.

It is important to realize that, if measurements of the water sorption characteristics are to be undertaken, it is necessary for samples to be extremely thin to be able to reach equilibrium water sorption in a realistic time. Also, for the comparison of water sorption data, the glass filler loading should be taken into account.

Coefficient of thermal expansion

To minimize the possibility of stresses being developed due to differential expansion and contraction, the coefficient of thermal expansion of the composite needs to be as close as possible to that of tooth tissue. The glass fillers have a low coefficient of thermal expansion, while the resin has a high coefficient of thermal expansion, so that the higher the inorganic filler loading, the lower the coefficient of expansion will be. Since the microfilled resins have a high resin content, with resin being present in both the matrix and the prepolymerized filler particles, these tend to have a high coefficient of expansion compared to the glass-filled composites.

Examples of the coefficient of expansion of some commercially available composites are presented in Table 2.2.2, which also shows the differential expansion factors when compared with enamel.

Table 2.2.1 Equilibrium water uptake for a number of composites

Material (manufacturer)	On material ($\mu g \cdot mm^{-3}$)	On resin* ($\mu g \cdot mm^{-3}$)	Volume of resin (%)
Occlusin (ICI Dental)	12.9	41.6	31
P-10 (3M Dental)	16.0	44.4	36
Profile (SS White)	16.3	37.0	44
Ful-Fil (LD Caulk)	20.3	63.4	32
Heliomolar (Vivadent)	20.6	43.6	47
Estilux (Kulzer)	23.1	82.4	28
P-30 (3M Dental)	36.9	119.0	31

*The uptake of water by the resin was based on the assumption that the glass does not absorb water and worked out using the volume % resin shown in the last column.

Adapted from the data of Oysaed and Ruyter (1986).

Table 2.2.2 The coefficient of thermal expansion (α) and the differential expansion factor (D) for some composites compared with enamel

Material (manufacturer)	Type	α (ppm$\times$°C^{-1})	D
Enamel		11.4	1.00
Z-100 (3M Dental Products)	Hybrid	22.5	1.97
Adaptic (Johnson & Johnson)	Traditional	25.7	2.25
Herculite (Kerr)	Small particle hybrid	32.6	2.86
Silux Plus (3M Dental Products)	Microfilled	41.6	3.65
Delton (Johnson & Johnson)	Unfilled	90.3	7.92

Data from Versluis A et al (1996) Thermal expansion coefficient of dental composites measured with strain gauges. Dent Mater **12(5)**: 290–294 (except for Delton).

Radiopacity

When composites are used as a posterior restorative material, their radiopacity is of the utmost importance. The detection of caries under a non-radiopaque composite is virtually impossible, and would allow the caries process to continue undetected for far too long. Some composites have a radiopacity lower than that of dentine, which is inadequate because an X-ray would not reveal the presence of caries. However, it is not clear what the optimum radiopacity for a composite is, since excessive radiopacity can potentially mask out caries lying behind the restoration. Nevertheless, the composite should at least be as radiopaque as the enamel. Some composites fall far short of this requirement, and should not be used for posterior restorations.

Colour match

The aesthetic qualities of composites are well recognized. The earliest composites suffered from discoloration, which can manifest itself in one of three ways:

- marginal discoloration
- general surface discoloration
- bulk discoloration.

Marginal discoloration is usually due to the presence of a marginal gap between the restoration and the tooth tissues. Debris penetrates the gap and leads to an unsightly marginal stain; elimination of the marginal gap would completely avoid this type of staining. If the margin is in enamel, it is possible to overcome this problem by employing the acid-etch technique of bonding to enamel. The bond between acid-etched enamel and composite is sufficiently strong and durable to achieve a good marginal seal, which avoids the ingress of debris. The use of an unfilled bonding resin is generally recommended, as this helps marginal adaptation.

General surface discoloration may be related to the surface roughness of the composite, and is more likely to occur with those composite resins employing large filler particles. Debris gets trapped in the spaces between the protruding filler particles and is not readily removed by tooth brushing. Polishing with a suitable abrasive, such as the aluminium oxide pastes available commercially, should remove this surface stain. It is important that a graded polishing process is carried out, such as, for example, 20 μm diamond instruments, followed by a 7 μm paste and finishing with a 1 μm paste. This will produce an optically smooth surface finish without any pits and grooves in the case of microfilled and small-particle hybrid composites. Sometimes a dark pitted discoloration can be observed, which is due to the exposure of trapped air bubbles as the composite wears away. Such discoloration cannot easily be removed, and it may be better to replace the restoration with a light-activated composite, which will have virtually no air trapped in it if it is placed sufficiently carefully.

Bulk, or deep, discoloration is a particular problem with the two-paste amine-cured composites. The colour of the restoration changes slowly over a long time period, giving the restoration a distinctly yellow appearance. This type of discoloration arises due to both the chemical breakdown of components within the resin matrix and the absorption of fluids from the oral environment. The visible light-activated composites seem to have much better colour stability.

Just as the introduction of packable and flowable composites being demand-driven, manufacturers have also introduced a range of highly aesthetic composites. These are composites with a maximum particle size of no more than 2 μm and an average of around 0.6 μm, making them highly polishable. The range is also broadened such that a veritable artist's palette of colours and translucencies is available.

Table 2.2.3 Compressive strength data for a variety of materials

Material (manufacturer)	Compressive strength (MPa)
Molar enamel	260
Molar dentine	305
Sybralloy (Kerr)	500
Dispersalloy (Johnson & Johnson)	440
Adaptic (Johnson & Johnson)	250
Silux (3M Dental Products)	286
Aurafil (Johnson & Johnson)	345
Occlusin (ICI Dental Products)	310
P-30 (3M Dental Products)	393

MECHANICAL PROPERTIES

Compressive strength

If one compares the compressive strengths of a number of composites and amalgams with those of enamel and dentine, the indications are that these materials are quite adequate (Table 2.2.3).

It is interesting to note that an anterior composite can have a similar compressive strength as a posterior composite, yet the recommendations for their uses are quite different. It is important to know the significance of this value.

Being relatively easy to measure, the compressive strength of a material is quoted frequently. Unfortunately, it is also a property that is difficult to interpret due to the possible modes of failure under compression:

- ductile materials can spread sideways, rather like putty
- brittle materials, like glass and stone, can explode in all directions
- buckling can occur in long, thin samples.

As can be imagined, highly complex stresses are generated in the specimen when testing compressive strength.

If we ask ourselves whether restorations fail in any of the modes described above, then the answer is that this would seem unlikely. It is much more likely that the restorations will fail under tension (due to the application of bending forces), as composites have a very low tensile strength.

Thus the compressive strength is but a poor indicator of a material's resistance to failure, as there is no simple relationship between a material's compressive and tensile strengths.

Diametral tensile strength

If restorative materials are more likely to fail in a tensile mode, then it would make more sense to measure their tensile strength than their compressive strength. Unfortunately, the measurement of the tensile strengths of brittle materials is extremely difficult, and gives rise to a great deal of scatter in the data. The reason for this is that such materials are highly susceptible to the presence of internal flaws or small cracks in their surfaces, which are impossible to eliminate. As a consequence, the tensile strengths of composites are dependent on the quality of surface finish.

Table 2.2.4 Diametral tensile strength of some composite restorative materials

Material (manufacturer)	Diametral tensile strength (MPa)
Adaptic (Johnson & Johnson)	51
Aurafil (Johnson & Johnson)	52
Occlusin (ICI Dental)	54
P-30 (3M Dental Products)	67

The *diametral tensile test* is an alternative method for measuring the tensile strength of a material. Again, complex stress patterns arise in the material, but the results are reasonably reproducible and it is an easy property to measure. For these reasons, the diametral tensile strength is often quoted for dental materials. It is interesting to note that this test is usually applied to brittle materials. Hence, if the diametral tensile strength is quoted rather than conventional tensile strength, this indicates that the material is brittle and therefore suffers from a lack of toughness.

Typical values for the diametral tensile strength of a number of composites are given in Table 2.2.4. From these figures, it can be seen that the traditional anterior composite has a similar diametral tensile strength to that of the current posterior composites. Yet, clinical experience has shown us that traditional composites do not perform well in the posterior situation. Thus, as for the compressive strength, it would seem that the diametral tensile strength alone gives no direct indication as to the particular use of a composite or its potential clinical performance.

As composites are used more and more widely for the restoration of posterior teeth, fracture of the restorations is likely to become an increasingly significant cause of failure; it may be that the above properties will then provide a useful indicator of the resistance to such fractures.

Hardness

The surface hardness of a dental material can be measured readily by a number of techniques, resulting in a hardness value that can then be used to compare different composites. At one time, it was thought that the hardness would provide a good indicator of the wear resistance of a composite, and this is true up to a point.

The original acrylic resins were very soft materials, but their hardness and wear resistance were much improved by the addition of a filler. Measurement of the hardness initially gave some indication of the wear resistance, but this relationship unfortunately breaks down at the high filler loadings used in the current generation of composites (see below).

Wear

Wear is the process by which material is displaced or removed by the interfacial forces which are generated as two surfaces rub together. Types of wear that occur in the oral environment are as follows.

Abrasive wear

When two surfaces rub together, the harder of the two materials may indent, produce grooves in or cut away material from the other surface. This direct contact wear is known as *two-body abrasion*, and occurs in

the mouth whenever there is direct tooth-to-tooth contact, in what most dentists would call *attrition*.

Abrasive wear may also occur when there is an abrasive slurry interposed between two surfaces such that the two solid surfaces are not actually in contact. This is called *three-body abrasion*, and occurs in the mouth during mastication, with food acting as the abrasive agent. Toothpastes also act as abrasive slurries between the toothbrush and the tooth.

Fatigue wear

The repeated loading of teeth produces cyclic stresses that can lead in time to the growth of fatigue cracks. These cracks often form below the surface, and initially grow parallel to it before veering towards the surface or coalescing with other cracks.

Corrosive wear

Chemical attack on composites can occur as hydrolytic breakdown of the resin, breakdown of the resin–filler interface or erosion of the surface due to acid attack.

It is likely that all of the above mechanisms are involved in wear of the composites. In occlusal contact areas, the main wear mechanisms are two-body abrasion and fatigue, whereas three-body abrasion dominates in non-contact areas. Corrosive wear can occur in either situation, and, when this takes place in combination with stressing conditions, can lead to stress corrosion cracking. This process involves the slow growth of a crack, which will eventually become sufficiently large to cause catastrophic fracture.

Since wear is such a multifaceted process, it does not lend itself to being measured by any single parameter. The poor correlation between mechanical properties and wear has already been noted, and some of the physical properties, such as a low water sorption, can only give an indication of potential wear resistance, particularly in relation to corrosive wear.

In general, a high filler loading, a smooth surface finish, a hydrolytically stable resin and a strong bond between the filler and the resin are desirable attributes in a posterior composite. However, it must be recognized that, by themselves, these do not guarantee that a material will be resistant to wear.

An alternative approach is the laboratory simulation of the clinical condition. Unfortunately, it is very difficult to simulate all of the conditions in the mouth that contribute to the wear process. Although a wide variety of in vitro methods for measuring the wear rate have been tried, none has been found to predict, with any measure of certainty, the in vivo rate of wear of the posterior composites.

Another major stumbling block in the development of a reliable laboratory wear test is that one needs to be able to correlate the results with clinical wear data, which are, in themselves, extremely difficult to acquire and interpret. From the many variables that have to be taken into account, the variation in wear from patient to patient is one of the more difficult to understand.

However, it has been shown that there is a marked difference in wear rates between occlusal contact areas and non-contact areas. Thus, any value quoted for a wear rate is meaningless unless it is supported with information on the methods used in determining it.

The size of the restoration can also affect the rate of wear, perhaps due to there being a greater likelihood of direct tooth-to-restoration contact with larger restorations. It must also be considered that larger restorations tend to occur more posteriorly, where the occlusal loads are higher.

Thus, even in vivo wear data are only a guide to the ability of posterior composites to resist wear. The situation is further complicated at present by the lack of a generally accepted method for the measurement of in vivo wear, and data have to be interpreted with a great deal of caution.

The best measure of the wear resistance of a posterior composite is its clinical performance and, despite the major improvements that have taken place over the years, the use of composites where there will be direct and heavy occlusal contact should be avoided. Hence the occlusion should be checked at the beginning of treatment and centric or sliding contacts avoided or at least minimized as much as possible.

DENTAL LABORATORY COMPOSITES

Indirect composite veneers, inlays and onlays

The clinical placement of multiple direct composite restorations poses a number of problems. These include the time-consuming nature of the placement itself, the difficulty of ensuring good tooth-to-tooth contact, the problems of marginal adaptation caused by polymerization shrinkage, and the risk of incomplete curing of the restoration due to the limited depth of cure. One way to overcome these problems is to use indirect composite restorations such as inlays, onlays and veneers.

Composite inlays are constructed in the dental laboratory by a dental technician, based on an impression prepared by the dental surgeon. Composite inlays are ideally suited to those situations where there is a need to carry out multiple posterior restorations in a single quadrant or the replacement of non-functional cusps. In all other respects, the indications for composite inlays are identical to those of direct posterior composites. The advantage with this type of restoration is that much of the work in achieving good anatomical contour and tooth-to-tooth contact is done by the technician in the dental laboratory.

Other benefits are that full depth of cure is assured, since the curing process is carried out in the laboratory and not in situ. Although it is suggested that problems associated with polymerization shrinkage are reduced, the experience is otherwise. Even the thin layer of luting resin used to fix the restoration to the tooth tissue can cause sufficiently high shrinkage stresses to lead to failure of the adhesive bond, especially the bond to the dentine. Thus, problems with polymerization shrinkage are not totally eliminated. There is also some doubt as to the quality of the bond between the luting resin and inlay itself. The laboratory curing process for the composite inlays is so effective that there are few unreacted methacrylate groups left on its surface to react with the resin luting agent (see Chapter 3.7).

Many laboratory composite resin systems use essentially the same composites that are used for direct placement. Consequently, they suffer from many of the same shortcomings as direct composites, which therefore limit their range of applications. Thus, laboratory-constructed composite restorations should only be used in those situations where a direct composite would also be considered acceptable.

Fibre-reinforced composites

Particulate-filled composite resins lack sufficient strength and toughness to be considered for the construction of crowns and bridges. Fibre-reinforced composites (FRC) offer enormous potential for producing high-strength and high-stiffness materials, but with a very low weight. During the 1990s, a number of fibre-reinforced resin systems became available, for use either in the dental laboratory or in the dental surgery. These are provided in a number of different forms, as

Table 2.2.5 Fibre-reinforced composite products

Product	Supplier	Fibre type	Fibre form
Pre-impregnated products			
Fibre-Kor	Jeneric/Pentron	Glass	Unidirectional
Splint-It	Jeneric/Pentron	Glass	Unidirectional
Splint-It	Jeneric/Pentron	Glass	Weave
Splint-It	Jeneric/Pentron	Polyethylene	Weave
Stick	Stick Tech	Glass	Unidirectional
Stick-Net	Stick Tech	Glass	Mesh
Vectris pontic	Ivoclar	Glass	Unidirectional
Vectris frame and single	Ivoclar	Glass	Mesh
Non-impregnated products			
Connect	Kerr	Polyethylene	Braid
Ribbond	Ribbond	Polyethylene	Weave

shown in Table 2.2.5. The unidirectional fibres allow the construction of long spans, while the mesh and weave patterns support stresses in different directions simultaneously. The FRCs have significantly better flexural strength and impact resistance compared with particulate-filled resins, as long as good fibre wetting and coupling by the resin and a high fibre content is achieved.

The range of applications suggested for these new materials are splints, bridges, crowns and removable dentures. Clinical experience with these materials is quite limited; it seems that FRC splints perform satisfactorily for at least 4 years but removable dentures have rather more variable outcomes.

CLINICAL CONSIDERATIONS FOR THE USE OF COMPOSITE RESTORATIONS

The indications for the use of composite restorations are primarily associated with their ability to achieve an excellent aesthetic result. These materials are therefore ideally suited for anterior applications, such as the restoration of proximal lesions, abrasion and erosion lesions and incisal tip fractures.

For the posterior region, the application of composites tends to be more limited due to such potential problems as a lack of marginal seal when the margin is not in enamel as in deep proximal boxes. Wear and fracture are also problems when the restorations are large and have to carry high occlusal loads due to direct contact with the opposing teeth. Composite restorative materials should ideally be considered as primary restorative materials for small early carious lesions.

The composite restoration should, at all times, be considered as an adhesive restoration. The advantages are manifold, but, principally, the reliance on adhesion rather than retention helps to conserve tooth structure, to improve the strength of the tooth crown and to provide a barrier to marginal leakage. It is therefore important that these materials are used only in situations where a good-quality adhesive bond can be achieved; the following contraindications are suggested.

Avoidance of large restorations

This problem is most likely to occur in the posterior application of composites, where these materials are frequently considered as a replacement for failed amalgam restorations. Since such cavities are generally much bigger than those of primary caries lesions, this is not the ideal circumstance in which to use composites. For a start, the cavity design has been largely dictated by the amalgam to be replaced, and was designed with retention in mind, rather than adhesion.

The larger the restoration, the greater the problem of polymerization shrinkage, and the lower the chances of achieving a good marginal seal. The shrinkage on polymerization causes the composite to pull away from the cavity walls, and, although acid-etch bonded enamel is sufficiently strong to resist the shrinkage forces generated, dentine-bonding agents may not have a sufficiently strong bond to dentine to do likewise. This can give rise to marginal leakage and postoperative sensitivity. Even when most or all of the margins are in enamel (where a good bond and seal is possible), the breakdown of the bond to dentine will result in a fluid-filled gap beneath the restoration. This too can give rise to postoperative sensitivity due to the movement of the fluid up and down the dentinal tubules when the restoration is subjected to a load or a change in temperature.

Another contributory factor to lack of marginal seal is the mismatch in the coefficient of thermal expansion of the restorative material and the tooth tissues. This is a problem with all composites, and, although it is minimized by having high filler loadings of low-expansion glasses, it has not yet been resolved.

With larger restorations, it is more likely that there will be occlusal contact between the restoration and the opposing tooth. As composites suffer from considerably higher rates of wear in contact areas than in contact-free areas, occlusal contact combined with the higher loads that are experienced posteriorly can give rise to unacceptable rates of wear. Hence, only non-functional cusps should be involved.

Composites are low-strength, brittle materials and do not have properties much better than amalgams in this respect. The restoration derives its strength from the ability to bond to the tooth tissues. If this bond breaks down, the potential for fracture is much increased, even more so if the occlusal loads are high. The reliability and durability of the adhesive bond are much reduced as the size of the restoration is increased.

Avoidance of deep gingival preparations

Proximal restorations, whether anterior or posterior, can extend subgingivally such that the base of the box extends into root dentine. In such circumstances, it is extremely difficult, if not impossible, to ensure close marginal adaptation and to obtain a perfect marginal seal, even with the use of dentine-bonding agents.

Microleakage and the associated problems of staining, caries and sensitivity are therefore likely to be a problem. Although it has been suggested that the base of such a box may first be filled with a GIC (see Chapter 2.3), there is the possibility that the cement will eventually erode, leaving the marginal ridge of the composite restoration unsupported and possibly causing it to fracture.

Lack of peripheral enamel

The acid-etch bond to enamel of composites is extremely effective, such that breakdown of these margins is unlikely.

When a tooth is badly broken down, there will be little enamel left to bond to and the restoration has to rely more and more on the bond to the remaining dentine. This bond is as yet highly unreliable and thus increases the possibility of a breakdown of the marginal seal

when subjected to stresses generated by polymerization shrinkage, thermal mismatch and occlusal loading.

Ideally, resin composites should only be used when all the margins are in enamel. The only exceptions to this are restorations of abrasion/erosion lesions, which tend not to be subjected to high stressing conditions and have proved reasonably effective clinically, although adhesive failures remain a problem.

Replacement or onlays of load-bearing cusps

As noted earlier, composites suffer from much higher rates of wear when they are in occlusal contact with opposing teeth. Anteriorly, this has not proved to be a major problem, but posteriorly, where the loads are generally much higher, excessive wear of the composite is likely to occur. This becomes more of a problem, the further posterior the restoration is placed. The increased loads experienced by the restoration will also increase the chances of cuspal fracture, especially if preceded by the breakdown of the adhesive bond.

Poor moisture control

Since it is impossible to obtain an adhesive bond between tooth tissues and composites when the tooth surfaces are contaminated with moisture, any situation in which moisture control is not possible should be avoided and an alternative approach must be adopted.

Habitual bruxism/chewing

The aggressive wearing action associated with bruxism will cause any composite restoration that is in occlusal contact, or one that is in contact with an implement such as a pipe, to wear down extremely rapidly. Thus, even incisal tip restorations, which do not normally suffer from high rates of wear, are contraindicated unless patients can be weaned off their habit.

CLINICAL SIGNIFICANCE

The introduction of resin-based composite restorative materials has had a major impact on the practice of restorative dentistry. Many of the advances in new techniques are based on the composite materials. Their clinical applications are many and varied, and will continue to grow as further improvements in their properties are achieved. However, there are certain limitations to the use of this group of materials and it is important that these are not disregarded.

POLYACID-MODIFIED RESIN COMPOSITES (COMPOMERS)

One of the major features of GICs is their ability to provide a sustained release of fluoride, which, it has been suggested, may contribute to the protection from caries attack of tooth tissues adjacent to the restoration. Composite resin restorative materials do not have this capacity to release fluoride over an extended period of time. The addition of fluoride (F)-containing compounds such as stannous fluoride to a composite resin will provide an initial release of fluoride over a period of a couple of weeks but this then tails off rapidly. This initial release is largely due to the presence of the F-compound being released from or near the surface of the restoration. However, very quickly, the

Table 2.2.6 Composition of a polyacid-modified resin composite

Component	Function
Fluoro-alumino-silicate glass	Filler and a source of fluoride
Dimethacrylate monomer (e.g. UDMA)	Forms the resin matrix
Special resin	Provides carboxyl groups
Hydrophilic monomers	Aid the transport of water and fluoride
Photoactivators/ photoinitiators	Provide cure by radical polymerization

Table 2.2.7 Spectrum of tooth-coloured filling materials

Glass-ionomer cements	Resin-modified glass-ionomer cements	Polyacid-modified resin composites	Resin composites
Chemflex[1]	Vitremer[2]	Dyract eXtra[1]	Spectrum TPH[1]
ChemFil Molar[1]			
Ketac-Fil Plus[2] Ketac-Molar[2]	Photac-Fil Quick[2]	Compoglass F[4]	Filtek P60[2]
Fuji II[3]	Fuji II LC Improved[3]	Freedom[6]	Tetric[4]
Fuji IX[3]		Luxat[7]	Prodigy[5]
Vivaglass Fil[4]		Glasiosite[8]	Glacier[6]
Ionofil[8]			Admira[8]
Opusfil[9]			

1 = Dentsply, 2 = 3M/Espe, 3 = GC, 4 = Ivoclar, 5 = Kerr, 6 = SDI, 7 = DMG, 8 = Voco, 9 = Schottlander.

surface layer of the restoration is depleted of the F-compound and the release virtually stops, as the F-compound cannot diffuse through the resin matrix at sufficient speed to maintain a reasonable level of release.

Polyacid-modified resin composites, commonly referred to as compomers, are in fact resin composite materials, which have been modified so as to be able to release significant amounts of fluoride over an extended period. In order to achieve this, some of the technology of GICs has been incorporated in the composite resin.

Composition

The composition of a typical compomer is presented in Table 2.2.6. Examination of the composition indicates that the material is essentially a resin-based system, with a radical polymerization process being activated by blue light acting on camphoroquinone. However, there are a number of important differences compared to composite resins.

One of the differences is the glass, which is similar to the composition of the fluorine-containing glasses used in GICs. This fluoro-aluminosilicate glass is thus susceptible to acid attack and provides the source of fluoride ions.

However, this would not be enough in itself, as some means is necessary for the fluorine to be released from the glass. This requires hydrogen ions able to attack and dissolve the glass in a manner similar to that occurring in the setting process of GICs. The source of these hydrogen ions is provided by a specially formulated carboxyl group (–COOH) containing polymerizable monomer, which copolymerizes with a dimethacrylate monomer such as UDMA (Figure 2.2.30). Alternatively, the methacrylated polycarboxylic acid copolymer employed in some resin-modified glass–ionomer cements (RMGICs) can be used (see Chapter 2.3).

The final ingredient that is required to provide the fluoride release is water. This is not present in the starting material but comes from being absorbed into the material from the oral environment. This water sorption allows an acid–base reaction between the glass and the polycarboxyl groups on the special resin, and provides the mechanism for a slow but continuous release of fluoride, which has not previously been possible with composite resins.

In order to aid the diffusion of water into the material through the matrix, and simultaneously aid the diffusion of the fluoride ions out of the matrix, some of the matrix resins used have a more hydrophilic characteristic than those normally used in composite resins (e.g. glycerol dimethacrylate).

Although compomers have both a radical polymerization and acid–base reaction, it is the former that drives the setting process of these materials. The contribution of the acid–base reaction is to provide the fluoride ions to be released over an extended period.

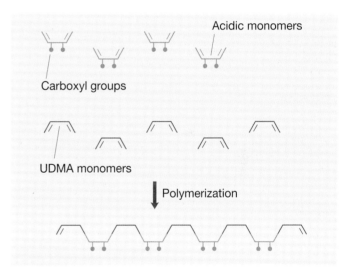

Figure 2.2.30 Copolymerization of an acidic monomer containing carboxyl groups and UDMA monomer in a compomer

CLINICAL SIGNIFICANCE

It should be stressed that, although the compomer may be considered a hybrid of a resin composite and a GIC, it is distinctively different from the RMGIC.

The starting material for a compomer is a composite resin, which is then modified, whereas for an RMGIC the starting material is a GIC. Thus we have a spectrum of materials from GICs to resins, as indicated in Table 2.2.7.

Properties

Fluoride release

Compomer products have been shown to be able to release fluoride over an extended period of time, but do not typically display as high an initial 'burst' of fluoride release as is seen with GICs. Modern compomers tend to have a similar fluoride release profile to GICs and RMGICs over the lifetime of a restoration. Fluoride release is highly variable from product to product and it is not yet known what the optimum release of fluoride is that is needed to induce an anticariogenic condition around the margins of a restoration. Also, the local conditions can have a significant influence on the amount of fluoride released, as some materials will be more susceptible to dissolution than others in an acid environment.

It has been shown that GICs have a capacity to reabsorb fluoride from the oral environment and release this at a later stage. Compomers can also be 'recharged' with fluoride in this way, although the process is typically less efficient than with GICs. Thus the restoration can act as a fluoride reservoir that is regularly replenished when exposed to topical fluorides. This may be a very important feature of the long-term anticariogenicity of fluoride-releasing restorative materials.

Handling characteristics

What makes a material with good handling characteristics is a complex issue, as this is governed by multiple interrelated features including rheology (e.g. flow and tendency to slump), stickiness, and working and setting times. Nevertheless, the general consensus among dental practitioners is that compomers have good handling characteristics and that compomers are easy to adapt to the cavity wall without sticking to the placement instruments, are easy to shape and do not slump.

Adhesion

Unlike GICs and RMGICs, compomers do not have a natural affinity for enamel and dentine and have to be used in conjunction with a dentine adhesive. In order to simplify the handling characteristics when using the dentine-bonding agent normally used with the composite resins, it is recommended that the acid etching of the enamel and dentine is omitted from the bonding procedure. This will result in a lower bond strength and should only be considered when using compomers in low-stress-bearing applications. Ultimately, this statement is confusing for the dental practitioner, as it is not easy to determine what constitutes a low-stress-bearing situation. Some compomers are provided with a proprietary adhesive, which have characteristics of the self-etching primers discussed in Chapter 2.5.

Polymerization shrinkage

Polymerization shrinkage is similar to that of the composite resins (~2–2.5 vol. %) and water sorption is not dissimilar to that of the composite resin, being in the region of 40 μg·mm^{-3}. Where the compomers differ from the composite resins is in their rate of water uptake. As noted earlier in this chapter, the diffusion of water through the resin matrix is very slow and it takes many years for the composite resin restoration to achieve equilibrium water content. For the compomer, the hydrophilic resin matrix provides a more rapid pathway for the absorption of water, with equilibrium water uptake possibly being reached in a matter of days rather than weeks, months or even years.

CLINICAL SIGNIFICANCE

The rapid water sorption by compomers provides compensation for the polymerization shrinkage of the resin matrix in a matter of days and helps to reduce any marginal gap that may have formed during placement of the restoration.

Mechanical properties

The mechanical properties of compomers would generally appear to be somewhat inferior to those of the composite resins, with a reduced compressive, diametral and flexural strength. This precludes their use in high-stress-bearing situations, such as the repair of the fractured incisal tip. Their wear resistance is better than that of the GICs and RMGICs. However, compared with composite resins, the wear resistance is reduced. It is possible that this may be due to use of slightly larger filler particles than normally used in composite resins, combined with a reduction in the interfacial integrity between the glass filler and the resin due to the ongoing acid–base reaction at this interface.

Applications

In order to have the benefit of fluoride release from the compomer, it would appear that the mechanical properties have had to be compromised to some degree compared to the composite resin. Therefore, the compomer does not have the same range of applications as the composite resin; in fact, the range of applications is similar to that of the GICs and the RMGICs. Since their mechanical properties and wear resistance tend to be inferior to those of composite resins, but better than that of GICs and the RMGICs, their use is limited to low-stress-bearing situations such as proximal and abrasion erosion lesions, permanent restorations in the primary dentition and long-term temporaries in the permanent dentition. Because of their aesthetic qualities still being comparable to that of the composite resins, combined with the fluoride release and the simpler bonding procedures, the compomers are a popular alternative to the glass–ionomer and RMGICs, showing excellent results after some 3–4 years of clinical use.

As with the RMGICs, there have been reports of excessive hygroscopic expansion associated with compomers, presumably due to their high content of hydrophilic resins. While such behaviour may be beneficial in reducing the marginal gap around a class V restoration, this expansion can also lead to fracture of all-ceramic crowns.

CLINICAL SIGNIFICANCE

Luting versions of the compomer are not recommended for all-ceramic restorations.

FURTHER READING

Boaro LC, Gonçalves F, Guimarães TC et al (2010) Polymerization stress, shrinkage and elastic modulus of current low-shrinkage restorative composites. Dent Mater 26(12): 1144–1150

Braga RR, Ferracane JL (2004) Alternatives in polymerization contraction stress management. Crit Rev Oral Biol Med 15: 176

Clelland NL, Pagnotto MP, Kerby RE et al (2005) Relative wear of flowable and highly filled composite. J Prosthet Dent 93: 153

Guggenberger R, Weinmann W (2000) Exploring beyond methacrylates. Am J Dent 13: 82D

Kumbuloglu O, Saracoglu A, Ozcan M (2011) Pilot study of unidirectional E-glass fibre-reinforced composite resin splints: up to 4.5-year clinical follow-up. J Dent 39: 871–877

Manhart J, Chen H, Hamm G, Hickel R (2004) Buonocore Memorial Lecture. Review of the clinical survival of direct and indirect restorations in posterior teeth of the permanent dentition. Oper Dent 29: 481

Moharamzadeh K, Brook IM, van Noort R (2009) Biocompatibility of resin-based dental materials. Materials 2(2): 514–548

Moszner N, Salz U (2001) New developments of polymeric dental composites. Prog Poly Sci 26: 535

Opdam NJ, Bronkhorst EM, Loomans BA, Huysmans MC (2010) 12-year survival of composite vs. amalgam restorations. J Dent Res 89(10): 1063–1067

Oysaed H, Ruyter IE (1986) Water sorption and filler characteristics of composites for use in posterior teeth. J Dent Res 65: 1315–1318

Peutzfeldt A (1997) Resin composites in dentistry: the monomer systems. Europ J Oral Sci 105: 97

Pye A (2009) How long do fibre-reinforced resin-bonded fixed partial dentures last? Evid Based Dent 10(3): 75

Roeters J, Shortall AC, Opdam NJ (2005) Can a single composite resin serve all purposes? Br Dent J 199: 73

Rueggeberg F (2002) From vulcanite to vinyl, a history of resins in restorative dentistry. J Prosthet Dent 87: 364

Schmalz G (1998) The biocompatibility of non-amalgam dental filling materials. Eur J Oral Sci 106: 696

Silikas N, Eliades G, Watts DC (2000) Light intensity effects on resin-composite degree of conversion and shrinkage strain. Dent Mater 16: 292

Soderholm KJ, Mariotti A (1999) BIS-GMA-based resins in dentistry: are they safe? J Am Dent Assoc 130: 201

van Heumen CC, Tanner J, van Dijken JW et al (2010) Five-year survival of 3-unit fiber-reinforced composite fixed partial dentures in the posterior area. Dent Mater 26(10): 954–960

Wiegand A, Buchalla W, Attin T (2007) Review on fluoride-releasing restorative materials – fluoride release and uptake characteristics, antibacterial activity and influence on caries formation. Dent Mater 23: 343

Glass–ionomer cements and resin-modified glass–ionomer cements

INTRODUCTION

Glass–ionomer cements (GICs), frequently also referred to as glass polyalkenoate cements, are restorative materials that consist of a powder and a liquid which are mixed to produce a plastic mass that subsequently sets to a rigid solid.

The GICs were first described by Wilson and Kent in 1972 and, at the time, presented a natural extension to the zinc–polycarboxylate cements that had become available in the late 1960s. The zinc–polycarboxylate cements had evolved from zinc–phosphate cement by the ingenious replacement of the phosphoric acid with polyacrylic acid (see Chapter 2.8).

The GICs were immediately seen as a potential replacement for the silicate cements that had been around for some 80 years and that were gradually being ousted by the resin-based composites.

The two main features of GICs that have allowed them to become one of the accepted dental materials are their ability to bond to enamel and dentine and their ability to release fluoride from the glass component of the cement. Thus, the GICs combine the adhesive qualities of the zinc–polycarboxylate cements with the fluoride release of the silicate cements. The relationship between the different materials is shown in Figure 2.3.1.

GICs were used mainly for the restoration of abrasion/erosion lesions and as a luting agent for crown and bridge reconstruction. Their clinical application has now been extended to include the restoration of proximal lesions, occlusal restorations in the deciduous dentition, cavity bases and liners and core materials by the introduction of a wide variety of new formulations.

A later innovation was the modification of the GIC by incorporating a resin, which allowed the material to be set by light activation. These new materials are, not surprisingly, known as resin-modified glass–ionomer cements (RMGICs), although sometimes they are also referred to as glass–ionomer–resin hybrids. However, the preferred description is RMGICs, in part to avoid confusion with compomers.

Thus, this group of materials deserves our closest attention.

CHEMISTRY OF GLASS–IONOMER CEMENTS

Composition

What makes the GIC such an interesting material compared to the zinc–phosphate cements is the enormous variety of compositions that can be achieved. The main components of a GIC are glass, polyacid, water and tartaric acid.

The composition of the glass can be varied widely, giving many different properties, and, to add to this, there are numerous combinations of polyacids that are suitable for copolymerization. In contrast, for the zinc–phosphate cements, once the composition is optimized in terms of the powder-to-liquid ratio and the concentration of the phosphoric acid, there is little scope for improvement.

Of course, such a variety can be as much of a hindrance as a help, and this is reflected in the development of the GICs, which began in the early 1970s.

It could never be claimed that the GICs have had a smooth passage since their inception. The proof of this statement is based on the observation that the materials currently marketed are quite different from those originally made available for clinical use. The early materials consisted of a glass powder to which a concentrated solution of a polyacrylic acid was added. ASPA (Dentsply De Trey Ltd, Weybridge, UK) was the first commercial product, and was made available in 1976.

Glass

The glasses for the GICs contain three main components: silica (SiO_2) and alumina (Al_2O_3) mixed in a flux of calcium fluoride (CaF_2), as shown in Figure 2.3.2. The composition of the glass is largely restricted to the central region of the phase diagram by the desire to have a translucent glass.

The mixture (which also contains sodium and aluminium fluorides and calcium or aluminium phosphates as additional fluxes) is fused at a high temperature, and the molten mass is then shock-cooled and finely ground to a powder before use.

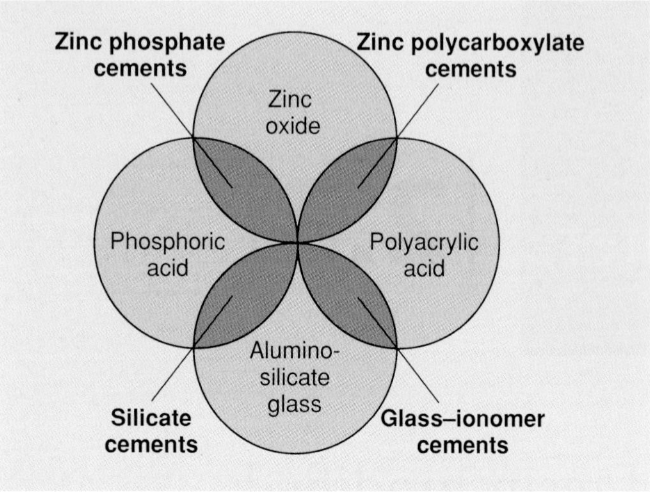

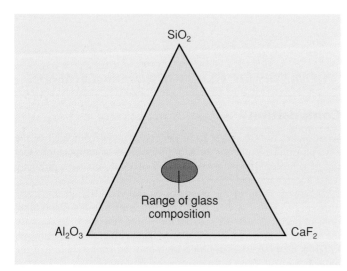

Figure 2.3.1 Schematic of the various dental cements based on powders of zinc oxide and alumino-silicate glass, and liquids consisting of phosphoric acid and polyacrylic acid

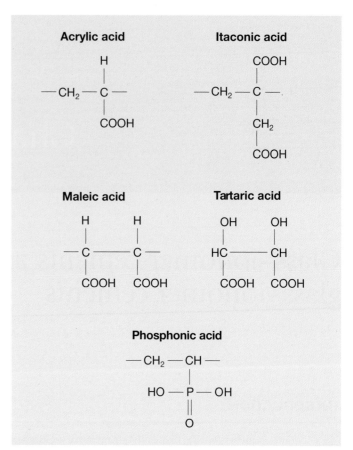

Figure 2.3.3 Acid components used in a GIC

Figure 2.3.2 Composition of glass used in GICs

The particle size of the powder is dependent on its intended application. For filling materials, the maximum particle size is 50 μm, while for the luting and lining materials it is reduced to less than 20 μm.

The rate of release of ions from the glass (which is an important factor in determining the setting characteristics, the solubility, and the release of fluoride) is a function of the type of glass employed (see below). The glass also plays a major role in the aesthetics of the restoration, as this is dependent on both the refractive index of the glass and the presence of pigments within it.

Polyacid

There are a wide range of polyacrylic acid analogues; when these are combined with variations in molecular weight and configuration, this means that a large variety of formulations are possible. The polyacids most used in current formulations are copolymers of acrylic and itaconic acid or acrylic and maleic acid (Figure 2.3.3).

A relative newcomer is a GIC based on a copolymer of vinyl phosphonic acid. This is a much stronger acid than the others

used in GICs, and the composition has to be carefully controlled to produce a cement with suitable handling properties. However, it is believed to give higher long-term strength and enhanced moisture resistance.

There is an optimum acid concentration in the case of the silicate cements, but the GICs are not so dependent on this. The strength and the resistance to aqueous attack both steadily increase with polyacid concentration, so the limiting factor is the consistency of the cement paste. The viscosity of the liquid depends on both the polyacid concentration and the molecular weight, which can vary from 10 000 to 30 000, depending on the formulation selected. Tartaric acid is an important component of the GIC, as it has a significant influence on the working and setting times.

Presentation

Powder–liquid

Many GICs consist of a glass powder to which a proprietary liquid is added. The powder is much as described above, and the liquid is an aqueous solution of polyacrylic or polymaleic acid and tartaric acid. A number of deficiencies were soon recognized with this mode of presentation and this brought about a change in formulation.

One of the problems is the excessive solubility of the cement in saliva, coupled with the slow setting reaction; another is concerned with judging the correct powder-to-liquid ratio. There is a tendency to reduce the powder content of the cement in order to obtain a smooth creamy paste, but this results in a slower-setting, weaker cement that is more susceptible to dissolution (Figure 2.3.4).

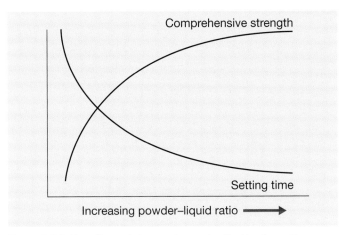

Figure 2.3.4 The effects of changes in powder–liquid ratio on the properties of GICs

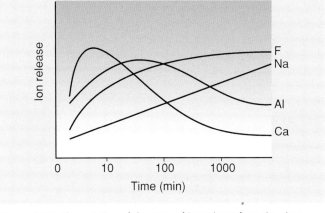

Figure 2.3.5 The variation of the rates of ion release from the glass

Anhydrous cements

Nowadays, many GICs are of a water-hardening type, and the cement is formed by the addition of the correct amount of distilled water. The glass powder is blended with freeze-dried polyacid and tartaric acid powder.

The first product that used this approach became available commercially in 1981. The new formulations, described as the *anhydrous systems*, present as a powder and a liquid. The powder contains aluminosilicate glass, polyacid powder and tartaric acid, and the liquid is just distilled water.

Capsules

It is well recognized that achieving the correct powder-to-liquid ratio can still be a problem, and a vigorous mixing process is required to ensure that all the powder is incorporated in the liquid. One way in which this may be overcome is by the use of preproportioned capsules.

The contents of different capsules do not necessarily have the same constituents, so it is inadvisable to mix them. For example, to ensure the most appropriate handling and physical properties, the filling materials have much larger glass filler particles than the luting agents. Similarly, the liquids used can vary in composition to suit the particular glass formulation and to give the correct working and setting times. This is dealt with in some detail later, in relation to the application of the different formulations.

CLINICAL SIGNIFICANCE

The difficulty of dispensing and mixing the correct amount of powder and liquid for these materials means that preproportioned capsules are preferable for consistency of performance, although they are usually more expensive and may lead to greater waste of the material.

Setting reaction

The setting reaction of the GICs is via an acid–base reaction:

$$MO \cdot SiO_2 + H_2A \rightarrow MA + SiO_2 + H_2O$$
$$\underset{glass}{} \quad \underset{acid}{} \quad \underset{salt}{} \quad \underset{silica\ gel}{}$$

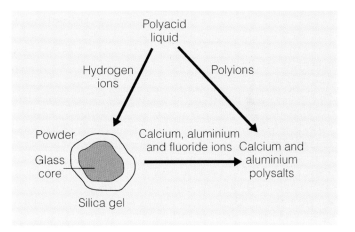

Figure 2.3.6 The initial stages of the setting reaction in a GIC

The setting process of a GIC involves three overlapping stages:

- dissolution
- gelation
- hardening.

This happens because of the different rates at which the ions are released from the glass and the rate at which the salt matrix is formed (Figure 2.3.5); as is apparent from this curve, the calcium ions are more rapidly released than the aluminium ions. This is because the calcium ions are only loosely bound in the glass structure, while the aluminium ions form part of the glass network, which is more difficult to break down. It is the calcium and the aluminium ions which will eventually form the salt matrix. The sodium and fluorine ions do not take part in the setting process but combine to be released as sodium fluoride.

Dissolution

When the proprietary solution or the water is mixed with the powder, the acid goes into solution and reacts with the outer layer of the glass. This layer becomes depleted in aluminium, calcium, sodium and fluorine ions, so that only a silica gel remains (Figure 2.3.6).

The hydrogen ions that are released from the carboxyl groups on the polyacid chain diffuse to the glass, and make up for the loss of the calcium, aluminium and fluorine ions. The setting reaction for the cement is a slow process, and it takes some time for the material to

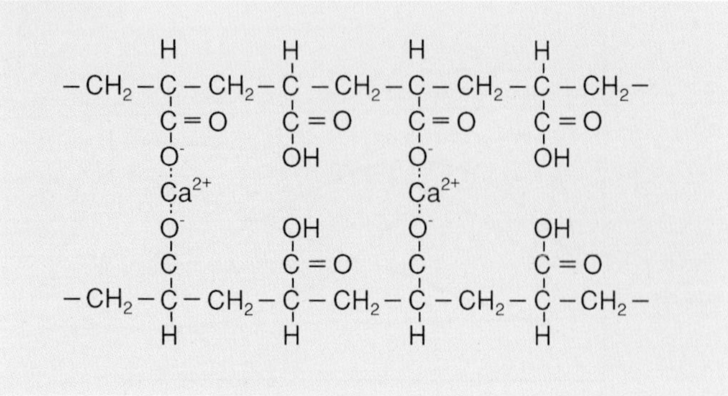

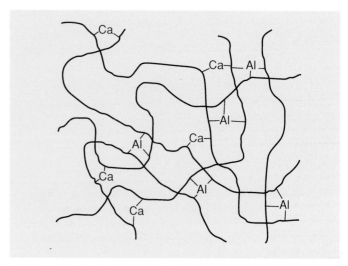

Figure 2.3.7 Gelation phase of the setting process

stabilize; the final translucency and colour of the material are not apparent until 24 hours after placement.

Although the material appears hard after its required setting time (usually 3–6 minutes, depending on whether it is a filling or a luting cement), it has still not reached its final physical and mechanical properties and will continue to set for up to 1 month.

Gelation

The initial set is due to the rapid action of the calcium ions, which, being divalent and more abundant initially, react more readily with the carboxyl groups of the acid than do the trivalent aluminium ions (Figure 2.3.7). This is the *gelation phase* of the setting reaction. The efficiency with which the calcium ions cross-link the polyacid molecules is not as good as it might be because they are also able to link carboxyl groups on the same molecule. A recent interesting development is the incorporation of zinc-containing fillers into GICs; the Zn^{2+} can also cross-link two polyacid molecules and may offer a more rapid set, although more data are needed before clinical conclusions can be drawn.

Various things can happen if the restoration is not protected from the outside environment during this critical phase. Aluminium ions may diffuse out of the material and be lost to the cement, thereby being unable to cross-link the polyacrylic acid chains. If the water is lost, the reaction cannot go to completion. In both instances, a weak material will result. Alternatively, additional moisture may be absorbed, which may be contaminated with blood or saliva, leading to compromised aesthetics, with the restoration looking exceptionally dull and white. The contaminating moisture will also weaken the material and may even cause it to crumble. Hence, it is essential that contamination by moisture and drying of the restoration are both avoided, at least during the initial period of setting when the material is at its most vulnerable.

Hardening

After the gelation phase, there is a hardening phase that can last as long as 7 days. It takes some 30 minutes for the uptake of aluminium ions to become significant, yet it is the aluminium ions that provide the final strength to the cement, as they are responsible for the introduction of the cross-links. In contrast to the calcium ions, the trivalent nature of the aluminium ions ensures that a high degree of cross-linking of the polymer molecules takes place (Figure 2.3.8).

There is a continuation of the formation of aluminium salt bridges, and water becomes bound to the silica gel, which now surrounds the residual core of each of the glass particles. Once the cement has fully reacted, the solubility is quite low. The final structure is as shown in Figure 2.3.9, and consists of glass particles, each of

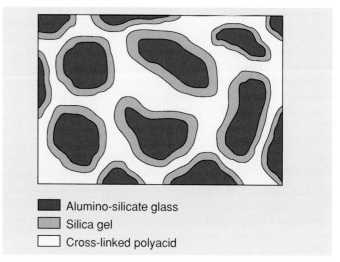

Figure 2.3.8 Hardening phase of the setting process

■ Alumino-silicate glass
■ Silica gel
□ Cross-linked polyacid

Figure 2.3.9 The structure of a GIC

which is surrounded by a silica gel in a matrix of cross-linked polyacrylic acid.

Whereas normally it is desirable for glasses to resist ion release, in the case of the GICs a controlled release of the ions of calcium and aluminium is essential. The skill in choosing the correct glass and the correct formulation is to balance the various requirements of good handling characteristics, low solubility, adequate fluoride release and aesthetics.

CLINICAL SIGNIFICANCE

GICs are slow to set and need protection from the oral environment in order to minimize dissolution or contamination.

PROPERTIES

Handling characteristics

The effects of the composition of the glass on the setting process are very pronounced and of considerable importance in determining the

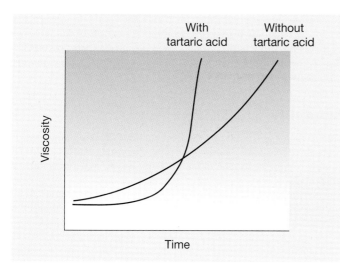

Figure 2.3.10 The effect of tartaric acid on the viscosity–time curve for a setting GIC

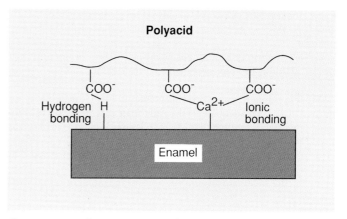

Figure 2.3.11 Adhesive mechanisms for GICs

Table 2.3.1 Handling characteristics of old and new GICs

Material	Mixing	Working	Setting	Finishing
ASPA	60 s	90 s	6 min	24 h
Modern GIC	20 s	75 s	2 min	7 min

Table 2.3.2 Effects of surface treatments on the tensile bond strength of GICs to enamel and dentine

Surface treatment	Bond strength (MPa)
Enamel	
None	3.2
Citric acid	5.6
Polyacrylic acid	7.1
Dentine	
None	3.1
Citric acid	3.7
Polyacrylic acid	6.8

acceptability of the final handling characteristics of the cement. The Al : Si ratio of the glass for the GICs is higher than that for the silicate cements because the polyacrylic acid and its analogues are much weaker than phosphoric acid. One of the effects of this increased ratio is that the working time is reduced.

However, GICs were inclined previously to have prolonged working and setting times. This was certainly a serious problem with the earliest formulations of this cement until it was overcome by the inclusion of the optimum concentration of tartaric acid. The tartaric acid is believed to have a twofold function. First, it reacts rapidly with the calcium ions being released from the glass with the formation of calcium tartrate, which has the effect of extending the working time. This is followed by an enhancement of the rate of formation of aluminium polyacrylate cross-links, which speeds up the set (Figure 2.3.10).

By manipulation of the glass composition and particle size, and the incorporation of tartaric acid, the handling characteristics have been much improved over the years, and are now far superior to those of the first commercially available products. These improvements are shown in Table 2.3.1. As a consequence of these changes, the GICs now have a much better defined snap set.

Adhesion

One of the most attractive features of GIC is that it is a bulk placement restorative material (no need for incremental placement), which is able to bond directly to dentine and enamel. It has been shown that the polyacrylate ions either react with the apatite structure (displacing calcium and phosphate ions, and creating an intermediate layer of polyacrylate, phosphate and calcium ions), or bond directly to the calcium in the apatite, as shown in Figure 2.3.11.

The bond to dentine may be a hydrogen bond type of adhesion to the collagen combined with an ionic bond to the apatite within the dentine structure. The bond strength, as measured in shear bond strength tests, would suggest that it is not particularly strong (2–7 MPa), but clinical experience would indicate that it is durable when the material is used for the restoration of erosion lesions. Whatever the details of the bonding process may be, the bond created is strong enough such that, when a GIC is debonded, the fracture will generally run through the GIC (cohesive failure) and not along the interface (adhesive failure). The major limitation on the bond strength of the GICs appears, therefore, to be its low tensile strength, which is only of the order of 7 MPa and is due to the brittle nature of these materials.

To obtain a good bond to dentine, it is advisable to treat the surface first with a dentine conditioner. The best conditioner appears to be a 20% aqueous solution of polyacrylic acid, although tannic acid has also proved to be effective. Typical tensile bond strengths that have been measured for the bond to dentine are presented in Table 2.3.2.

The major purpose of the surface treatment is to remove debris and to produce a smooth, clean surface. Citric acid should not be used, as it opens up the dentinal tubules, increasing the dentine permeability and the potential for pulpal reaction. Additionally, it demineralizes the dentine, which may compromise the bond to the apatite component.

Aesthetics

A major requirement of any restorative material intended for use in anterior teeth is that it must blend in well with the surrounding tooth tissues, so as to be barely distinguishable. The factors governing this are the colour and the translucency of the restorative material.

In GICs, the colour is produced by the glass. This can be controlled by the addition of colour pigments such as ferric oxide or carbon black.

Whereas colour does not present a major problem, the translucency of the GICs was inadequate in the early materials, being more comparable to that of dentine than enamel. This lack of translucency has meant that the aesthetic appearance of GICs has always been considered inferior to that of composite resins. The cements appeared dull and lifeless, and this limited their application to that of a filling material for the treatment of erosion lesions and non-critical class III cavities.

There are essentially two causes of the opacity of GICs:

1. *Phase separation of the glass.* To some extent, this problem can be overcome by reducing the aluminium, calcium and fluorine content of the glass, but this reduces the strength of the material and extends the working and setting times.
2. *Mismatch of refractive index.* This problem can be minimized by reducing the aluminium content and increasing the fluorine content; however, the latter leads to phase separation. In general, optically good GICs tend to have poor setting characteristics.

The translucency of a restorative material can be described and measured by considering its inverse – *opacity*. Opacity is defined as being 0 for a transparent material and 1.0 for a white opaque material. The opacity, or *contrast ratio*, is defined as the ratio between the intensity of the light reflected from the material when placed against a dark background and that obtained for a white background of known reflectivity (70% in the case of dental cements).

This is not an absolute property of the material, as it depends on the thickness of the material and the spectral distribution of the incident light. This property, denoted by $C_{0.70}$ (see Chapter 1.7), gives mean values for enamel and dentine of 0.39 and 0.70 respectively. The early formulations of the GICs gave $C_{0.70}$ values in the range 0.7–0.85. These have been improved and are now approaching those of enamel, with $C_{0.70}$ values of 0.4 for some formulations.

The opacity is affected by the absorption of water, causing a decrease in the opacity. Thus, clinically, the restoration can darken when it comes in contact with saliva.

Selecting the appropriate colour and translucency is a difficult problem, as these are affected by the optical properties of the underlying material. On some occasions, the translucency has to be forsaken, and a relatively opaque material must be used in order to mask out a particularly dark substructure. In these cases, the GICs can prove to be particularly beneficial.

While the initial match in colour and translucency between the enamel and the GIC is important, it is also important that this close match is maintained in the severe environment of the oral cavity. A loss of aesthetic quality of the restoration can arise from staining, and, if excessive, would be considered a clinical failure and would need replacement.

The GICs appear less susceptible to staining than the silicate cements that preceded them. This has been ascribed to the superior adhesion between the matrix and the glass in the GIC when compared to the bond between the resin and filler in the composite. However, the composites have been improved considerably in recent years and are now far less susceptible to surface staining. Staining of the margins around GICs has also been found to be far less pronounced than for the composite resins. This may be a reflection of the excellent bond that can be achieved between a GIC and the tooth tissues. Another contributory factor may be that shrinkage on setting for GICs should be considerably less than that for composite resins. In effect, GICs set by an acid–base-mediated cross-linking reaction of the polyacid chains, which inherently produces less shrinkage than polymerization. Hence the local interfacial stresses generated will be less and the bond stands a better chance of survival.

Solubility

Due to their high solubility, the dental silicates had a reputation for loss of material in the mouth. To some extent, this can be attributed to incorrect preparation and handling, but it is an inherent feature of all dental cements; as such, the GICs are no exception.

Nevertheless, this negative aspect of the material's behaviour can be minimized by an appreciation of the mechanisms involved and the adoption of proper clinical technique. The processes giving rise to loss of material are complex, as there are many variables involved, such as the cement composition, the clinical technique used and the nature of the environment. The loss of material from a GIC can be classified into three main categories:

- dissolution of the immature cement
- long-term erosion
- abrasion.

Dissolution of the immature cement occurs before the material is fully set, which can take up to 7 days, although the dissolution rate drops dramatically in the first 24 hours. The temporary protection of a layer of nitro-cellulose, methyl methacrylate or amide resin acting as a varnish should be sufficient to minimize this effect. This protection must survive for at least 1 hour, as it takes this much time for the GIC to approach the properties that are achieved when it is fully set. At present, there is some controversy as to the quality and duration of protection offered by the different varnishes available, and some clinicians advocate the use of an unfilled light-activated resin, as this will give longer protection. A high powder-to-liquid ratio helps because it accelerates the setting process, whereas a thin mix has the opposite effect, and also adversely affects the mechanical properties (see Figure 2.3.4).

Once the cement has fully set (usually within 7 days; manifested by a dramatic drop in the amount of water-leachable material), this particular form of material loss will stop. From this point onwards, loss of material can be considered long-term, and is a function of the conditions in the oral environment.

Loss of material in the long term may arise either from acid attack or from mechanical abrasion. This is hardly surprising, given that the main application of GICs is the restoration of lesions, which have themselves arisen because of the combined effect of acid and abrasion. The potential for acid attack tends to be very marked in stagnation regions, such as around the gingival margin. Here, plaque accumulates and a highly acidic environment develops due to the formation of lactic acid. The GICs are more resistant to this form of attack than the silicate cements, as indicated by a reduction in the extent of surface markings.

GICs are extensively used in applications where they will be subject to mechanical abrasion, such as tooth brushing. Their resistance to abrasion is poor, which limits their application to low stressing conditions and certainly prevents their use as permanent posterior restorative materials.

An in vitro test, in which cement samples are arranged in small holders and subjected to a jet of liquid consisting of a dilute acid, attempts to assess loss of material by a combination of abrasion and acid attack. If this method is used, the indications are that the polyacrylic acid-based cements are more resistant to abrasion/erosion than the polymaleic acid-based cements. However, it is important to remember that this observation is based on a laboratory test and would need to be confirmed clinically before its validity can be established.

Fluoride release

The fact that dental cements dissolve in the oral environment is usually regarded as an adverse effect, since it leads to degradation of the material. However, whereas degradation by acid dissolution is a potential problem with GICs, fluoride released by an ion exchange mechanism is believed to increase significantly the caries resistance of enamel adjacent to the restoration. Whether fluoride release or other factors (e.g. the release of other ions, antibacterial properties and adhesive capabilities) have a role to play in the anticariogenic characteristics of GICs is still a matter of debate. Nevertheless, attempts have been made to impart this property to amalgams and composites, as well as the GICs.

This presents the dentist with an interesting dilemma in making the choice between a GIC or a composite, with the former being most definitely weaker but potentially providing some protection of the surrounding tissues, and the latter being more stable and stronger but not providing such protection.

CLINICAL SIGNIFICANCE

GIC is a fluoride-releasing, intrinsically adhesive, bulk-filling material.

CLINICAL APPLICATIONS

It must be appreciated from the outset that the GICs are designed to suit a wide variety of applications, their range encompassing materials with widely different properties.

Hence, although they are all based on the same principles outlined above, each formulation has features that make it more suited to a particular application, and it is important that these are not confused. The various applications are listed in Table 2.3.3, but only the tooth-coloured filling materials will be considered in this chapter.

Tooth-coloured filling materials

Presentation

The materials are available in three formulations:

- the traditional powder–liquid systems with the polyacids in an aqueous solution
- the anhydrous systems with the dried acid incorporated in the powder
- encapsulated versions.

Table 2.3.3 Clinical applications of GICs: tooth-coloured filling materials

Abrasion and erosion lesions
Class III lesions involving exposed root dentine
Occlusal lesions on deciduous dentition
Temporary anterior and posterior restorations
Repair of crown margins
Cavity bases and liners
Cement base under composites, amalgams and ceramics
Blocking out undercuts
Cementation of crowns and bridges

Table 2.3.4 Compressive and diametral tensile strengths of a range of commercially available GIC filling materials

Material (manufacturer)	Compressive strength (MPa)	Diametral tensile strength (MPa)
Chemfill-II (De Trey)	230	19
Ketac-Fil (ESPE)	170	10
Legend (SS White)	220	16
Opus-Fil (DSD)	220	18
RGI (Rexodent)	220	16

The latter requires activation of the capsule, and mixing in an amalgamator, which ensures an accurate powder-to-liquid ratio, not unlike the amalgam capsules.

Some of the properties of a number of tooth-coloured GICs are presented in Table 2.3.4. The differences are not really sufficient to suggest that one material is superior to another.

The main feature of all of these materials is their low diametral tensile strength, which is an indication of the low tensile strength of these materials. Thus, GICs should not be used where they are going to be subjected to high tensile loads, such as incisal tip restorations, cuspal replacement or pin-retained cores. In situations where the restoration is supported all around by tooth tissue, the GIC is protected (to some degree) from tensile loading conditions.

The size of the glass powder particles ensures that a very high powder-to-liquid ratio can be achieved, and this is reflected in the compressive and diametral tensile strengths of these materials. (These strengths are much higher than for the luting and lining cements described later.) It also affects the solubility, which is reduced as the powder-to-liquid ratio is increased.

There are differences in the working and setting times of the different cements; some have much shorter setting times than others (which is desirable in limiting the early solubility), but the working time is also much reduced (which may present a problem to some clinicians).

Shade selection

The aesthetic quality of the tooth-coloured GICs has long been considered a drawback, but recent changes in formulation have resulted in a marked improvement.

The choice of shade of the restorative material should be carried out prior to the isolation of the tooth or any other form of preparation. The colour of rubber dam, if used, alters the colour of the tooth. This change in shade is increased still further when the enamel is allowed to dehydrate during isolation.

For the restoration of lesions that involve an extensive amount of the labial surface, the use of GICs may not give an aesthetically adequate result, and the use of composites should be considered. Nevertheless, for those patients who are known to have a high caries rate, it may be better to forsake some of the aesthetic quality of the composites in preference to the fluoride release provided by the GICs.

Another aspect of the aesthetics of GICs is the observation that there is a colour change during the setting process. Generally, the shade is somewhat darker after the material has fully set than at the time of placement. This darkening is believed to be associated with an increase in translucency on setting and may take up to 24 hours to develop.

Cavity preparation

The adhesive quality of the GICs dictates that an ultra-conservative approach should be adopted. This means that minimal removal of tooth substance is required, and it should be stressed that the excessive removal of tooth tissues for the provision of undercuts or dovetails is not necessary. However, for situations where the restoration may be subjected to high stresses, some undercut may be advantageous. In the case of a replacement restoration, the original restoration should be carefully removed without removing any tooth tissues unless they are carious. The cavo-surface margins should be butt-jointed and not bevelled.

Isolation

Although the GICs are hydrophilic materials, it is recommended that careful isolation of the field of operation is carried out. The presence of blood or saliva will not only impair the formation of a strong bond but may also lead to contamination of the restoration, thereby reducing both bond strength and aesthetics. A well-placed GIC should not fail adhesively, as the bond to dentine and enamel is at least as strong as the cohesive strength of the cement.

Preparation of the dentinal surfaces

The nature of the dentine surface varies from site to site, with the major distinction being between cut dentine after caries removal and sclerotic dentine.

Abrasion/erosion lesions

Lesions at the cervical margin need to be restored to provide direct protection of the pulp, to prevent the development of pulpal sensitivity and to improve appearance. Since the GICs are adhesive, it should not be necessary to cut any finishing lines or undercuts in the dentine. Preparation prior to placement of the material should only involve the cleaning and conditioning of the dentine surface. The cleaning procedure should be carried out by scrubbing for a few seconds only with a slurry of pumice and water in a soft rubber cup or bristle brush, and is aimed at removing any surface contaminants, such as plaque or pellicle, which obscure the dentine surface. The surface should be thoroughly washed to remove any debris. A conditioner consisting of an aqueous solution of polyacrylic acid may then be applied to the surface for 10 seconds for a concentration of 20–25%, or 20 seconds for a concentration of 10%, using a pledget of cotton wool and a light rubbing action. This procedure will ensure that the surface is clean, but will also result in some opening of the dentinal tubules. Some argue that exposure of the dentinal tubules is contraindicated, as it increases the dentine permeability and thus raises the likelihood of a pulpal reaction. This is probably not a problem in the case of patients who have no history of sensitivity, since the tubules will have sclerosed and secondary dentine will have been laid down. However, for those patients with sensitivity, acid treatment of the dentine surface should not be undertaken. There is still some controversy as to the need for the prior application of polyacrylic acid to the dentine surface. Some studies have shown that this will improve the dentine bond strength, whereas others have shown that it has no effect.

Class III, class V and other carious lesions

It is not necessary to clean the cavities with pumice and water in the case of carious lesions, as the surface will consist of freshly exposed dentine. However, there is still the dentine smear layer to consider, which is present in any cavity preparation. While the smear layer is strongly bonded to the underlying dentine, surface debris needs to be removed in such a way as to avoid opening of the dentinal tubules.

Again, the use of polyacrylic acid is recommended. A variety of other dentine conditioners have been advocated from time to time (e.g. citric acid, EDTA (ethylenediaminetetraacetic acid) and ferric chloride), but these should not be applied to freshly cut dentine for the reasons already mentioned. The simplest and most effective dentine surface conditioner appears to be polyacrylic acid.

Pulpal protection

The increased application of GICs in recent years has raised some interesting problems, not least being the pulpal toxicity associated with these materials and whether or not a lining material should be used. If the cement is in direct contact with the pulp, this will result in a localized zone of pulp necrosis, which inhibits calcific repair. However, in those instances where there is a residual dentine layer, dentine bridge formation will occur. If the cavity is very deep and there may even be a micro-exposure of the pulp, then it is recommended that a calcium hydroxide lining is placed on the pulpal aspects of mechanically prepared cavities prior to the insertion of the GIC.

The potential cause of pulpal sensitivity when using GICs has been suggested to be differences in techniques of manipulating the cement or some other, unknown, patient-related factors. As yet, it is not clear what gives rise to the small number of cases of pulpal sensitivity; nor is it clear what the role of bacterial contamination or invasion may be.

Lower levels of bacteria are associated with GICs rather than with zinc–phosphate or zinc–polycarboxylate cements. This may be because glass–ionomer lining cements have a pronounced antimicrobial effect. Nevertheless, for all types of GIC (including the silver cermets), lining the dentine is recommended, especially if the tooth is symptomatic or the cavity preparation is particularly deep.

There are situations where a small amount of affected soft dentine, which has the potential to remineralize, may be left in the deepest portions of the preparation since there is the danger of a microscopic pulpal exposure if it were removed. The ability of calcium hydroxide to activate the formation of secondary dentine and its alkalinity are of great value under these circumstances. However, this material should be used sparingly to ensure that the maximum amount of dentine remains exposed for bonding to the GIC.

In general, if there is any doubt about the thickness of the remaining dentine, it is advisable to line the cavity of freshly prepared dentine with calcium hydroxide. For sclerotic dentine, it is not usually necessary to use a calcium hydroxide cavity base, but the use of citric or phosphoric acid should be avoided.

Dispensing, mixing and insertion

For the powder–liquid systems, great care must be exercised to ensure that the correct amount of powder is mixed with the liquid. It is important that the manufacturer's instructions are carefully followed.

Tapping the bottle prior to use will ensure that the powder is not compacted. Any excess powder should be scraped off with a spatula and not against the side of the bottle. The powder should be spatulated quickly into the liquid in no more than two increments. The maximum mixing time is 20 seconds. The incorporation of a large amount of powder initially should be avoided, as this will appear to give a satisfactorily thick mix, even though the powder-to-liquid ratio may be too low.

In the case of the preproportioned capsules, the capsule should be shaken before activation. The mixing should be carried out in a high-speed amalgamator, typically operating at around 4000 rpm, for a period of 10 seconds. The whole process of activation, mixing and application should be carried out without any delays.

Contamination of the filling materials with saliva should be avoided during insertion, setting and finishing. The cavity and surrounding area should be dry, although excessive desiccation must not occur.

Finishing and polishing

After the material has been allowed to set for the required time, the matrix can be removed and the restoration should be protected immediately from contamination or dehydration, by placing a waterproof varnish. The best surface finish is achieved at this stage, and the removal of excess material will be detrimental to the finish. However, it is virtually impossible to place a GIC without having to do some trimming and polishing.

Gross excess may be trimmed with a sharp blade. As the material is still fairly weak and the bond to the tooth tissues tenuous, the trimming process should be performed from the restoration towards the tooth and not the other way round. It has been shown that the use of hand instruments for carving can damage the marginal integrity of the restoration. In fact, one manufacturer specifically recommends that hand instruments are not used.

It has been suggested that, after the initial set, finishing may be performed with rotary instruments such as a white stone or with flexible discs lubricated with a grease such as Vaseline or petroleum jelly. The use of a water spray at this stage is not recommended since the material is still highly soluble. Final finishing should not be attempted and is best left till a later visit by the patient, preferably within 24 hours.

A number of studies have shown that, if finishing is carried out after only 8 minutes, the resultant surface finish is very poor when using either abrasive discs, impregnated rubber wheels, tungsten carbide blanks or white stones, even in the presence of petroleum jelly. This situation may change with the more recent rapid-setting materials, but so far the early finishing of GICs is contraindicated.

After 24 hours, the material is set sufficiently for final finishing to be carried out using either a fine diamond or a 12-bladed tungsten carbide bur. This should be carried out in the presence of a copious supply of water to avoid dehydration, and is now possible as the early susceptibility to dissolution in water has subsided. Final polishing can be performed with the range of abrasive discs, again in the presence of water.

Whichever method is used, it is not possible to obtain a smooth surface finish for a GIC. This is due to the large particle size of the glass used in the production of these cements.

Surface protection

The use of a varnish is extremely important. Solutions of natural (Copal) and synthetic resins (cellulose acetate), dissolved in an organic solvent such as ether, acetone or chloroform, are generally recommended. Polyurethane varnishes, which polymerize on contact with water and nitro-cellulose (nail varnish), are a less permeable and less soluble alternative.

The light-activated enamel-bonding resins or dentine-bonding agents that are supplied with the composites provide a particularly effective seal and last sufficiently long to offer the necessary protection. The disadvantage with their use is that a small ledge may be left, especially at the gingival margin, which has to be dealt with at a later stage. Also, they suffer from an oxygen-inhibited set, so that the surface layer remains tacky. However, if only a thin layer is applied, it is removed too readily. The problem can be overcome by the use of a matrix strip but this is very cumbersome to use. Further finishing should be carried out within 24 hours.

The use of greases or gels such as Vaseline offers little protection, as these are rapidly removed by the action of the lips and the tongue.

Glass–ionomer restorations that have been in place for some time still need to be protected from dehydration during any prolonged isolation of the dentition when carrying out other restorative procedures. This is especially the case when using rubber dam, when dehydration of the cement can be very pronounced and the resultant shrinkage can lead to fracture of the restoration. Thus, all known or suspected GIC restorations, crowns, inlay margins and cermets should be protected with a layer of varnish.

Clinical performance

The primary applications of the GICs have always been as a filling material for the treatment of abrasion and erosion lesions, and as a luting agent for crowns, bridges and inlays. With the advent of newer and better materials, their use is being extended to include class III restorations, occlusal restorations (particularly in deciduous teeth), a core material, and a dentine adhesive lining cement under composite restorations.

Most of the interest in the clinical evaluation of GICs has centred around their use as restorative filling materials. Their ease of placement in bulk, their adhesive qualities and their fluoride protection are seen as important advantages over the aesthetically more pleasing composites.

Whilst there have been quite a few publications on the clinical performance of GICs for class III and class V restorations, it would be difficult, if not impossible, to draw many conclusions from the data. A compilation of results for the performance of class V restorations is given in Figure 2.3.12.

In many of the studies undertaken, there was little appreciation of the exacting requirements of the early materials in terms of powder-to-liquid ratio or the need for protection during the long setting period. Thus, high failure rates reported in these studies may have been a consequence of using techniques inappropriate or inadequate for these particular materials.

More recent studies have reported a consistently high retention rate for GIC restorations where there is primarily reliance on their adhesion to enamel and dentine, confirming the tenacious bond that is formed between a GIC and tooth tissues.

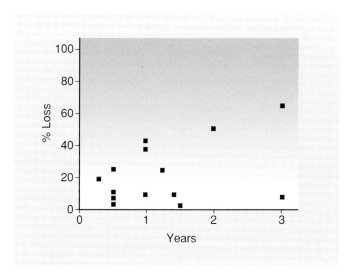

Figure 2.3.12 A compilation of survival data for class V restorations restored with ASPA cement taken from publication during the period 1977–1983

Table 2.3.5 Some commercial examples of the new high-viscosity GICs

Product	Manufacturer
CHEMFLEX	Dentsply, Weybridge, UK
Fuji IX	GC UK Ltd, Newport Pagnell, UK
HI-FI	Shofu, Tonbridge, UK
KETAC-MOLAR	ESPE UK Ltd, Knutsford, UK

CLINICAL SIGNIFICANCE

With regard to clinical retention rates of class V adhesive restorations, the GICs have shown a consistently durable bond to tooth tissues.

Although not recommended for class II restorations for adults, GICs have been used with some success in deciduous posterior teeth. Minimal cavity preparation is required, and the marginal seal and the release of fluoride compensate to some degree for the limited lifespan of such restorations, which is acceptable when used to fill a short-term need. Very promising results are being obtained in the primary dentition with the new high-viscosity GICs, sometimes also referred to as condensable GICs. The higher viscosity has been attributed to the addition of polyacrylic acid to the powder and a reduced grain size (~3 μm). One of the main attractions of these materials is their amalgam-like handling characteristics. Although their strength properties are little changed from those of the conventional GICs, their abrasion resistance does appear to be superior to that of the conventional GICs, which has been attributed to the reduced particle size of the glass. Some commercial examples of these materials are shown in Table 2.3.5.

SILVER CERMETS

By its nature, glass is extremely brittle, and tends to fracture relatively easily compared to metals. The idea behind the silver cermets is that the incorporation of silver in the glass will increase the toughness of the resultant material by acting as a stress absorber and will improve wear characteristics. This has been attributed both to the increase in toughness of the material and to the very low coefficient of friction of the surface, with the silver imparting a polished metallic finish.

In terms of the other properties of the material, such as compressive strength, flexural strength and solubility, the silver cermets seem no better than the GICs.

Naturally, the silver cermets have the ability to bond to enamel and dentine to the same degree as the GICs. As with the GICs, it is recommended that a surface conditioner such as polyacrylic acid is applied to the dentine before placing the cement.

Composition and presentation

The silver cermets are available either as a powder–liquid composition, presented in two separate bottles which have to be mixed by hand, or are dispensed in a preproportioned capsule which has to be placed in a high-speed amalgamator. In some formulations, the powder is presented as a simple mixture of glass and silver, whereas in others the silver is incorporated in the glass powder.

The latter is produced from a mixture of glass and silver of equal volumes (17.5/82.5 wt %). The particle size of the silver is approximately 3–4 μm. The mixture is formed into pellets and then sintered at 800°C until the glass and the silver fuse together and form an intimate mixture. The sintered solid substance is then ground to produce the right particle size for mixing and manipulation. The particles are rounded by the grinding process, which aids mixing with the polyacid.

Thus, each particle consists of a mixture of glass and silver particles tightly bonded to each other by the sintering process. In addition, approximately 5% Ti_2O is added to improve the aesthetics by acting as a whitening agent. The liquid consists of an aqueous solution of a copolymer of acrylic and/or maleic acid (37%) and tartaric acid (9%).

The wear resistance of the silver cermets is adequate for small class I cavities, but anything bigger should be treated with caution. Unpublished information would suggest that the cermets do not stand up to the wear in large multiple surface restorations. Thus, its use is very much limited to the treatment of the early carious lesion. Because of the large amount of silver in the powder particles, the final restoration is sufficiently radiopaque to allow ready detection of recurrent caries.

As with the GICs, the release of fluoride also occurs with the cermets, which should provide protection to the enamel adjacent to the restoration. However, there is evidence to suggest that the fluoride release from silver cermets is not as high as that for GICs and that these materials do not provide the same degree of protection from caries as do the GICs. The silver cermets have not lived up to expectations, especially as an occlusal restorative in the deciduous dentition. Their performance has been such that their continued use is highly questionable, especially in light of the continuing improvements made to the conventional GICs and the introduction of the resin-modified GICs, and they have disappeared from the commercial dental materials market.

CLINICAL SIGNIFICANCE

The clinical performance of silver cermets has been such that their continued use is contraindicated.

RESIN-MODIFIED GLASS–IONOMER CEMENTS

Some of the major disadvantages of GICs are:

* short working time and long setting time
* low strength and low toughness
* cracking on desiccation
* poor resistance to acid attack.

With the advent of the light-activated resin composites, dental practitioners have complained that the handling characteristics of the GICs are far from ideal. Yet, the material continues to be used because of its fluoride release and adhesive properties. The manufacturers have sought to improve the handling properties of GICs by incorporating a resin, which will polymerize under the action of a blue-light curing unit. These are the materials known as resin-modified GICs. Although sometimes also referred to as hybrid GICs or light-curing GICs, such terms should be discouraged as they are insufficiently specific and can be confused with some of the compomer materials.

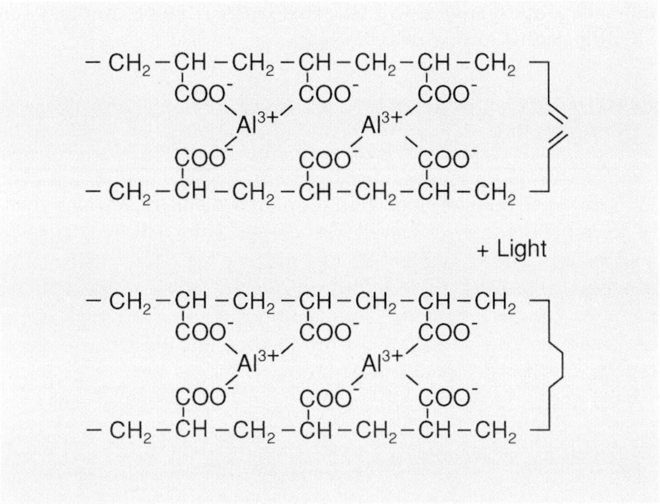

Figure 2.3.13 Combined light-activated cross-linking and hardening during the setting process for a resin-modified GIC

Table 2.3.6 Relative properties of a glass–ionomer cement (GIC) and a resin-modified glass–ionomer cement (RMGIC)

Property	GIC	RMGIC
Working time	2 min	3 min 45 s
Setting time	4 min	20 s
Compressive strength	202 MPa	242 MPa
Diametral tensile strength	16 MPa	37 MPa
Shear bond strength to bovine enamel	4.6 MPa	11.3 MPa
Shear bond strength to bovine dentine	4.3 MPa	8.2 MPa

Composition

The material is presented either as a powder–liquid system, with the powder consisting of a radiopaque fluoroaluminosilicate glass and a photoactive liquid kept in a dark bottle (to protect it from ambient light) or in capsule form. The liquid composition varies from product to product, but in general it is an aqueous solution of hydrophilic monomers, e.g. hydroxyethyl methacrylate (HEMA), polyacrylic acid or a copolymer of polyacrylic acid with some pendant methacryloxy groups and a photoinitiator. The choice of resin is limited by the fact that GICs are water-based materials and so the resin needs to be water-soluble. HEMA is a very effective hydrophilic monomer in this respect, as it readily dissolves in water.

Setting reaction

The acid–base setting reaction is essentially the same as for the GICs, and is initiated when the powder and liquid are mixed. The material differs from other GICs in that this reaction is much slower, giving a considerably longer working time.

The rapid set is provided by the light activation mechanism, causing polymerization of the HEMA and, for the copolymer-containing materials, additional cross-linking through the pendant methacrylate groups, as shown in Figure 2.3.13. Once mixed, the material can be made to set hard after just 30 seconds of exposure to light. If not exposed to the light, the material will eventually set in some 15–20 minutes. It should be appreciated that the light-activated curing reaction precedes the formation of the aluminium salt bridges. Hence these materials will continue to set via the acid–base reaction for some time after the polymerization process has been completed.

Some systems are also known to contain a redox reaction curing process, providing an activator and an initiator, in one case using micro-encapsulation technology. This has the advantage that, if the light from the curing unit is not able to penetrate to the full depth of the restoration, the redox reaction will ensure full depth of cure of the resin component. This means that incremental placement of the RMGIC is not necessary for the redox-reaction-containing systems. One disadvantage with this system is that it cannot be provided in encapsulated form, as the shear stresses during capsule mixing, as distinct from hand mixing, are insufficient to break the glass microspheres.

As a note of caution, it is important to remember that one may also inherit some of the problems associated with light-cured composites, such as limited depth of cure, which requires incremental packing, and polymerization shrinkage, which may compromise the bond to the tooth.

Properties

The addition of resin chemistry to the GICs has significantly improved many of the properties. Using this approach, the advantages of GICs, such as the ability to bond to dentine and enamel and to release fluoride, are combined with a prolonged working time and a rapid set, once irradiated with visible light. The restoration can also be polished immediately.

Their strength and their resistance to desiccation and acid attack are believed to be much improved. The bond to enamel and dentine is as good as, if not superior, to that of the GICs, since the resin component imparts additional tensile strength to the set cement. A typical example of the differences in properties between a GIC and RMGIC from one and the same manufacturer is shown in Table 2.3.6.

One potential drawback with the incorporation of HEMA in these systems is that HEMA has been reported to be cytotoxic when it comes into contact with dental pulp tissues and osteoblasts. Thus it is very important that the necessary procedures are followed that will ensure that all the HEMA will have polymerized.

Applications

The resin-modified GICs have been designed specifically as direct restorative materials or as bases or liners for use under composites, amalgams and ceramic restorations. When used in conjunction with composites, a strong bond is obtained between the liner and the composite and there is no need to etch the surface of the resin-modified GIC.

These materials have become very popular, and have the potential to replace GIC restorative materials and many types of cavity bases and liners. Whether or not they are superior to and will replace the GICs, only time will tell. However, early indications are that these materials are more popular than GICs for liners. RMGICs also perform better than the traditional GICs as posterior restorative materials in the deciduous dentition and are comparable to the new condensable GICs. Some of the latest restorative materials are listed in Table 2.3.7.

There are significant differences in the composition and properties of these materials. The RMGICs behave quite differently from one another, depending on the amount and type of resin element incorporated and the curing mechanisms employed. Thus, each product will have handling properties that are best suited to only a selection of dental practitioners.

Table 2.3.7 Some of the latest restorative RMGICs

Product	Manufacturer
FUJI-II-LC Improved	GC UK Ltd, Newport Pagnell, UK
VITREMER	3M/ESPE, Loughborough, UK
PHOTAC-FIL QUICK	3M/ESPE, Loughborough, UK
RESTORE-PF VLC	First Scientific Ltd, Abertillery, UK

Nano-ionomers

There has recently been interest in the development of 'nano-ionomer cements', via the incorporation of nanoscale fillers in RMGICs, although the commercial availability of these materials is much less than nanofilled composite materials. A product has recently been launched by 3M ESPE, called Ketac Nano; it contains the same silica and zirconia nanoparticles and nanoclusters as used in the company's nanocomposite material. Data are, as yet, sparse on this new development in GICs, and although claims have been made for an improved wear resistance and increased fluoride release in the laboratory, only time and clinical studies will tell what benefits nanotechnology can offer the dentist in this area.

SUMMARY

GICs have had a major impact on restorative dentistry. A wide variety of formulations are now available, designed for a broad range of applications. The new RMGICs have produced materials with superior properties. However, these improvements are as yet insufficient for them to compete with the resin composites in such high-stress-bearing situations as incisal tip restorations and posterior occlusal restorations in the permanent dentition.

CLINICAL SIGNIFICANCE

GICs have improved immensely compared to the original ASPA cements. GICs have shown themselves to be efficacious dental restorative materials and are still evolving dental materials, as shown by the recent introduction of condensable GICs and RMGICs, which suggests that more improvements can be expected.

FURTHER READING

Billington RW, Williams JA, Pearson GJ (1990) Variation in powder/liquid ratio of a restorative glass–ionomer cement used in dental practice. Br Dent J **169**: 164

Chen H, Banaszak Holl M, Orr BG et al (2003) Interaction of dendrimers (artificial proteins) with biological hydroxyapatite crystals. J Dent Res **82**: 443

Espelid I, Tveit AB, Tornes KH, Alvheim H (1999) Clinical behaviour of glass ionomer restorations in primary teeth. J Dent **27**: 437

Inoue S, Van Meerbeek B, Abe Y et al (2001) Effect of remaining dentin thickness and the use of conditioner on micro-tensile bond strength of a glass–ionomer adhesive. Dent Mater **17(5)**: 445–455

Kilpatrick NM, Murray JJ, McCabe JF (1995) The use of a reinforced glass–ionomer cermet for the restoration of primary molars: a clinical trial. Br Dent J **179**: 175

Nicholson JW, Czarnecka B, Limanowska-Shaw H (2003) The interaction of glass–ionomer cements containing vinylphosphonic acid with water and aqueous lactic acid. J Oral Rehabil **30(2)**: 160–164

Peumans M, Kanumilli P, De Munck J et al (2005) Clinical effectiveness of contemporary adhesives: a systematic review of current clinical trials. Dent Mater **21**: 864

Qvist V, Manschert E, Teglers PT (2004) Resin-modified and conventional glass ionomer restorations in primary teeth: 8-year results. J Dent **32**: 285

Smales RJ, Ng KK (2004) Longevity of a resin-modified glass ionomer cement and a polyacid-modified resin composite restoring non-carious cervical lesions in a general dental practice. Aust Dent J **49**: 196

Wilson AD, Kent BE (1972) A new translucent cement for dentistry. Brit Dent J **132**: 133–135

Intermediate restorative materials

INTRODUCTION

A wide variety of direct restorative materials (e.g. amalgams, composite resins, glass–ionomer cements and resin-modified glass–ionomer cements) are placed in dentine in close proximity to the pulp.

Since the presence of a restoration may have an adverse effect on the pulp, a range of materials, termed *intermediate restorative materials* (IRMs), has been developed to be applied to the dentine prior to the placement of the restorative material. These materials include cavity varnishes, bases and liners, and, as they are intended to remain in place permanently, these materials should not be confused with temporary restorative materials.

The distinction between cavity bases and liners is that the former consist of a thick mix of material that is placed in bulk in the cavity, while the latter is only applied as a thin coating over the exposed dentine. A definition of a *cavity liner* is a dentine sealer that is less than 0.5 mm thick and is able to promote the health of the pulp by adhesion to the tooth structure or by antibacterial action. In contrast, a *base* is a dentine replacement used to minimize the bulk of the restorative or block out undercuts.

Their role may be protective, palliative or therapeutic when they are applied to vital dentine. The choice of a cavity varnish, base or liner requires an appreciation of the need for pulpal protection, and how the agents may interact with the restorative material chosen for a particular clinical situation.

PULPAL PROTECTION

In order to make the correct choice of which intermediate restorative material to use for a particular restorative procedure, it is important to understand the nature and mechanisms by which adverse factors affect the pulp. Three possible sources of pulpal irritation have been identified:

- thermal stimuli
- chemical stimuli
- bacteria and endotoxins.

The importance of the first two factors has been well recognized for some time, but more recently it has been shown that the latter factor is probably the most important in producing pulpal irritation.

Thermal stimuli

In the intact tooth, temperature changes are conducted through the enamel and dentine to the pulp. Here, nociceptive afferent fibres may be thermally stimulated, eliciting a painful response. Such a direct thermal stimulus of the pulp is, however, unlikely except when cutting a cavity or direct heat is generated due to an exothermic reaction on the part of the restorative material when in close proximity to the pulp. When dentinal tubules are exposed, it is possible for fluid to flow into and out of the tubules, commonly referred to as the hydrodynamic effect. This is the process responsible for exposed root surface sensitivity and is readily dealt with by sealing the root surface. The hydrodynamic effect is almost certainly also responsible for the short-latency pain produced by thermal stimulation of some minimal-amalgam restorations. If the dentinal tubules are patent and a small gap has been allowed to form under the amalgam restoration, possibly due to inadequate adaptation to the cavity wall, fluid movement down the tubules can occur because of the opening and closing action of this gap. This can happen as a consequence of the amalgam expanding or contracting when exposed to extremes of temperature or the application of an occlusal load. Thus, the placement of a cavity varnish or thin lining in a cavity is done in order to protect against fluid movement through the dentine, and not to act as a thermal insulator, as was thought at one time.

Chemical stimuli

Many of the dental materials that come into contact with dentine may release compounds that are thought to be toxic to the pulp because of either their organic structure or their pH.

Acrylic resins have been cited as examples of materials that will cause a pulpal reaction when placed without a lining. However, toxicity tests suggest that these materials are well tolerated by the soft tissues. Acrylic resins are extensively used as bone cements in hip replacements without any adverse inflammatory reaction. This would suggest that other factors are responsible for the pulpal reaction associated with these materials.

Until recently, most studies of the pulpal toxicity of restorative materials have not considered the influence of bacterial contamination, which is now believed to play a major role in the production of pulpal inflammation, as considered below. This does *not* mean that we need not worry about chemical toxicity, as the low pH of some materials, such as zinc–phosphate cements and zinc–polycarboxylate cements, may well have an effect on the pulp.

Bacteria and endotoxins

A matter of considerable interest and debate is the effect of *micro-leakage*. This term loosely describes the penetration of oral fluids and small numbers of bacteria and their toxic by-products between the filling material and the cavity walls. This percolation has been shown to be a potential source of pulpal irritancy.

In experiments that use germ-free animals, it has been shown that the pulpal response to some materials is considerably different to that seen in animals with a normal microbiological flora.

For example, zinc–phosphate cements do not show pulpal inflammation (and may even show some dentine bridge formation) when placed on exposed pulps in the absence of bacteria. In contrast, control animals showed severe pulpal inflammation and abscess formation. Other materials do show an inflammatory response, even in the germ-free animals, demonstrating that chemical toxicity may still be an important factor in some instances.

Our increased understanding of the mechanism of pulpal toxicity does not change the fact that some materials will damage the pulp if not separated from the overlying dentine by a suitable lining. However, whereas in the past it was thought that the primary role of an intermediate restorative material was to protect the pulp from the toxic action of restorative materials, this view has had to be modified to take account of the role of bacterial toxins. The use of intermediate restorative materials is now aimed at:

- eliminating the potential for bacterial micro-leakage by the use of adhesive techniques so that no gap exists between the restorative material and the tooth
- presenting an antibacterial barrier to the infiltrating bacteria so as to protect the pulp from their toxins.

The adhesive approach is now so important that it has been dealt with separately in Chapter 2.5; here we will consider only the cavity varnishes, bases and liners. We will first discuss the chemistry of these materials and then consider which may be the most appropriate for various clinical applications.

CLINICAL SIGNIFICANCE

The primary role of a lining material is to protect the pulp by providing a bacterial barrier and preventing fluid movement down the dentinal tubules.

CAVITY VARNISHES, BASES AND LINERS

The main groups of materials that fall into the category of cavity bases and liners are:

- varnishes
- calcium hydroxide cements
- zinc oxide-based cements

- glass–ionomer cements
- resin-modified glass–ionomer cements
- visible-light-cured resins.

Cavity varnishes

Presentation and constituents

Cavity varnishes consist of a clear or yellowish liquid that contains natural resins such as copal, colophony and sandarac, or synthetic resins such as polystyrene. The resins are dissolved in a solvent such as alcohol, ether or acetone, and are applied to the cavity floor with a brush or cotton pledget. The solvent is allowed to evaporate, leaving behind a thin coating of the resin. This process may have to be repeated up to three times to ensure a uniform coating of resin.

Applications

Their main uses are:

- to present a barrier to the penetration of chemicals
- to act as a temporary barrier to the loss of constituents from the surface of a filling material.

Calcium hydroxide cements

Presentation and constituents

This material is supplied as two white or light yellow pastes. One paste consists of a mixture of calcium hydroxide (50%), zinc oxide (10%) and sulphonamide (40%). The other paste consists of butylene glycol disalicylate (40%) with varying amounts of titanium dioxide and calcium sulphate.

Setting process

Equal volumes of the two pastes are mixed together for about 30 seconds; the cement will then set in approximately 2 minutes. The setting process for these materials has not been fully elucidated but is believed to involve a chelating reaction between the zinc oxide and butylene glycol disalicylate.

Properties

These materials have a low compressive strength, typically 20 MPa, but this is sufficient to withstand the condensation pressures of dental amalgam filling materials.

The freshly mixed cement is highly alkaline, with a pH of 11–12. It is believed that this is responsible for an important feature of calcium hydroxide cements: their ability to cause the pulp of the tooth to lay down secondary dentine. When the paste is placed in contact with the pulp, possibly in the presence of a microexposure, it will cause a three-layer necrosis of some 1.5 mm thickness. This eventually develops into a calcified layer.

Once the bridge becomes dentine-like in appearance and the pulp has been isolated from any irritant, hard tissue formation ceases.

Zinc oxide-based cements

The zinc oxide-based cements used in dentistry are powder–liquid systems, with the powders being bases and the liquids being acids. When they are mixed, there is an acid–base reaction with the general formula:

$$\underset{\text{base}}{MO} + \underset{\text{acid}}{H_2A} \rightarrow \underset{\text{salt}}{MA} + \underset{\text{water}}{H_2O}$$

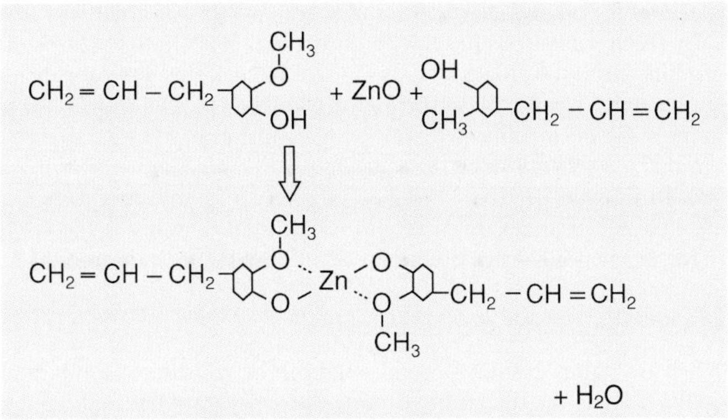

Figure 2.4.1 Chelating reaction of zinc oxide with eugenol to form a zinc eugenolate

In these dental cements there is a surplus of powder, such that the final material consists of unreacted powder particles held together by a salt matrix.

Zinc oxide–eugenol cements

Within the group of zinc oxide–eugenol cements, there are a wide variety of different formulations for different applications.

Unmodified zinc oxide–eugenol

This comes as a white powder which is mainly zinc oxide, but contains up to 10% magnesium oxide that is mixed with a clear liquid, which is eugenol mixed with either olive oil or cotton seed oil. The oils are added to mask the taste of the eugenol and modify the viscosity.

Setting process

The cement is mixed by adding the powder to the liquid in small increments until a thick consistency is obtained; this should take about 1 minute, and the powder-to-liquid ratio is about 3 : 1.

The zinc oxide initially absorbs some eugenol, which is confined to the surface layer of the powder particles and reacts to form an amorphous zinc eugenolate, as shown in Figure 2.4.1. This binds the unreacted portion of the powder together. A trace of water is needed to initiate the reaction, but, once started it is a by-product of the setting reaction. The set material contains both unreacted zinc oxide and eugenol.

The material is available as a slow-setting or a fast-setting cement. The slow-setting cement takes some 24 hours to set hard, with the fast-setting cement taking as little as 5 minutes, although this depends on the nature of the powder, its particle size and the addition of accelerators such as zinc acetate or acetic acid.

Properties

The set cement has a pH of 6.6–8.0, and has little or no effect on the pulp when placed in deep cavities. The presence of free eugenol has an obtundent effect on the pulp, and reduces pain that may be associated with the antibacterial properties of the cement. However, its use is not recommended when there is a suspected pulpal exposure, since it is mildly irritant to the pulp when in direct contact with it.

One of the main failings of zinc oxide–eugenol cements is their high solubility in the oral environment. Eugenol is constantly released and, as it dissolves, the cement gradually disintegrates. It also has poor mechanical properties, with a compressive strength of only 15 MPa. This, combined with the high solubility, makes it unsuitable as a cavity base or liner material. The eugenol is also known to inhibit the set of resins, so eugenol-containing cements can not be used in conjunction with resin-based restorative materials.

Applications

The slow-setting version is most commonly used as a root canal sealing material, with its various modifications being discussed in more detail in Chapter 2.6. The fast-setting version is mainly used in periodontal dressings.

Modified zinc oxide–eugenol

In order to overcome some of the shortcomings of the above cement, modified versions have been introduced. These are aimed at raising the compressive strength and reducing the solubility. These modifications take the form of resins added to the powder and/or the liquid, such as:

- hydrogenated rosin 10%, which is added to the powder
- polystyrene or methyl methacrylate, which is dissolved in the liquid.

Properties and applications

The added resin raises the compressive strength to 40 MPa. This is sufficiently high for the material to be used as a cavity base or liner. The material can also be used as a temporary filling material since it is less soluble in the oral cavity than the unmodified cements.

EBA cement

EBA cement is another modified zinc oxide–eugenol cement, presented as a white powder and a pinkish-coloured liquid. The powder consists of zinc oxide (60–75%), fused quartz or alumina (20–35%) and hydrogenated rosin (6%). The liquid is 37% eugenol and 63% ethoxybenzoic acid (EBA). The EBA encourages the formation of a crystalline structure, which imparts greater strength to the set material.

Properties and applications

With the above additions and modifications, a considerable improvement in the compressive strength (60 MPa) and a reduction in the solubility are achieved. This makes EBA cements suitable for use as liners and temporary filling materials.

Glass–ionomer and resin-modified glass–ionomer lining cements

In recent years, the concept of using glass–ionomer cements (GICs) as a lining under composite restorations has gained widespread acceptance. The glass–ionomer liner is able to bond to the dentine, and the composite can be bonded to the GIC and the etched enamel. The ability to release fluoride is believed to provide added protection to the enamel and dentine that is adjacent to the restoration.

A wide selection of glass–ionomer lining cements is now available. Their chemistry has already been discussed in detail in Chapter 2.3. These materials are all radiopaque, which is especially important when used in the posterior situation. They tend to have shorter working and setting times than the filling versions, which is appropriate to their application as a liner under composites or amalgams, as the rapid set reduces the waiting time before placing the restorative material. A slow set would be a disadvantage, especially in the case of the composite placement technique, which is already quite time-consuming.

It is important to know what quality of bond between the GICs and the composites can be achieved. For those liners that require etching of the glass–ionomer base with phosphoric acid in order to obtain a bond to the composite resin, the etching process should be undertaken for no more than 20 seconds. The best method of etching is to employ a viscous etchant gel in a syringe. This can then be applied carefully to the enamel surfaces for a period of 20 seconds; thereafter the whole surface (including the GIC) is exposed to the etchant for an additional 20 seconds. Excessive exposure of the GIC to etchant will cause crazing of the surface and acid penetration that is impossible to remove on washing; this may develop into pulpal pain or sensitivity. It can also cause extensive fracture and is best avoided. It is preferable to use a low-viscosity resin in order to obtain a good bond between the composite and the GIC.

The practical problems generated by the need for differential etching can be avoided completely by using resin-modified glass–ionomer (RMGIC) liners, which do not require etching in order to achieve a bond to the composite resin. Examples of currently available RMGICs are Vitrebond (3M/ESPE) and Vivaglass Liner (Ivoclar-Vivdent). These liners have the added advantage that they provide a stronger adhesive between the tooth and the composite resin due to their greater cohesive strength compared to the GICs. The RMGIC has become so popular that the use of GIC liners is on the wane.

Visible-light-cured resins

A variety of resin-based cavity bases and liners have appeared on the market, whose role is somewhat obscure. The objective with these materials seems to be to combine the advantages of light activation with some of the therapeutic effects of calcium or fluoride release.

Materials included in this group are Bis-GMA resins containing calcium hydroxide, phosphonated resins containing a fluoride-releasing glass, and Bis-GMA resins containing calcium hydroxide and a fluoride-releasing glass. How these materials differ from light-activated composites (other than in the nature of the filler) is not clear.

Since the fillers are encased in resin, their effect on the surrounding tissues is debatable, although the resins may be sufficiently permeable to allow the release of some fluoride and calcium hydroxide. As yet, these materials have not shown any particular advantage over the many other cavity bases and liners available, and it is unlikely that they will replace them, especially since these have been superseded by the RMGICs and the latest dentine-bonding agents.

CHOICE OF INTERMEDIATE RESTORATIVE MATERIALS

Amalgams

The choice of intermediate restorative material prior to the placement of an amalgam restoration depends on whether the cavity is a minimal-depth, moderate-depth or deep-caries cavity.

Minimal-depth cavities

For minimal-depth caries, the cavity should be prepared only to a depth sufficient to provide adequate bulk of amalgam. Dentine should not be removed unnecessarily (to create space for a lining material), as there is sufficient dentine to act as thermal insulator. Neither should a lining material be placed in the cavity in such bulk that the amalgam will be thin in section, which will make the amalgam prone to gross fracture.

In this situation, the pulp requires protection only from fluid movement down the dentinal tubules arising from occlusal pressure, from thermal expansion of the metal, and from the ingress of bacteria down the dentinal tubules.

The most common method is to apply a thin layer of varnish over the whole of the dentine surface. The varnish effectively seals the dentinal tubules, preventing fluid movement and also reducing the

potential for micro-leakage. Although the varnish will eventually dissolve (being only a few μm thick), the gradual deposition of corrosion products from the amalgam helps to seal the margins and provide an antibacterial barrier. Nevertheless, the kinetics of this process have never really been confirmed and cavity varnishes have been criticized for giving poor insulation, not providing an even film, and having a lack of biological activity, a lack of adhesion, and high solubility. For a well-adapted amalgam restoration with tight margins, it has been suggested that any form of base under the amalgam is unnecessary.

Moderate-depth dentine caries

When the caries extends beyond what can be considered a minimal cavity, there is the possibility of direct thermal stimulus of the pulp; this is especially so in the case of an inflamed pulp as temperature thresholds are reduced.

There is no need to encourage the growth of reparative dentine, as this will have occurred in response to the caries attack. Also, any inflammation will subside if the irritating stimulus (i.e. bacteria and toxins in the caries) is removed. A modified zinc oxide–eugenol cement would be a good choice in such situations, because the eugenol has an obtundant effect on the inflamed pulp and kills off any residual bacteria in the cavity. The thermal insulating properties of these materials are more than adequate. Finally, a cavity varnish is applied, as not all the exposed dentine is necessarily covered by the lining material.

Deep caries

In situations of near-exposure of the pulp, it is generally considered desirable to leave some caries in the floor of the cavity rather than risking an exposure. However, this is not possible if the caries has progressed to the stage where it cannot remineralize. It is possible to distinguish between carious dentine that will remineralize and irreversible dentine caries, as the former is more difficult to remove with hand instruments or can be visualized by using a caries-disclosing solution. Calcium hydroxide cement must first be placed in the deepest parts of such a cavity. This will encourage the formation of reparative dentine and help to remineralize the carious dentine. A thermal insulating base of zinc oxide–eugenol can then be placed over the top, followed by a cavity varnish. However, one problem is that, in due course, oral fluids can penetrate through the interface and start to dissolve the calcium hydroxide cement. The gap that forms will increase the risk of sensitivity and marginal leakage.

Despite all that has been said above, the use of liners under amalgam has become a topic of considerable controversy. As far back as 1980, Osborne suggested that bases and liners under amalgam restorations are unnecessary. Yet, many studies have shown recurrent decay to be one of the most significant contributors to the failure of amalgam restorations. It is possible that the aetiology of recurrent dental decay associated with amalgam restorations has changed over the years. Any such change in the pattern of dental decay could reasonably be expected to occur as a result of better oral hygiene awareness and the greater use of topical fluorides and access to fluoridated water supplies in the last 20 years. Also, it has been reported by Mahler and Marantz that almost no recurrent caries is observed around high-copper-content amalgam restorations. Is it possible that the pattern of decay has also altered because of the improvements in high-copper amalgams compared with the traditional amalgams?

Composites

A fully set composite has little cytotoxicity, and pulpal inflammation under restorations of these materials is due primarily to the leakage of microorganisms and endotoxins. To overcome the problem of micro-leakage, a variety of adhesive techniques have been developed, three of which are in current use:

- acid etching of enamel
- GIC/RMGIC-bonded base
- dentine-bonding agents.

Acid etching the enamel will ensure a good marginal seal and is now routine when placing a composite resin restorative material. In order to avoid postoperative sensitivity, it is important not only to obtain a marginal seal but also that the restoration is bonded to the cavity walls and floor; otherwise there is the possibility of postoperative sensitivity due to the presence of a gap that gives rise to the hydrodynamic effect. This can be overcome by bonding the composite resin to the dentine, either by using a GIC or RMGIC in the so-called sandwich technique or by employing a dentine-bonding agent.

Incisal-tip restorations and fissure sealants

If the restorative procedure involves enamel only, such as for small incisal-tip restorations or fissure sealants, a cavity base or liner is not necessary. The cavity preparation involves only the use of the acid-etch technique, which virtually eliminates any micro-leakage and is described in more detail in Chapter 2.5.

Preventive resin restoration

This is a minimal restoration, where there may be a small amount of exposed dentine. As the margins of this restoration are wholly within enamel, the use of the acid-etch technique will ensure that there is a good marginal seal. Although it might appear that there is no need to protect the dentine surface from the effects of micro-leakage and the composite is an excellent thermal insulator, so that there is no need to worry about thermal stimulus of the pulp, the use of phosphoric acid-etchant on exposed dentine without the subsequent application of a dentine-bonding agent is not recommended. When the protective smear layer that is formed on cut dentine (blocking many of the dentinal tubules) is removed by the acid solution, this reopens the dentinal tubules. The consequence of this is a greatly increased permeability of the dentine and, if the tubules are not resealed, this can give rise to postoperative sensivity problems. It is therefore wise to seal the dentine surface with a dentine-bonding agent. Another option is the use of a GIC or RMGIC lining, the latter generally being the more popular choice because of its command set. With the improvements in dentine-bonding agents, more and more dentists employ this procedure as their preferred method. The combination of enamel bonding with the acid-etch technique and dentine bonding with a dentine-bonding agent should eliminate any possibility of micro-leakage occurring in these minimal restorations. The different types of dentine-bonding agents and their modes of action are dealt with in more detail in the next chapter.

Proximal and occlusal caries lesions

Due to the size of these restorations and the fact that not all of the margins may be confined to enamel, there is an increased likelihood of micro-leakage leading to pulpal inflammation. The provision of a marginal seal becomes much more difficult when the margin goes subgingival and involves root dentine.

Whilst the acid-etch technique for enamel bonding of composites is very effective, the same cannot be said for dentine-bonding procedures. Thus, it would be unwise to rely solely on the adhesive bond of dentine-bonding agents to provide a hermetic seal around all of the margins of the restoration. In fact, it has to be assumed that micro-leakage *will* occur and is unavoidable. Calcium hydroxide is the best lining material to use in such situations. However, it should be used sparingly so that only a small amount of dentine is covered, leaving more available for bonding. Glass–ionomer lining materials present a problem, as they may produce a mild pulpal inflammation in freshly cut cavities. A more popular option in recent years has been the use of a resin-modified, glass–ionomer liner cement.

Although the adhesive bond to dentine limits micro-leakage, bacteria have been found in voids beneath the material. These bacteria are not affected by the material, as it has little or no antibacterial action. It is therefore prudent to protect any areas close to the pulp with a calcium hydroxide cement prior to the placement of the glass–ionomer liner and the composite restorative material.

Abrasion/erosion lesions

Since this type of lesion involves a large expanse of dentine, the composite resin needs to be bonded to the dentine via a dentine-bonding agent or a GIC liner. When a glass–ionomer liner is applied to dentine that has been exposed for some time (as in abrasion lesions), the secondary dentine that is laid down seems to protect the pulp. In this situation, GIC can be applied directly to the dentine and then overlaid with composite resin in the sandwich technique. Until recently, this appeared to be a more effective means of bonding composite resin to dentine than the use of a dentine-bonding agent. It should be noted, however, that there have been rapid improvements in dentine-bonding agents and the quality of the adhesion, as indicated by retention rates of three-stage dentine-bonding agents, is beginning to match that of GICs.

Glass–ionomer cements and resin-modified glass–ionomer cements

The same arguments as outlined above for GIC and RMGIC lining materials apply to the filling materials. A liner is not generally required, except in cases where the cavity is very deep and there may be the possibility of micro-exposures of the pulp, in which case a calcium hydroxide cement may be indicated (see Chapter 2.6).

FURTHER READING

Baratieri LN, Machado A, Van Noort R et al (2002) Effect of pulp protection technique on the clinical performance of amalgam restorations: three-year results. Oper Dent **27**: 319

Fisher FJ, McCabe JF (1978) Calcium hydroxide base materials: an investigation into the relationship between chemical structure and antibacterial properties. Brit Dent J **144**: 341

Gordan VV, Mjor IA, Hucke RD, Smith GE (1999) Effect of different liner treatments on postoperative sensitivity of amalgam restorations. Quintessence Int **30**: 55

Hilton TJ (1996) Cavity sealers, liners and bases: Current philosophies and indications for use. Oper Dent **21**: 4

Mahler DB, Marantz RL (1980) Clinical assessments of dental amalgam restorations. Int Dent J **30**: 327

Øilo G (1984) Early erosion of dental cements. Scand J Dent Res **92**: 539

Osborne JW (1980) Dental amalgam: Clinical behaviour up to eight years. Oper Dent **5**: 9

Peumans M, Kanumilli P, De Munck J et al (2005) Clinical effectiveness of contemporary adhesives: a systematic review of current clinical trials. Dent Mater **21**: 864

Smith DC (1971) Dental cements. Dent Clin N Am **15**: 3

Wilson AD (1978) The chemistry of dental cements. Chem Soc Revs **7**: 265

Chapter |2.5|

Enamel and dentine bonding

INTRODUCTION

The development of an adhesive approach to restorative dentistry has brought many advantages, such as:

- better aesthetics
- conservation of tooth tissue
- reinforcement of weakened tooth structure
- reduced marginal leakage
- reduced potential for pulpal sensitivity
- a wider range of techniques.

A wide variety of adhesive systems have been introduced in recent years, many of which have not survived the test of time. Such adhesives were unable to satisfy the stringent requirements that are placed on a dental adhesive.

A dental adhesive should:

- provide a high bond strength to enamel and dentine
- provide an immediate and durable bond
- prevent the ingress of bacteria
- be safe to use
- be simple to use.

The bonding systems that have survived the test of time include:

- the acid-etch technique for bonding resins to enamel, now extensively used in the placement of anterior and posterior composite resins and compomers, resin-bonded bridges, veneers and orthodontic brackets
- the glass–ionomer cements (GICs) and resin-modified glass–ionomer cements (RMGICs), with their abilities to bond to both enamel and dentine as direct adhesive restorations, to act as dentine-bonded bases under composite restorative materials and as luting cements for indirect restorations.

By comparison, the dentine-bonding agents have had a turbulent history. Many have come and gone, but at each stage of their development there has been an encouraging improvement. Perhaps some of the dentine-bonding agents now being marketed will survive the test of time.

Why some materials and techniques should have survived and others waned is due to the requirement that the adhesive needs to be able to bond to a variety of materials (e.g. composites, metals, ceramics) and to two very different substrates: namely, enamel and dentine.

The principles of adhesion have already been discussed in Chapter 1.9 and the adhesive aspects of GICs have already been dealt with in Chapter 2.3. Hence, in this chapter, the methods of bonding composites and resins to enamel and dentine with dentine-bonding agents only will be considered.

ENAMEL BONDING

Structure of enamel

Enamel is the most densely calcified tissue of the human body, and is unique in the sense that it is formed extracellularly.

It is a heterogeneous structure, with mature human enamel consisting of 96% mineral, 1% organic material and 3% water by weight (Table 2.5.1). The mineral phase is made up of millions of tiny crystals of hydroxyapatite, $Ca_{10}(PO_4)_6(OH)_2$, which packed tightly together in the form of prisms, held together by an organic matrix. Due to ionic substitution (e.g. fluoride), the enamel apatite does not have the calcium-to-phosphate ratio of theoretically pure hydroxyapatite (1.6:1) and is usually in the ratio 2:1 by weight.

The prisms are long, rod-like shapes of approximately 5 μm in diameter, having a distinctive keyhole cross-section with a head and a tail. The prisms are aligned perpendicular to the tooth surface, as shown in Figure 2.5.1.

The crystals of hydroxyapatite are flattened hexagonals, as shown in Figure 2.5.2, and, because of their structure, it is not possible to obtain a perfect packing. The spaces left between the crystals are occupied by water and organic material. Much of the water is tightly bound within the enamel structure and not easily removed on drying. The surface layer of enamel tends to have a higher organic content than the deeper layers, and is protected by a layer of pellicle, which is about 1 μm thick.

Table 2.5.1 Typical composition of enamel and dentine

	Enamel		Dentine	
	Wt %	Vol %	Wt %	Vol %
Organic	1	2	2	30
Inorganic	95	86	70	45
Water	4	12	10	25

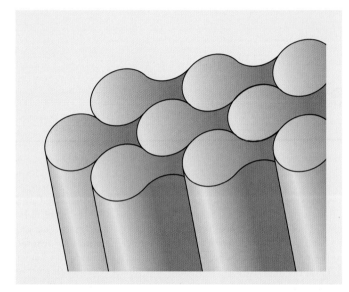

Figure 2.5.1 The prismatic structure of enamel

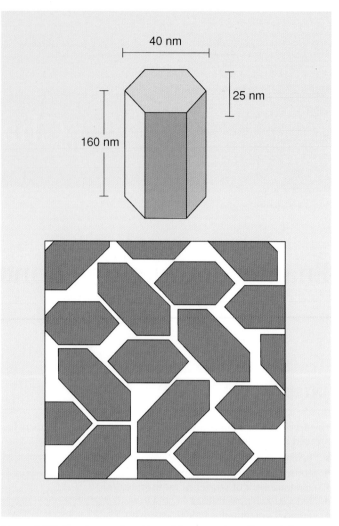

Figure 2.5.2 Structure and packing of the enamel apatite crystals

Acid-etch technique

Due to its composite structure, the surface of enamel can be modified by the application of acid primers. The importance and potential exploitation of this were first appreciated by Buonocore in 1955, when he found that he could make the surface of enamel more amenable to adhesive techniques by modifying it with the application of a solution of phosphoric acid. Thence, the acid-etch technique for the bonding of composite restorative materials to enamel was developed. Its main effect is that of increasing the surface roughness of the enamel at the microscopic level (Figure 2.5.3) and raising the surface energy, which improves wettability (see below).

A major shortcoming of composites is that they have no intrinsic adhesive qualities to tooth tissues, as the resins are essentially non-polar. The acid-etch modification of the enamel surface allows the formation of an intimate micro-mechanical bond between enamel and the resin component of the composite, as long as there is close adaptation at the molecular level.

This discovery has allowed the introduction of a wide variety of restorative techniques that were not previously possible, such as fissure sealants, directly bonded orthodontic brackets, resin-bonded bridges and laminate veneers. Many studies have contributed to our understanding of the relationship between etched enamel and resins, such that now the acid-etch technique forms an integral part of restorative procedures using composites.

As mentioned, the application of a strongly acidic solution (such as phosphoric acid) to enamel has the effect of modifying the surface characteristics. It does this in two important ways.

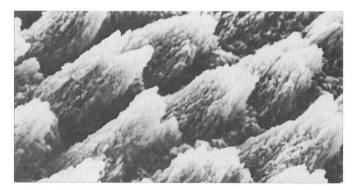

Figure 2.5.3 Scanning electron micrograph (SEM) of the enamel surface after etching for 40 seconds with 35% phosphoric acid solution

1. The etching process increases the surface roughness of the enamel. When the phosphoric acid is applied to the enamel surface, an acid–base reaction is initiated, which causes the hydroxyapatite to go into solution and different topical features can develop. These include a predominant loss of enamel prism periphery, as shown in Figure 2.5.3, a predominant loss of prism core constituents, and a pattern in which there is no specific evidence of a prism structure. These etch patterns are

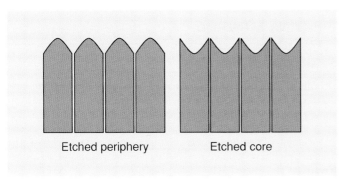

Etched periphery   Etched core

Figure 2.5.4 The effect of phosphoric acid on enamel in removing prism periphery or core

shown schematically in Figure 2.5.4. The overall effect is that of increasing the surface roughness and, hence, the bonding area. It is possible to bond to this surface by a process of micro-mechanical interlocking. The increased surface roughness provides the added advantage that the surface area for bonding by chemical means, be it only through secondary bonding, is much enhanced.

2. The acid has the effect of raising the surface energy of the enamel by removing surface contaminants. This provides for a better wettability of the enamel by the adhesive (see Chapter 1.9). Typically, the surface tension of an adhesive resin is in the range of 34–38 mJ·m^{-2}. Untreated enamel has a surface energy lower than this, and thus the conditions for perfect wetting to take place are not complied with. Normally, the surface of enamel is covered with a layer of pellicle, which has an extremely low surface energy (28 mJ·m^{-2}). This layer is removed by the acid and exposes the underlying surface of the enamel with its high surface energy and thus high reactivity (42 mJ·m^{-2}). The resin will adapt well to this high surface energy, as long as it is thoroughly dry. The micro-mechanical interlocking will ensure that the resin will not separate from the enamel. Thus, the acid-etch bond to enamel is essentially mechanical in nature.

Clinical procedure

The features of increased surface roughness and raised resin wettability using the acid etching of the enamel surface combine to offer the opportunity for an excellent bond between a composite and the enamel. However, as with any seemingly simple technique, mistakes are easily made unless the operator adheres strictly to the rules for achieving a bond. The various stages of the acid-etch technique can be identified as follows:

- patient selection
- enamel prophylaxis
- application of the etchant.

Patient selection

The first rule of achieving a good adhesive bond is that the surfaces to be bonded to must be kept free of contaminants. If the surface becomes contaminated with water or saliva, a good bond between the composite and enamel will not be obtained. The highly polar nature of the surface contaminants will prevent the non-polar resin from closely adapting to the enamel surface.

The best approach to the prevention of contamination of the surface of the enamel is to use rubber dam. This may not always be possible,

and in those cases where rubber dam cannot be used, it is inadvisable to adopt an adhesive approach.

Appropriate patient selection can avoid these problems. In particular, the use of the enamel acid-etch technique should not be used in patients with mental health issues, children and very elderly or frail patients.

CLINICAL SIGNIFICANCE

The acid-etch technique should not be attempted with patients for whom the procedure is too time-consuming.

Enamel prophylaxis

As with any other adhesive joint, it is important that the surface of the substrate is thoroughly cleaned. The surface of enamel is covered with a layer of pellicle and possibly a layer of plaque as well. Such layers need to be removed before the etching process.

Whereas a thin layer of pellicle may be stripped off by the acid, it is not possible to remove thick deposits of plaque in this way. If this cleaning is not done, the resin will effectively bond to the surface contaminants and not the enamel. Cleaning of the enamel surface is best performed with a slurry of pumice and water, applied with a bristle brush for some 30 seconds. It is best to avoid proprietary brands of prophylactic pastes, as these may contain components such as oils which are left behind on the enamel surface. These will have the effect of reducing the wettability of the enamel surface by the resin.

Once the surface has been cleaned, it should be thoroughly washed and dried to remove all the debris.

Application of the etchant

Considerable research has been undertaken to evaluate the best method of etching the surface of enamel.

With the teeth dried and properly isolated from the saliva, the aqueous solution of phosphoric acid-etchant can be applied to the enamel with a cotton pledget. An interesting and important observation is that there is an inverse relationship between the etching efficiency and the concentration of the phosphoric acid. High concentrations of phosphoric acid are not as effective at producing the ideal etch pattern as low concentrations. The optimum concentration appears to be in the range of 30–50%. Excessively high concentrations of phosphoric acid tend to show minimal change of the enamel surface, possibly because the low pH causes a rapid saturation of the solution with the reaction by-products, slowing down the rate of dissolution. Hence, the use of phosphoric acid solutions supplied with zinc–phosphate cements should not be used, as the concentration is too high (approximate acid concentration 65%).

It is important that the surface of the enamel is not rubbed during the etching process, as the enamel prisms that stick up from the surface are extremely friable and will break under even the slightest load. A rubbing action will have the effect of breaking all of these prisms, and the crevices and cracks for resin tag formation will be lost.

It is also important that all of the phosphoric acid and the reaction products produced during the etching process are removed. Too often this is dealt with in a cursory and dismissive manner. The procedure to adopt is to wash the enamel surface with copious amounts of water, and to follow this with a water–air spray for no less than 20 seconds. If cotton rolls are used to isolate the teeth, these will have to be replaced in order to ensure a dry field.

The drying process is equally critical, as the objective is to achieve a perfectly dry enamel surface.

The removal of surface hydroxyl groups in the drying procedure will enhance the wettability of the resin on the surface and allow it to flow readily over the surface and into all the little cracks and crevices generated by the etching process. It is important to ensure that the air-hose that is used for drying is free of any contaminants such as oils and water. The etched and dried enamel should have the appearance of a dull, white, slightly frosted surface finish.

Application of unfilled resins

When the resin is applied to a dry and well-etched enamel surface, it will readily invade all the surface irregularities and form resin tags that penetrate the enamel to a depth of up to 30 μm. This produces a very effective bond, by the mechanism of micro-mechanical interlocking.

Although opinions are divided, it is recommended, on balance, that a low-viscosity resin (i.e. either an unfilled Bis-GMA resin or one of the many dentine adhesive resins) is applied to the enamel surface prior to placement of the composite. The rationale for the use of such an intermediate bonding resin is that the low viscosity of the bonding agent facilitates a better penetration into the microscopic spaces in the etched enamel than would be achieved by the direct placement of the composite.

The wettability of the resin composite is as good as that of low-viscosity resin, but the high viscosity of the composite prevents it from spreading easily over the surface of the enamel. Also, the viscosity of the composite is sufficiently high that it can actually bridge across the recesses in the enamel and cause entrapment of air. This has the dual effect of creating a zone of inhibition of the cure of the resin and an interfacial defect, which may be the source of subsequent bond breakdown.

Bond strength

If the above procedure is carried out with diligence, an extremely effective bond between the enamel and the composite is created. In those situations where failure of the adhesive bond has occurred, it can usually be ascribed to poor clinical technique.

Clinically, bonding to enamel should not present a problem. The intimate micro-mechanical interlocking between the etched enamel and the resin will be such that it should be impossible to separate the resin from the enamel without causing the resin or the enamel to fracture. However, this does not mean that failure of enamel bonded restorations will not occur, since cohesive failure of the adhesive or the restoration can still take place. Equally, metallic or ceramic restorations can fail adhesively due to a lack of bonding between the resin and these restorative materials. When a bond failure occurs, it is very important to establish where the fracture has arisen, as this will tell you which component represented the weakest link in the bonding system.

DENTINE BONDING

Structure of dentine

Dentine is composed of approximately 70% inorganic material, 20% organic material and 10% water by weight (see Table 2.5.1). The inorganic material is mainly hydroxyapatite and the organic material is predominantly collagen. A characteristic feature of dentine is the arrangement of dentinal tubules that traverse its entire thickness. The presence of these tubules makes the dentine permeable to drugs, chemicals and toxins, which can diffuse through the dentine and injure the pulp.

The heterogeneous composition of dentine makes it a particularly difficult substrate to bond to with an adhesive. A second problem is that the differential pressure between the pulp and the dentine floor causes fluid to pump out of the dentinal tubules, such that it is not possible to create a dry dentine surface. Excessive desiccation of the dentine is likely to result in irreversible damage of the vital pulp and is thus not an option.

In the case of an abrasion/erosion lesion, the dentine surface usually consists of sclerotic dentine that is covered with a layer of pellicle, plaque and possibly calculus. It is important that these surface contaminants are removed prior to the use of a dentine-bonding procedure. This removal is very readily achieved with the application of pumice and water. A surface is then available that should be free of any contaminants and ready for the bonding procedure. However, the dentine surface is still covered with a layer of disorganized dentine known as the smear layer (Figure 2.5.5).

The smear layer essentially consists of a gelatinous surface layer of coagulated protein, some 0.5–5 μm thick. It is generally highly contaminated with bacteria from the caries process and contains cutting debris. The problems with dentine bonding can thus be summarized as follows:

- dentine is hydrophilic whereas most adhesives are hydrophobic
- dentine is a vital tissue
- dentine consists of both inorganic and organic material
- dentine is covered by a smear layer.

Components of dentine-bonding agents

Based on the concepts of primers and coupling agents as discussed in Chapter 1.9, dentine-bonding agents can be considered to consist of three essential components, namely:

- a primer
- a coupling agent
- a sealer.

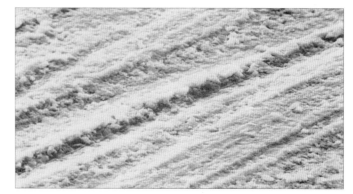

Figure 2.5.5 SEM of the dentine smear layer

In the dental literature, the primers are commonly called *dentine conditioners*, and consist of a variety of acids that alter the surface appearance and characteristics of the dentine. The coupling agents are, in effect, the components that do the bonding, but are generally described in the dental literature and by the manufacturers as *primers*. The function of the *sealer* is to flow into the dentinal tubules and seal the dentine by producing a surface layer rich in methacrylates that will ensure bonding to the resin in the composite. This component is variously referred to as the bond, the resin or the *adhesive*. This last term is especially confusing since it is the coupling agent that provides the bond. This mixing of terminology for the various components of dentine-bonding agents adds to the general confusion surrounding them. In further discussions of dentine-bonding agents we will use the terminology that is commonly used in the dental literature – dentine conditioners, primers and sealers – so as hopefully not to add to the confusion. Besides, later we will discuss how these various components can be mixed up in order to produce formulations that are easier to use.

Role of the dentine conditioner, primer and sealer

Dentine conditioners

The role of the dentine conditioners is to modify the smear layer that is formed on the dentine due to the cutting action of the bur when preparing a cavity or during exposure to abrasives such as tooth pastes in smooth surface caries and abrasion/erosion lesions. One of the major distinguishing features of dentine-bonding agents is the variety of dentine conditioners that have been used over time. These include maleic acid, EDTA (ethylenediaminetetraacetic acid), oxalic acid, phosphoric acid and nitric acid. What these substances have in common is that they are all acids and they modify the smear layer to varying degrees. The application of an acid to the dentine surface induces an acid–base reaction with the hydroxyapatite. This causes the hydroxyapatite to be dissolved and results in an opening of the dentinal tubules and the creation of a demineralized surface layer of dentine that is generally up to 4 μm deep (Figure 2.5.6). The stronger the acid, the more pronounced these effects. Thus, for EDTA, which is a mildly acidic chelating agent, only partial opening of the tubules occurs (Figure 2.5.7), whereas for nitric acid, which is a strong acid, extensive opening of the dentinal tubules occurs (Figure 2.5.8). The effect of this is shown schematically for a cross-sectional view of the dentine in Figure 2.5.9.

Some of the dentine conditioners may contain glutaraldehyde. The incorporation of glutaraldehyde is also aimed at modifying the dentine. Glutaraldehyde is a well-known cross-linking agent for collagen and is widely used for the tanning of hide to produce leather.

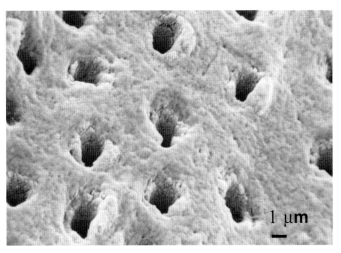

Figure 2.5.7 SEM of the dentine surface after application of EDTA primer

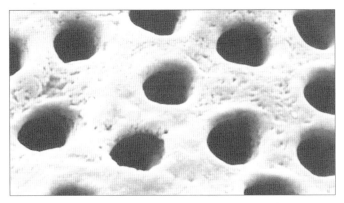

Figure 2.5.8 SEM of the dentine surface after application of a nitric acid primer

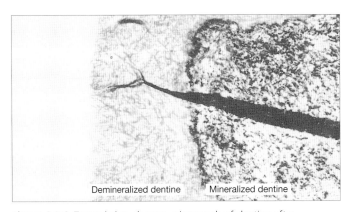

Figure 2.5.6 Transmission electron micrograph of dentine after application of a nitric acid primer to the surface

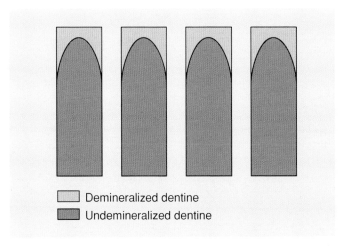

Figure 2.5.9 A cross-sectional view through dentine after application of an acid primer

The cross-linking process is said to produce a stronger dentine substrate by improving the strength and stability of the collagen structure. One reservation about the use of glutaraldehyde is that tissue necrosis has been observed in other areas where it has been used.

Primers

The role of the primer is to act as the adhesive in dentine-bonding agents since it provides a means of bonding hydrophobic composites and compomers to hydrophilic dentine. Thus, primers act as an intermediary, and consist of bifunctional monomers dissolved in a suitable solvent. The bifunctional monomer is, in fact, a coupling agent that is able to combine with two distinctly different materials. The situation is analogous to that of bonding resin to glass in the composites, where a silane coupling agent is used (see Chapter 1.9). The general formula for the coupling agent in dentine primers is as follows:

Methacrylate group–Spacer group–Reactive group
M–S–R

The methacrylate group (M) has the ability to bond to the composite resin and provide a strong covalent bond. The methacrylate group must be able to provide a satisfactory means for polymerization with the resin of the composite.

The spacer group (S) must be able to provide the necessary flexibility to the coupling agent to enhance the potential for bonding of the reactive groups. If the molecule is excessively rigid (due to steric hindrance), the ability of the reactive group to find a satisfactory conformational arrangement may be jeopardized, leading, at best, to a strained bond arrangement and, at worst, to only limited sites for bonding being available.

The reactive groups (R) are polar pendant- or end-groups. A variety of polar functional groups are shown in Table 2.5.2. The bond polarity is a consequence of asymmetric electron distribution in the bond. Polar reactions occur as the result of attractive forces between positive and negative charges on the molecules (see Chapter 1.2). Thus, the polar pendant- and end-groups on the coupling agent can combine with similar polar molecules in the dentine, such as hydroxyl groups

on the apatite and amino groups on the collagen. The attraction may be purely physical but can, in some instances, result in the formation of a chemical bond. The nature of this reactive group will determine whether the bond will be to the apatite in the dentine or to the collagen. In some cases, both may be involved.

Although all of the coupling agents used in dentine primers have polar reactive groups, these vary from one dentine-bonding agent to another. All have the objective of producing a strong bond to the dentine, but manufacturers and researchers are not agreed on which coupling agent may be the best. A small selection of these coupling agents is shown in Table 2.5.3, with hydroxyethylmethacrylate (HEMA) in particular being a very popular choice.

HEMA is able to penetrate the demineralized dentine and bond to the collagen via the hydroxyl and amino groups on the collagen. The action of the coupling agent in the primer solution is therefore to create a molecular entanglement network of poly(HEMA) and collagen (Figure 2.5.10).

It is very important that the primer is able to penetrate fully into and saturate the demineralized collagen layer. If this does not happen, then a thin layer of demineralized collagen will remain. This layer will not be reinforced by the resin and will form a weak interfacial region. In order to achieve good depth of penetration, the coupling agent is therefore dissolved in a solvent, such as ethanol or acetone. The solvents are extremely effective at seeking out water and displacing it ('water-chasing'), carrying the coupling agent along with it as it penetrates the demineralized dentine. However, it is important that the dentine is not excessively demineralized, as the depth of demineralization may become too much for complete penetration by the primer to occur.

In order to saturate the demineralized dentine, it is important that enough of the dentine-bonding agent is applied to the dentine surface. This may require multiple coatings, and also sufficient time should be allowed for the primer to penetrate and absorb. Excessive air thinning with an air-stream should also be avoided, as all that is needed is to evaporate the solvents gently.

CLINICAL SIGNIFICANCE

The method of application of the primer will largely determine whether or not micro-leakage will develop.

Sealers

The earliest dentine sealers were simply light- or dual-cured unfilled Bis-GMA or UDMA resins. Although the direct application of an unfilled resin such as Bis-GMA to an acid-treated dentine surface would result in the formation of resin tags, this has been shown not to result in an adequate bond between the resin and the dentine. The major difference is that, by not using the primer, the hydrophobic resin will adapt poorly to the hydrophilic dentine. When a primer is employed, its action is to make the dentine surface more hydrophobic, thus preventing the resin from shrinking away from the walls within the dentinal tubules, and ensures the formation of a tightly fitting resin-tag structure. For example, the methacrylate ends of the HEMA coupling agent are available for bonding to the resin sealer when this is subsequently placed on to the prepared surface of the dentine.

The dentine surface is thus thoroughly sealed with a resin, which is bonded to the dentine via the coupling agent in the primer. This sealer will now readily bond to the composite resin. The resulting interpenetrating layer of dentine and resin is commonly referred to as the *hybrid zone*, as shown schematically in Figure 2.5.11.

Most of the recent dentine sealers are a mixture of Bis-GMA and HEMA. This helps to improve the adaptation of the sealer to the

Table 2.5.2 Polarity patterns in some common functional groups	
Compound type	**Functional group structure**
Alcohol	$\overset{\delta+}{-\!\!-}C\!-\!OH^{\delta-}$
Amine	$\overset{\delta+}{-\!\!-}C\!-\!NH_2^{\delta-}$
Carboxylic acid	$\underset{OH^{\delta-}}{\overset{O^{\delta-}}{-\!\!-C^{\delta+}}}$
Aldehyde	$\underset{H}{\overset{O^{\delta-}}{-\!\!-C^{\delta+}}}$

Table 2.5.3 Coupling agents used for dentine bonding

Hydroxyethylmethacrylate (HEMA)	$C = C - C - O - CH_2 - CH_2 - OH$
Dimethacryloxyethyl phenol phosphate (MEP-P)	structure
N-Phenylglycine glycidyl methacrylate (NPG-GMA)	structure

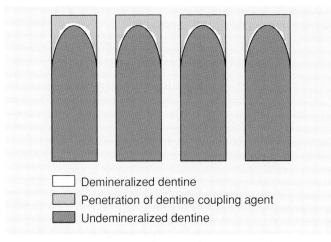

Figure 2.5.10 The penetration of the coupling agent into the demineralized dentine

Demineralized dentine
Penetration of dentine coupling agent
Undemineralized dentine

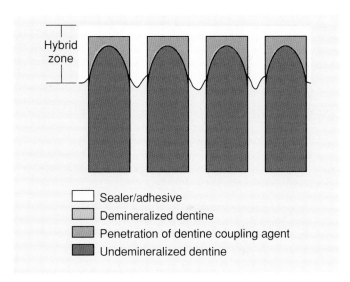

Figure 2.5.11 The hybrid zone created with a dentine-bonding agent

Sealer/adhesive
Demineralized dentine
Penetration of dentine coupling agent
Undemineralized dentine

dentine surface. There has been recent interest in filled sealers, particularly those containing nanoscale silica particles. Larger, 'micro' filler particles such as those used in some composites and GICs would not be appropriate for dentine sealers, as they would interfere with the penetration of the dentine tubules and collagen network by the resin. It is plausible that the addition of nanoscale filler particles to dentine sealers would increase the compressive strength of these materials, although it is not yet clear what clinical advantage this offers.

CLINICAL SIGNIFICANCE

Although some penetration of the sealer down the dentinal tubules will occur, providing additional micro-mechanical bonding, it is the primer that will determine the quality of the final bond.

Wet dentine bonding

The coupling agent component of the dentine-bonding agents is carried in a volatile solvent such as ethanol or acetone. Such solvents

are very effective at displacing the water in the dentine, and, in the process, pull the adhesive into the dentine with them. Therefore, it is not necessary – in fact, it may be detrimental – to dehydrate the dentine surface excessively. If the dentine is dried excessively, the consequence of this is that the demineralized collagen layer will collapse down on to the mineralized dentine, producing a dense structure which is difficult for the primer to penetrate (Figure 2.5.12). If the dentine has dehydrated excessively, then the collapsed collagen can be rehydrated with water.

In contrast, if the demineralized collagen layer is kept moist, a porous structure is maintained and the primer can readily infiltrate this layer and form a molecular entanglement bond (Figure 2.5.13). Thus it is only necessary to remove excess surface moisture. However, manufacturers' instructions will vary, depending on the composition of the primer. Some primers contain water as a carrier and for those it is possible that the demineralized collagen will rehydrate sufficiently after drying for the primer to penetrate the collagen structure.

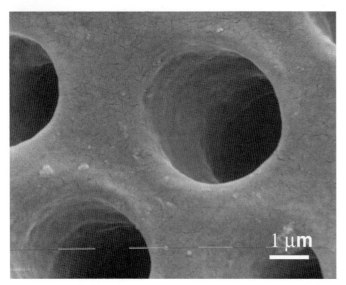

Figure 2.5.12 Demineralized surface of dentine after air drying

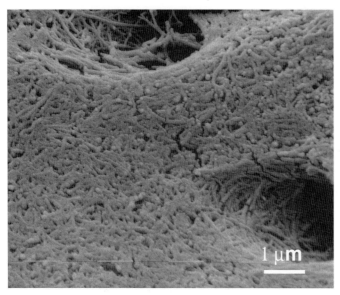

Figure 2.5.13 Demineralized surface of dentine that has been kept moist to prevent the collapse of the collagen structure

CLINICAL SIGNIFICANCE

The efficacy of the primer in dentine-bonding agents in producing a hybrid zone depends not only on the bifunctional monomers used and the solvents incorporated, but also on the water content of the dentine.

Total-etch technique

When dentine-bonding agents were first introduced, there was concern about etching the dentine surface. Before the advent of dentine-bonding agents, the dental practitioner's experience was that, when the phosphoric acid from the enamel etching procedure was allowed to flow on to the dentine, patients would return complaining of postoperative sensitivity. It was thought that this was due to the increased permeability of the dentine after acid etching resulting in the hydrodynamic effect and possibly penetration of the acid into the pulp. Hence there was a reluctance to etch dentine.

The development of dentine-bonding agents meant that the dentine surface could be sealed and postoperative sensitivity due to the hydrodynamic effect could be avoided as long as the bond between the dentine and restoration was maintained. Gradually, it was also realized that the use of a solution such as 35% phosphoric acid resulted in minimal penetration of the dentine (4–5 μm) and thus it was unlikely that the acid would contact the pulp. A differential etching technique began to be used, which involved etching the dentine separately with a low concentration of phosphoric acid or using a mild acid such as EDTA. However, this process of differential etching was both cumbersome and time-consuming. Eventually, the concept of the total-etch technique evolved; this involves etching both the enamel and the dentine simultaneously, typically for 10–15 seconds with a 35% phosphoric acid solution. This procedure is only applicable to freshly cut enamel, and unprepared enamel still needs to be etched in the conventional way.

PRESENTATION OF DENTINE-BONDING AGENTS

Three-stage etch and rinse systems

Some of the earliest dentine adhesives tried to bond directly to the dentine smear layer. However, the smear layer is a disrupted surface layer of dentine, which is not the ideal surface to bond to directly with an adhesive. The first dentine-bonding agents to prove reasonably effective were those that developed a hybrid zone for bonding; these were developed in the mid-1980s. They were presented as *three-stage systems*, consisting of a dentine conditioner, primer and dentine sealer, and functioned in the way described above. Examples of some commercially available systems are presented in Table 2.5.4. The dentine conditioner is generally a 35% phosphoric acid solution, while the primer either can be a single-component, light-activated, bifunctional monomer in a solvent or may require mixing of two components to be chemically cured. The dentine sealer also may be a single-component, light-activated resin or chemically and often dual-cured. Thus the number of syringes/bottles can be as many as five.

The problem with these three-stage bonding systems is that they not only involve many bottles, which can be confusing, but also require many bonding steps, typically 8–10. Both dental practitioners and the manufacturers wanted to see a reduction in the number of steps involved in the bonding process.

CLINICAL SIGNIFICANCE

It is a reasonable premise to expect that simplification of the bonding process would produce more consistent results and thus would be more reliable.

The development of new dentine-bonding agents has produced a wide variety of bonding systems, which have sought to simplify the bonding procedure while maintaining a good bond between the dentine and the restorative materials. This has resulted in a plethora of two-stage dentine-bonding agents.

Table 2.5.4 Components of a number of commercially available three-stage dentine-bonding agents

Product (Manufacturer)	Stage 1 Dentine conditioner	Stage 2 Primer	Stage 3 Sealer	No. of steps
Scotchbond multipurpose (3M/ESPE)	35% H_3PO_4	PCA copolymer HEMA Water	Bis-GMA HEMA	7
Optibond FL (Kerr Corp)	35% H_3PO_4	GPDM HEMA Ethanol	Bis-GMA HEMA	8
All-Bond 2 (Bisco)	32% H_3PO_4	Bottle 1: NTG-GMA acetone, ethanol, water Bottle 2: BPDM CQ, acetone	Bis-GMA UDMA HEMA	12

BPDM, biphenyl dimethacrylate; CQ, camphorquinone; GPDM, glycerophosphoric acid dimethacrylate; HEMA, hydroxyethylmethacrylate; NTG-GMA, *n*-tolyglycine-glycidyl methacrylate; PCA, polycarboxylic acid.

Table 2.5.5 Components of a number of commercially available two-stage dentine-bonding agents of the one-bottle bond variety

Product (Manufacturer)	Stage 1 Dentine conditioner	Stage 2 Primer/sealer	No. of steps
Scotchbond One (3M/ESPE)	35% H_3PO_4	PCA copolymer HEMA Bis-GMA Ethanol and water	7
Optibond Solo Plus (Kerr Corp)	35% H_3PO_4	GPDM HEMA Bis-GMA Ethanol	5
One-Step (Bisco)	32% H_3PO_4	BPDM HEMA Bis-GMA Acetone	8

Abbreviations: see Table 2.5.4.

Two-stage etch and rinse systems

Since the three-stage systems consist of a dentine conditioner, primer and sealer, one way of reducing the number of components, and possibly the number of steps, is to combine the action of some of these components. In order to simplify the presentation and use of dentine-bonding agents, essentially two different approaches can be adopted. New two-stage dentine-bonding agents were developed, where in some cases the primer and sealer are combined (Table 2.5.5), or the dentine conditioner and primer are combined (Table 2.5.6). The former are frequently referred to as *one-bottle bond* systems and the latter as *self-etching primers*.

The one-bottle bonding systems continue to use a separate acid-etch step before infiltration with the primer/adhesive. In this instance, the objective is for the process of hybridization of the demineralized dentine and the sealing of the dentinal tubules to take place simultaneously. In order to achieve this, many of the one-bottle bonding systems require multiple applications of the primer/adhesive. This will ensure complete saturation of the demineralized dentine with the mixture of resins provided in the primer/adhesive.

The benefits of the one-bottle bond systems are:

- The dental practitioner only needs to consider two components ('one bottle' and acid-etchant), compared with the myriad of bottles usually associated with the three-stage bonding systems.
- The order in which the components are to be used is less likely to be confused.
- Inventory control is kept very simple.

One limitation of the one-bottle bonding systems is that they cannot be used in situations where access of the light from the light-curing unit is compromised, such as for resin-bonded posts or amalgam bonding.

Some manufacturers have proposed that, when the one-bottle bonding systems are used in conjunction with compomers, it is possible in certain low-stress-bearing situations to omit the acid-etch step and thus use the one-bottle bond systems directly on the enamel and dentine. Although this approach may not be too detrimental to the bond to the dentine, it will compromise the bond to enamel.

At least one manufacturer (Dentsply) has produced a dentine conditioner to be used with compomers. The conditioner consists of an aqueous solution of itaconic and maleic acid, and does not require to be rinsed off. This two-stage system has the advantage of reducing the steps involved, but has the disadvantage that it still has to compete with other dentine adhesives used with compomers that are single-stage systems (see below). Also, it is not clear when the adhesive can be used on its own, when it should be used with a rinse-free conditioner and when the acid conditioner should be used.

Two-stage self-etching systems

The self-etching primers work on the premise that these will carry out both the demineralization and the infiltration process simultaneously and thus form the hybrid layer. This has the advantage that the ambiguous drying step for the dentine is avoided. The second-stage application of the unfilled resin(s) will ensure that the dentinal tubules are sealed and a methacrylate-rich surface layer is formed. It has been suggested that the two-stage self-etching systems should be further

Table 2.5.6 Components of two commercially available two-stage dentine-bonding agents of the self-etching primer variety

Product (Manufacturer)	Stage 1 Dentine conditioner/primer		Stage 2 Primer/sealer		No. of steps
Clearfil Liner Bond II (Kuraray Dental)	LB-Primer A:	Phenyl-P 5-NMSA CQ	LB-Bond:	MDP HEMA Bis-GMA Silanized colloidal silica photoinitiators	7
	LB-Primer B:	HEMA Water			
Clearfil SE Bond (Kuraray Dental)	SE-Primer:	MDP HEMA Hydrophilic dimethacrylate CQ N,N-Diethanol p-toluidine Water	SE-Bond:	MDP Bis-GMA HEMA Hydrophylic dimethacrylate CQ N,N-Diethanol p-toluidine Silanized colloidal silica photoinitiators	6

5-NMSA, N-methacrylaxyl-5-aminosalicylic acid; MDP, 10-metacryloyloxy methacrylate; phenyl-P, 2-methacryloyloxyethyl-phenyl hydrogen phosphate (see also Table 2.5.4).

subdivided into a 'strong' (pH <1), an 'intermediately strong' (pH ≈ 1.5), a 'mild' (pH ≈ 2) and an 'ultra-mild' (pH ≥2.5) self-etch approach, depending on the self-etching or demineralization intensity. The self-etching systems do not involve a rinsing step and thus the dissolved calcium phosphates remain in the hybrid layer. The lower the pH, the more intense is the dissolution process, such that more of the calcium phosphates remain embedded in the hybrid layer. Since these calcium phosphates are rather soluble, they may leach out and compromise the long-term durablity of the bond to dentine. However, it is possible that the bond to enamel is better with the low pH systems due to the more aggresive etching of the enamel.

Single-stage self-etching systems

The simplest adhesive would be the one that is applied in a single-stage procedure. The manufacturers have not quite gone to the lengths of simply putting all the components into a single bottle. Although this might seem to be the logical next step, lack of compatibility between the components does not allow this. The closest they have come to developing a single-stage dentine-bonding agent is to present the adhesive as two components that have to be mixed prior to application to the enamel and dentine surface, without the prior need to treat the enamel or dentine (Table 2.5.7). The bonding procedure involves four steps, consisting of (1) dispensing and/or mixing the two components, (2) application to the enamel and dentine surface, (3) drying and (4) light curing. The advantage with this approach is not only its simplicity but also the avoidance of the ambiguous drying step for the dentine.

The single-stage dentine-bonding agents are generally indicated in low-stress-bearing areas, as the bond strength – to enamel in particular and, to a lesser degree, to dentine – is possibly not as good as that obtained with the three-stage or two-stage bonding systems.

Single-stage dentine-bonding agents can also be used to overcome sensitivity by simply painting them on to the affected surface.

Read the instructions

A full classification of dentine-bonding agents is provided in Table 2.5.8. It must be stressed that different dentine-bonding agents have distinctive and different detailed instructions on how they should be used to best effect. It is not possible here to cover each and every one of the subtleties and nuances of the application procedure for each.

Table 2.5.7 Components of commercially available single-stage dentine-bonding agents

Product	Stage 1 Dentine conditioner, primer and sealer	No. of steps
Prompt-L-Pop (3M/ESPE)	Part one: methacrylated phosphates, photoinitiators and stabilizers	4
	Part two: fluoride complex, water and stabilizers	
iBond (Heraeus Kulzer)	UDMA, 4-META, glutardialdehyde, acetone, water, photoinitiators and stabilizers	3

4-META, 4-methacryloxy ethyl trimellitate anhydride; UDMA, urethane dimethacrylate

Nevertheless, it should be clear from the above description of dentine-bonding agents that there is no universal technique for producing a bond to dentine and that each system has its own unique procedure.

CLINICAL SIGNIFICANCE

It is extremely important that careful note is taken of the instructions for use of individual dentine-bonding agents, as these will differ widely, depending on the components used and how these are presented to the user.

Selection of a dentine-bonding agent

Biocompatibility

The way in which the pulp may react to the procedure adopted (particularly the application of acid to dentine) is an important consideration. It is apparent that these dentine adhesives rely, to varying degrees, on the formation of resin tags in order to achieve a bond to dentine.

Table 2.5.8 Classification of dentine-bonding agents

Stage	Type	Description	Brand (Manufacturer)
Three-stage etch and rinse	1	1. Application of etchant and washed off to create demineralized dentine layer 2. Application of primer 3. Application of sealer	All-Bond 2 (Bisco) Optibond FL (Kerr) Scotchbond Multipurpose (3M/ESPE)
Two-stage etch and rinse	2	1. Application of etchant and washed off to create demineralized dentine layer 2. Application of primer and sealer in single solution	Excite (Ivoclar/Vivadent) Gluma Comfort Bond (Heraeus Kulzer) One-Step (Bisco) Optibond Solo Plus (Kerr) Prime & Bond NT (Dentsply) Scotchbond One (3M/ESPE)
Two-stage self-etching	3	1. Application of self-etching primer 2. Sealer applied separately	Clearfill Liner Bond 2V (Kuraray Dental) Clearfill SE Bond (Kuraray Dental) AdheSE (Ivoclar-Vivadent)
Single-stage self-etching	4	1. Self-etching primer and sealer applied as a single solution	One-Bond F (J. Morita) Prompt-L-Pop (3M/ESPE) G-Bond (GC) Xeno III (Dentsply) I-Bond (Heraeus Kulzer)

One potential problem is that opening the dentinal tubules can cause fluids from within the tubules to rise to the surface under the influence of the pulpal pressure. This will prevent good bonding, as it prevents the adhesive from penetrating the dentinal tubules and from adapting to the dentine surface. Whilst this may be overcome by thorough drying of the dentine surface prior to the application of the bonding agent, excessive desiccation of the dentine is likely to result in post-operative pulpal sensitivity and a poor bond.

There has been a considerable degree of reticence within the dental profession as regards the use of these adhesive systems, since the opening of dentinal tubules and the consequent increase in dentine permeability can present a problem, as noted previously. Concern has also been expressed about the possible pulpal response to the application of acids to the dentine surface. Some consideration is given to this with regard to direct pulp capping in Chapter 2.6.

In the case of sclerotic dentine, as is found in cervical abrasion lesions on mature patients, the application of acids to the dentine is felt to be acceptable, as the dentine is highly mineralized and an open pathway to the pulp is not created. This would not be so in the case of carious dentine, although a number of studies have indicated that dentine-bonding agents and their associated acid primers will not have an adverse affect on the pulp.

Thus, pulpal inflammation will only recur if there is a bond failure resulting in bacterial leakage. Whether or not this is likely to happen depends on the strength and durability of the bond to dentine, how easy it is to achieve this bond clinically, and the restorative material used. Dentine-bonding agents do not have any intrinsic antibacterial activity to counter the bacterial invasion, although in some cases attempts have been made to incorporate antibacterial agents.

CLINICAL SIGNIFICANCE

A very important point to appreciate is that, should the adhesive bond fail, there is a ready route for bacterial invasion through the permeable dentine.

With all dentine-bonding agents, it is important to avoid direct skin contact with the primer/adhesive liquids, as regular contact may result in a type IV sensitization (delayed allergic reaction) or contact dermatitis.

Strength and durability

A breakdown of the adhesive bond can have serious consequences, as it allows the reintroduction of bacteria and debris into the cavity margins. This will cause unsightly marginal staining and can result in the development of pulpal sensitivity. Alternatively, the restoration may simply be lost due to a lack of adhesion, unless some form of retention has been provided.

There are a number of potential causes for breakdown of the bond between the restoration and the dentine:

- polymerization shrinkage
- differential thermal expansion and contraction
- internal stresses from occlusal loading
- chemical attack, such as hydrolysis.

The possible consequences of polymerization shrinkage of the composites have been discussed already (see Chapter 2.2). As it can take up to 24 hours before the full bond strength for the dentine-bonding agents is achieved, the polymerization shrinkage may cause disruption of the bond before it has had a chance to establish itself.

CLINICAL SIGNIFICANCE

It is prudent to recommend to patients that they try to place minimal stress on a newly bonded restoration, at least for the first 24 hours.

The breakdown of the dentine bond due to polymerization shrinkage is also dependent on the cavity shape. This is defined by the so-called C-factor, which is the ratio of bonded surface area to the free surface area. If the free surface for contraction is very small compared to the surface area of the interface between the tooth and the restoration, then disruption of the composite/dentine bond is favoured over contraction towards the surface. This means that a bond may only be achievable on a flat surface or in very shallow cavities, unless the bond is sufficiently strong to resist the stresses generated by the polymerization contraction of the resin. Should this be the case, then the cusps of the tooth will need to deform to compensate for the shrinkage effect.

In situations of heavily undermined cusps, as may be the case in large mesial occlusal distal restorations, this could result in fracture at the base of the cusp. Even if this does not occur, the stress generated within the tooth crown may give rise to pulpal sensitivity.

In situations of stress-induced lesions, such as cervical abfraction lesions, the application of eccentric or high occlusal forces can cause the restoration to debond and eventually to be dislodged. It has been suggested that this problem can be overcome to some degree by employing a restorative material with a low elastic modulus (e.g. micro-filled resins), since this prevents stresses from being transferred across the tooth–restoration interface. This concept is essentially the same as the idea of applying a thick layer of a relatively low-elastic modulus resin (such as a dentine sealer) to the dentine surface prior to the application of the composite resin. If this layer is of sufficient thickness, it would then act as a stress breaker by absorbing the polymerization shrinkage strains by elastic elongation. However, this does mean that the stresses have to be supported elsewhere in the tooth structure and this may not be the most benign situation.

Number of bonding steps

If the choice between dentine-bonding agents were simply based on their complexity of application, then the single-stage dentine-bonding agents would be the preferred option. However, fewer steps do not necessarily mean better performance.

CLINICAL SIGNIFICANCE

The clinical efficacy of dentine-bonding agents with a reduced number of steps still requires to be established.

There are also situations in which some of the dentine-bonding agents would be inappropriate. For example, when a dentine-bonding agent is to be used in conjunction with an indirect restoration, those that have to be light-cured immediately can give rise to problems of seating of the restoration, as there is a tendency for the resin to pool at the internal line angles. In those situations, a dentine-bonding agent with a two-component, chemically cured primer would be indicated. As mentioned previously, in situations where access of light is a problem, such as resin-bonded metal posts and amalgam bonding, a chemically cured primer is also indicated.

Clinical performance

For small restorations with margins wholly in enamel, direct composites with dentine-bonding agents are acceptable, as long as suitable techniques are adopted to minimize the effects of polymerization shrinkage. For large restorations involving extensive areas of exposed dentine, and especially where the cavity extends subgingivally, the use of direct composites in conjunction with dentine-bonding agents is contraindicated. The problem of polymerization shrinkage can be overcome, to some degree, by the use of composite inlays. However, the mismatch in the coefficient of expansion still presents a problem, and resin-bonded ceramic restorations may be preferred since these will place less stress on the dentine bond.

It is in the particular area of long-term bond durability that the newer two- and single-stage dentine-bonding agents still need to prove their clinical efficacy. Unfortunately, the in vitro measurement of tensile or shear bond strength has been shown to be a poor indicator of clinical performance. Only a few dentine adhesives being promoted have been adequately evaluated clinically and not all dentine-bonding agents can be recommended for widespread clinical use. A comprehensive review of the performance of dentine-bonding agents with regard to their retention rates was carried out by Peumans et al (2005), and showed that the three-stage dentine-bonding agents had an average failure rate of $4.8 \pm 4.2\%$, as compared with the two-stage etch and rinse systems ($6.2 \pm 5.5\%$), the two-stage self-etch systems ($4.7 \pm 5.0\%$) and the single-stage dentine-bonding agents ($8.1 \pm 11.3\%$). Yet the most striking outcome was that for the GICs and RMGICs at $1.9 \pm 1.8\%$. Thus, the use of GICs and RMGICs as a dentine-bonded base underneath the composites would appear to continue to be a highly acceptable alternative approach to the use of dentine-bonding agents.

SUMMARY

There are many different dentine adhesives and each appears to be unique in its properties. The latest generation of dentine-bonding agents is very promising, such that loss of retention is no longer a major factor in causing failure. However, it is not yet possible to guarantee a marginal seal with dentine-bonding agents in all clinical situations.

CLINICAL SIGNIFICANCE

The clinical performance of dentine-bonding agents has significantly improved, such that clinical success with adhesive restorations has become much more predictable.

FURTHER READING

Armstrong SR, Keller JC, Boyer DB (2001) The influence of water storage and C-factor on the dentine-resin composite microtensile bond strength and debond pathway utilizing a filled and unfilled adhesive resin. Dent Mater 17: 268–276

Bouillaguet S, Gysi P, Wataha JC et al (2001) Bond strength of composite to dentine using conventional, one-step, and self-etching adhesive systems. J Dent 29: 55–61

Choi KK, Condon JR, Ferracane JL (2000) The effect of adhesive thickness on polymerization contraction stress of composite. J Dent Res 79: 812–817

Davidson CL, de Gee AJ, Feilzer A (1984) The competition between the composite-dentine bond strength and the polymerisation contraction stress. J Dent Res 63: 1396–1399

Erickson RL (1992) Surface interactions of dentine adhesive materials. Oper Dent 5: 81–94

Finger WJ, Balkenhol M (1999) Rewetting strategies for bonding to dry dentine with an acetone-based adhesive. J Adhes Dent 2: 51

McLean JW (1996) Dentinal bonding agents versus glass–ionomer cements. Quintessence Int **27**: 659

Moll K, Haller B (2000) Effect of intrinsic and extrinsic moisture on bond strength to dentine. J Oral Rehabil **27**: 150–165

Nakabayashi N, Kojima K, Masuhara E (1982) The promotion of adhesion by the infiltration of monomers into tooth substrates. J Biomed Mater Res **16**: 265–273

Nakabayashi N, Watanabe A, Arao T (1998) A tensile test to facilitate identification of defects in dentine bonded specimens. J Dent **26**: 379–385

Pashley DH, Carvalho RM (1997) Dentine permeability and dentine adhesion. J Dent **25**: 355–372

Perdigão J, Frankenberger R, Rosa BT et al (2000) New trends in dentine/enamel adhesion. Am J Dent **13**: 25D-30D (special issue)

Peumans M, Kanumilli P, De Munck J et al (2005) Clinical effectiveness of contemporary adhesives: a systematic review of current clinical trials. Dent Mater **21**: 864

Tay FR, Sano H, Carvalho R et al (2000) An ultrastructural study of the influence of acidity of self-etching primers and smear layer thickness on bonding to intact dentine. J Adhesive Dent **2**: 83–98

Van Meerbeek B, Peumans M, Poitevin A et al (2010) Relationship between bond-strength tests and clinical outcomes. Dent Mater **26(2)**: 100–121

van Noort R, Noroozi S, Howard IC et al (1989) A critique of bond strength measurements. J Dent **17**: 61–67

Endodontic materials

INTRODUCTION

Endodontics is concerned with the morphology, physiology and pathology of the human dental pulp and periradicular tissues. Endodontic treatment is aimed at saving the tooth when injury to the pulp and associated periradicular tissues has occurred. Treatments involving the use of dental materials include capping of an exposed vital pulp, sealing of the root canal space when the pulp has had to be removed and, in the case of badly broken down teeth, reconstruction with endodontic post and core systems (Figure 2.6.1).

VITAL PULP CAPPING

Two main causes of pulpal exposure are:

- dental decay and tooth wear
- accidental exposure during operative procedures or due to trauma.

In each of the above instances, remedial treatment is necessary to save the tooth. The nature of this treatment depends on which of the above causes of pulpal injury applies.

Indirect pulp capping

Sir John Tomes stated in 1859 that 'It is better that a layer of discolored dentine be allowed to remain for the protection of the pulp rather than run the risk of sacrificing the tooth.' He had observed that discoloured and demineralized dentine could be left behind in deep cavities of the tooth before restoration, often with highly satisfactory results. This is especially applicable if micro-exposures of the pulp are suspected. The removal of this dentine may lead to exposure of the pulp, thus impairing its prognosis. It has been shown that demineralized dentine, if it is free of bacteria, will remineralize once the source of the infection has been eliminated. The diagnosis of the presence of demineralized dentine that is caries-free can be assisted by using a caries-disclosing solution. The placement of a suitable material directly on this demineralized dentine is commonly called *indirect pulp capping* (IPC) and it has to be said that there is as yet no clear consensus for the acceptance of this clinical procedure.

IPC has been defined as the steps undertaken to protect a vital tooth where removal of all affected tissues would result in a pulpal exposure. In this context, a non-exposed pulp is one that exhibits no signs of haemorrhage at or near the pulp chamber. When carrying out such a procedure, it is vitally important that the infection is removed and is not allowed to recur. This can be achieved with the placement of an antibacterial liner such as calcium hydroxide or zinc oxide–eugenol cement, which is aimed at stimulating secondary dentine formation. Of course, resin composites should not be placed directly on eugenol-based liners because they interfere with the polymerization of the resin.

With the advent of adhesive dental materials, another possible restorative option is the placement of calcium hydroxide cement, followed by an adhesive liner such as glass–ionomer (GIC) or resin-modified glass–ionomer cement (RMGIC). Yet another option is the use of resin composites in conjunction with a dentine-bonding agent. The aim is to provide a combination of an antibacterial barrier and an adhesive seal against the further ingress of bacteria, thus removing the pulpal antagonist and allowing the pulp to heal. When calcium hydroxide is used in this way, it should be applied sparingly so as to ensure that as much dentine is available for further bonding with the GIC/RMGIC or dentine-bonded resin composite.

More recently, an adhesive approach involving the direct application of a dentine-bonding agent has been proposed. This is aimed at sealing the remaining dentine by the creation of a hybrid zone, thus preventing immediate postoperative sensitivity and protecting the tooth from the ingress of bacteria. There are those who have serious reservations about acid etching dentine so close to the pulp, but as Figure 2.6.2 shows, the demineralization of the dentine by the penetration of acid is only a matter of a few micrometres. Further evidence exists to support the position that acid etching of dentine will not kill the underlying pulp. With regard to the stimulation of secondary dentine, more evidence has been gathered to suggest that this is not a feature unique to calcium hydroxide cement.

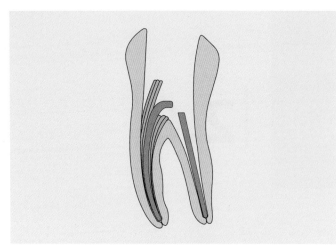

Figure 2.6.1 Schematic of a root-filled tooth

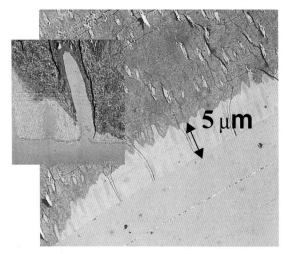

5 µm

Figure 2.6.2 Transmission electron micrograph showing the extent of acid penetration into dentine

---

CLINICAL SIGNIFICANCE

The important points to appreciate are that many dental materials:
- are biologically compatible with the pulp for indirect pulp capping, as long as there are no bacteria present and coronal micro-leakage is prevented
- will stimulate the formation of reparative dentine.

Direct pulp capping

Direct pulp capping can be described as the dressing of an exposed pulp with the objective of maintaining pulp vitality. If a pulpal exposure occurs as a consequence of tooth preparation or trauma, it is important that steps are taken to avoid bacterial contamination. If one can be sure that this is the case, then the procedure of direct pulp capping carries a good prognosis for saving the pulp; although views vary, the general consensus is that calcium hydroxide cement is the choice of pulp-capping material in such situations. However, this view is now being challenged, with some clinicians promoting the merits of mineral trioxide aggregate.

Nevertheless, many clinicians believe that the long-term success rate with root-canal therapy does not warrant the treatment of traumatic pulp exposures with the more unpredictable pulp-capping procedures, especially as unsuccessful pulp capping may lead to resorption, calcification, pulpitis, pulp necrosis or periapical involvement. However, the advantages of a successful pulp-capping procedure are that young vital teeth have an opportunity to continue to develop and the tooth-weakening effects of root-canal treatment are avoided.

If direct pulp capping as a clinical procedure is controversial, then so is the choice of materials for pulp capping. A pulp-capping material can be considered to behave as a wound dressing for the exposed pulp. Such a material can passively wall off the pulp from the outside environment so as to prevent bacterial invasion and/or can induce some change in the pulp.

There is evidence to suggest that the pulp has the capacity to wall itself off by forming a connective tissue barrier that eventually changes into hard tissue. The induction of hard tissue formation needs to be preceded by a low-grade irritation that results in superficial coagulation necrosis. On this basis, a pulp-capping material must:

- have a superficial effect on the pulp tissue, thereby inducing a biological encapsulation process that results in hard tissue formation
- cause no adverse effects, whether systemically or locally, such that the pulp is kept alive
- protect the pulp from the coronal ingress of bacteria.

In other words, a pulp-capping material needs to be able to interact with the pulp to initiate hard tissue formation and, once this process has been triggered, should adopt a passive role.

If the pulp is exposed due to the presence of caries, the procedure for pulp capping is contraindicated; the infiltration of bacteria that will have occurred into the pulp cannot be reversed, and the only solution is a full pulpectomy.

Pulp-capping materials

Until recently, the only material that appeared to satisfy the requirements for pulp capping was calcium hydroxide cement, which was first used for this purpose in the 1930s. However, as already mentioned, the dominant position of calcium hydroxide as the preferred pulp-capping material is now being challenged by MTA and, to some degree, by the dentine-bonding agents.

Calcium hydroxide cements

The first use of $Ca(OH)_2$ was in the form of a slurry, consisting of no more than a mixture of calcium hydroxide in water. This was changed to a paste using methyl cellulose, being somewhat easier to handle. In the early 1960s, the hard-setting calcium hydroxide cements were introduced, in which the calcium hydroxide reacts with a salicylate ester chelating agent in the presence of a toluene sulphonamide plasticizer (see Chapter 2.4). The hard-setting cements are either two-paste systems or are single-paste systems consisting of calcium hydroxide-filled dimethacrylates, polymerized by light.

The problem with the non-setting versions is that these will gradually dissolve and disappear from underneath the restoration, which can undermine the restoration's function. The hard-setting versions are therefore generally preferred, as these are less soluble. The difficulty for the manufacturer is to achieve a balance between a material that is sufficiently soluble to be therapeutic and not so soluble as to dissolve away, although whether the pulp-capping material needs to release anything to stimulate dentine bridge formation is arguable.

When the paste is brought in contact with the pulp it causes a layer of necrosis some 1.0–1.5 mm thick, which eventually develops into a calcified layer. Experiments using radioactive calcium in the paste have shown that the calcium salts necessary for mineralization of the bridge are not derived from the cement, but are instead supplied by the tissue fluids of the pulp. Once the bridge has become dentine-like in appearance and the pulp has been shut off from the source of the irritation, the hard tissue formation ceases. It is believed that the high pH of the calcium hydroxide cement is responsible for this type of pulpal response, and that this is also closely associated with its antibacterial properties.

Mineral trioxide aggregate

Mineral trioxide aggregate (MTA) is a cement composed of tricalcium silicate, dicalcium silicate, tricalcium aluminate, tetracalcium aluminoferrite, calcium sulphate and bismuth oxide. Its composition is not unlike that of Portland cement, except for the addition of bismuth oxide. The latter is added in order to improve its radiopacity.

MTA is very alkaline (pH ~12.5) and has biological and histological properties similar to those of calcium hydroxide cement. It has been shown that MTA can induce bone deposition with a minimal inflammatory response, as it is less cytotoxic than reinforced zinc oxide–eugenol cements.

The material is mixed with sterile water to provide a grainy, sandy mixture and then can be packed gently into the desired area. The material is not the easiest to handle, although some clinicians claim that calcium hydroxide cement is technically more difficult to place. The powder-to-liquid ratio (3 : 1) is critical if one is to achieve appropriate hydration of the powder. MTA requires moisture to set, such that absolute dryness not only is unnecessary but also is contraindicated. On occasion, it may be necessary to place a moist cotton pellet directly in contact with the material in order to allow proper setting; however, excessive moisture softens the material. It takes an average of 4 hours for the material to solidify completely and, once the cement has set, it has a compressive strength comparable to that of reinforced zinc oxide–eugenol cement. It should be noted that a low pH environment can prevent the material from setting.

MTA has also been recommended for use as a root-end-filling material, a retrograde root-filling material, to seal perforations or open apices, or to cap vital pulps.

Dentine-bonding agents

The use of dentine-bonding agents is even more controversial than the use of calcium hydroxide as a direct pulp-capping agent, but is an area being extensively researched. As stated by Stanley (1998), the research data on pulp capping are, at times, inadequate, confusing, misleading or even incorrect, and diminish the confidence of practitioners in performing pulp capping. At best, the situation is confusing and more research is needed to make any definitive statement. Haemostasis seems to be essential and, for this, cleaning with a dilute solution of sodium hypochlorite (1.0% or less) has been recommended. If bleeding cannot be controlled within a matter of a minute, endodontic treatment is indicated.

What continues to remain controversial is the practice of total-etch direct bonding with dentine-bonding agents, and more research needs to be focused on this area. Some successes have been claimed for direct pulp capping with dentine-bonding agents when the acid-etch step is omitted, or for bonding systems not requiring a separate acid-etch step, such as the self-etching primers, despite the observation that phosphoric acid can act as an effective haemostatic agent. Hence, the results obtained with one dentine-bonding agent may be different from those obtained with another dentine-bonding agent, such that clinical experience cannot be extrapolated from one to the other. It is, therefore, not surprising that most general dental practitioners continue to use a minimal quantity of calcium hydroxide, before placing a dentine-bonding agent.

Failure after direct pulp capping

Failure after direct pulp capping can be due to three reasons:

1. *Chronically inflamed pulp.* There is no healing effect on inflamed pulp, and, in such situations, a full pulpectomy is indicated.
2. *Extra-pulpal blood clot.* Such a blood clot prevents contact between the healthy pulpal tissue and the cement, and interferes with the wound-healing process.
3. *Restoration failure.* If the restoration fails to provide a bacterial seal, then coronal ingress of bacteria can lead to failure.

It is important to distinguish the last of these failures from the others, as it is not, strictly speaking, a failure of pulp capping. The outcome of direct pulp capping with calcium hydroxide cement can be unpredictable, which may be related to the importance of achieving direct contact between the sealant and the pulp tissue without any intervening blood clot. It has been found that iatrogenic pulp exposures treated with MTA are generally free from inflammation 1 week after placement and a hard tissue bridge will form over a period of about 3 weeks. Thus it would appear that MTA has excellent sealing abilities and prevents pulpal inflammation by providing a predictable secondary barrier under the surface seal provided by the restorative material.

CLINICAL SIGNIFICANCE

The long-term success of direct pulp capping not only depends on the reactions induced local to the pulp by the pulp-capping material, but also is crucially dependent on the practitioner being able to make certain that micro-leakage will not occur and the marginal seal is maintained.

ROOT CANAL FILLING MATERIALS

The objectives of modern non-surgical endodontic treatment are:

- *to provide a clean canal.* The aim is to produce a reduction of bacteria to a non-pathogenic level.
- *to provide an 'apical seal'.* This prevents the ingress of fluids that will provide nutrients for canal bacteria and also prevents irritants leaving the canal and entering the periapical tissues.
- *to provide a 'coronal seal'.* This prevents recontamination due to the ingress of oral microorganisms.

A wide variety of materials have been used in an attempt to produce an impervious seal of the tooth root apex. The most widely used root-canal-sealing materials are a combination of root-obturating points and canal-sealer cements.

Obturating points

Gutta percha

Gutta percha is a rubber that is tapped from the Taban tree. It was introduced into the UK in 1843 and has been used in endodontics for over 100 years. Rubbers are polymers of isoprene (2-methyl-1,3-butadiene), and isoprene is a geometric isomer, which means that it can have different structural arrangements despite having the same composition, as depicted in Figure 2.6.3. When the CH_3 group and the H atom are positioned on the same side of the isoprene mer, this is termed a *cis* structure and the resulting polymer, *cis*-isoprene, is known as *natural rubber*. When the CH_3 group and the H atom sit on opposite sides of the isoprene mer, this is termed the *trans* structure

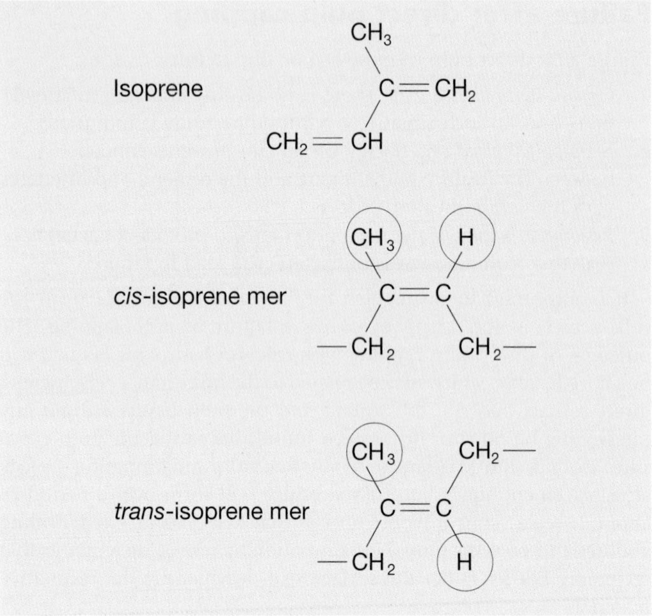

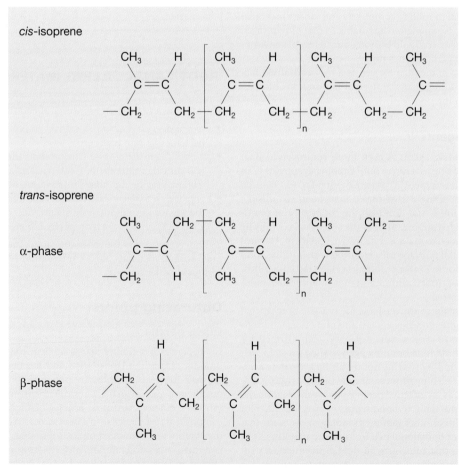

Figure 2.6.3 The structure of isoprene and the *cis*-mer and *trans*-mer of isoprene, on which natural rubber and gutta percha are based

and *trans*-isoprene polymer is commonly referred to as *gutta percha* (Figure 2.6.4). The effect on the properties of these different configurations of the polymer is quite profound. In the *cis* form, the hydrogen atom and methyl group prevent close packing such that the natural rubber is amorphous and consequently soft and highly flexible, whereas the gutta percha crystallizes, and usually becomes about 60% crystalline, forming a hard, rigid polymer.

The natural rubbers are soft and tacky unless they are hardened by *vulcanization*, a process discovered by Charles Goodyear in 1839 (see page xii). Vulcanization involves heating the polymer with a few percent by weight of sulphur. The hardening occurs because *sulphur bridges* or *cross-links* form between the polymer chains, preventing the polymer molecules from slipping over one another. This cross-linked rubber is used to produce rubber dam and rubber gloves.

Gutta percha is a thermoplastic material and softens at 60–65°C; it will melt at about 100°C, so it cannot be heat-sterilized. If necessary, disinfection can be carried out in a solution of sodium hypochlorite (5%). The use of solvents such as acetone or alcohol should be avoided, as these are absorbed by the gutta percha, causing it to swell. Eventually, the gutta percha will return to its unswollen state, thus compromising the apical seal. On exposure to light, gutta percha oxidizes and becomes brittle. It is therefore important to check that the points have retained their flexibility before using them.

The gutta percha is able to take up two distinct conformations. At high temperature, the gutta percha chains take on an extended

Figure 2.6.4 The structure of *cis*-isoprene (natural rubber) and the α-phase and β-phase of *trans*-isoprene of gutta percha

Table 2.6.1 Composition of gutta percha points

Constituent	Amount (%)	Purpose
Gutta percha	19–22	Rubber
Zinc oxide	59–75	Filler
Heavy metal salts	1–17	Radio-opacifier
Wax or resin	1–4	Plasticizer

conformation, which can be preserved if cooled rapidly so that it forms the crystalline β-phase, whereas when the gutta percha is cooled more slowly, the denser α-phase is formed (see Figure 2.6.4). The α-phase gutta percha has better thermoplastic characteristics and is therefore preferred for use in hot gutta percha application systems, where heat-softened gutta percha is injected into the root-canal filling. This technique was first developed by Johnson in 1978 and further improvements of the original technique include the use of plastic carriers (Thermofil) and injection guns (Obtura) for the delivery of softened gutta percha. However, in the presence of a patent apical foramen, there may be a predisposition for extrusion of filling material beyond the apex.

An alternative approach is to dissolve the gutta percha in a chemical solvent such as chloroform or xylene. This softens the gutta percha and allows it to be adapted closely to the canal wall and duplicate the intricate canal morphology. However, as the solvent is lost, so the dimensional stability may be compromised, and concerns have been expressed regarding the possible cytotoxic effects of using these solvents.

One of the main uses is the gutta percha point, which is softened and compacted by warm vertical and lateral condensation. The composition of commercially available gutta percha obturating points will vary from product to product, but typical values are shown in Table 2.6.1. The additional ingredients are added to overcome the inherent brittleness of the rubber and to make it radiopaque.

Metal points

Metals, including gold, tin, lead, copper amalgam and silver, have long been used as root-canal filling materials. Silver points were used extensively at one time because of their bactericidal effect. Silver is a more rigid and unyielding material than gutta percha and was used when access and instrumentation were difficult due to a small cross-section or awkward anatomy. Unfortunately, the rigidity of silver made it impossible to adapt it closely to the canal wall and greater reliance had to be placed on the cements used to provide the seal. Other disadvantages with silver points were that they tended to corrode, which could give rise to apical discoloration of the soft tissues, and they were problematic to remove. Corrosion can be limited by sealing the entire point within the root canal, such that it is totally surrounded by the sealer cement. However, acrylic and titanium points are now available as alternatives to silver points in order to avoid the problems of corrosion, and silver points are perhaps now only of historical interest.

Thermoplastic polymer points

In an interesting departure from gutta percha, which has been around for a very long time, a new root-canal point consisting of a thermoplastic polyester polymer has recently become available. It forms part of a system that comprises the polymer point, a resin composite that acts as the sealant, and a dentine primer that aids in providing good contact between the sealer and the tooth wall (Resilon-Epiphany system, Resilon Research LLC, Madison, CT, USA). The detailed composition is as follows:

- *Core material*: organic part: thermoplastic synthetic polymer – polycaprolactone; inorganic part: bioactive glass, bismuth oxychloride, barium sulphate
- *Sealer*: organic part: Bis-GMA, ethoxylated Bis-GMA, urethane dimethacrylate (UDMA), hydrophilic difunctional methacrylates; inorganic part: calcium hydroxide, barium sulphate, barium glass, bismuth oxychloride, silica
- *Primer*: sulphonic acid terminated functional monomer, hydroxyethylmethacrylate (HEMA), water, polymerization initiator.

The thermoplastic polymer handles like gutta percha and is consequently referred to as 'resin percha'. It is available in a range of sizes that fit endodontic instruments and in various tapers, as well as in accessory points and pellets. Various techniques can be employed to place this material in the canal (single-cone method, cold lateral condensation and thermoplastic techniques), with the same instruments and devices that are used for gutta percha condensation. This system allows formation of a so-called mono-block made up of root dentine, sealer and resin percha, which has the potential to strengthen the structure of the tooth that has been compromised by endodontic treatment, at the same time ensuring complete sealing of the root canal. However, as it is relatively new, any claims for this system need to be treated with a degree of circumspection.

ROOT CANAL SEALER CEMENTS

The ideal properties of a root canal sealer are that it should:

- be easy to use
- be free of air bubbles and homogeneous when mixed
- flow to a thin film thickness
- be insoluble
- adapt well to the canal wall and the obturating point
- be radiopaque
- be biocompatible
- be bacteriocidal, or at least bacteriostatic
- be easy to remove in case of failure.

It is well accepted that the sealing properties of a conventionally applied and laterally condensed gutta percha are such that it is essential to use it in conjunction with a root canal sealer cement. The function of the cement is to fill the spaces between the obturating point and the wall of the root canal, producing an antibacterial seal. It also lubricates the gutta percha points during compaction and will fill canal irregularities and lateral canals.

Conversely, the use of root-canal cements without obturating points is also contraindicated. When used in bulk, the cements either are too soluble or shrink excessively on setting. Additionally, it is difficult to gauge when, or if, the canal is adequately filled, and there is a danger that the cement may pass beyond the root apex into the surrounding tissues.

It is interesting to note that a similar approach with root canal sealers has been adopted as with cavity liners. It is now accepted that the root canal sealer cement is unable to provide an impervious seal and most of the attention has been focused on incorporating antibacterial properties, with the emphasis on providing an antibacterial seal.

A wide variety of materials are used as root canal sealers and these include:

- zinc oxide–eugenol cements (e.g. Tublseal, Kerr)
- resins (e.g. AH Plus, Dentsply; Diaket, 3M/ESPE; Resilon-epiphany, Resilon Research LLC)

Table 2.6.2 Composition of a zinc oxide–eugenol cement based on Rickert's formulation

Powder	%	Liquid	%
Zinc oxide	34–41	Oil of cloves	78–80
Silver	25–30	Canada balsam	20–22
Oleoresin	16–30		
Dithymoliodide	11–13		

Table 2.6.3 Composition of Grossman's Sealer (Grossman)

Powder	%	Liquid	%
Zinc oxide	42	Eugenol	100
Staybelite resin	27		
Bismuth subcarbonate	15		
Barium sulphate	15		
Sodium borate	1		

Table 2.6.4 Composition of Tubli-seal (Kerr Mf. Co., USA)

Base	%	Catalyst
Zinc oxide	57–59	Eugenol
Oleoresin	18–21	Polymerized resin
Bismuth trioxide	7.5	Annidalin
Thymol iodide	3–5	
Oils and waxes	10	

Table 2.6.5 Composition of AH Plus (Dentsply De Trey GmbH, Germany)

Paste A	Paste B
Epoxy resin	1-adamantane amine
Calcium tungstate	N,N′-Dibenzyl-5-oxanonane-diamine-1,9
Zirconium oxide	Tricyclodecane (TCD)-diamine
Aerosil	Calcium tungstate
Iron oxide	Zirconium oxide
	Aerosil
	Silicone oil

- calcium-hydroxide-containing cements (e.g. Apexit, Ivoclar; Sealapex, Kerr)
- GICs (e.g. Ketac Endo, 3M/ESPE; Endion, Voco)
- polydimethyl siloxanes (e.g. RSA RoekoSeal, Roeko)
- MTA (e.g. Pro-Root MTA, Dentsply).

First, the composition of the most widely used sealer, zinc oxide–eugenol cements, will be described. Then, the characteristics which make them suitable as sealers will be discussed, and finally, the clinical data on their performance will be assessed.

Zinc oxide–eugenol-based cements

There are many cements based on zinc oxide, used with eugenol, to which are added a variety of other substances to modify them for use as root canal sealers (see Chapter 2.4). There are three major reasons for the additives in root canal sealers:

- to impart bacteriocidal properties
- to increase their radiopacity
- to improve the adhesion to the canal wall.

As with zinc oxide–eugenol cements used for cavity liners and temporary fillings, some of the sealers consist of a powder that is mixed with a liquid. The complete list of ingredients of one widely used material (based on a formulation originally proposed by Rickert in 1931) is presented in Table 2.6.2. The powder is predominantly zinc oxide, to which silver is added to increase the radiopacity. The resin acts as a plasticizer and the iodide as an antiseptic agent.

The problem with this formulation is that the silver is prone to causing discoloration of the dentine. This is problematical particularly in the coronal access cavity, and affects the appearance of the tooth. Formulations such as Grossman's Sealer (Table 2.6.3) have replaced the silver with barium or bismuth compounds.

The particle size of the above preparations is fairly large and tends to produce a gritty texture to the resultant mix unless it is thoroughly spatulated. To overcome this, paste–paste systems have been developed and have become very popular. The typical constituents of such a root canal sealer are presented in Table 2.6.4.

Resins

The attraction of resin systems is that these materials can readily be formulated in such a way that they have a rapid setting time and yet maintain a sufficiently long working time. Also, these products do not contain any coarse powders so they have a very smooth texture.

There are two resin systems that have been around sufficiently long for some clinical data to have been gathered on them. These are an epoxy–amine resin (AH Plus, De Trey, Germany) and a polyvinyl resin (DIAKET, 3M/ESPE, Seefeld, Germany). Both have very complex formulations; the composition of AH Plus is shown in Table 2.6.5. The resin sets by an addition polymerization reaction after the two pastes are mixed. The diepoxide, a diglycidyl ether of bisphenol-A, and an amine, either 1-adamantane amine or N,N′-dibenzyl-5-oxanonane-diamine-1,9, react to form oligomers with epoxy and amino end-groups, which can then react with other monomers or oligomers, as shown in a simplified form in Figure 2.6.5. This produces a highly flexible thermoplastic polymer of high dimensional stability, although still subject to polymerization shrinkage. The addition polymerization reaction takes several hours and thus provides a long working time. The radiopaque fillers ensure that the material has a high radiopacity, even when applied in thin layers. Viscosity is controlled by the amount (>76% by weight) and type of filler. Filler particle size averages out at less than 10 µm to ensure a thin film thickness and provide a smooth consistency. The main problem with these resins is the amount of shrinkage that takes place on setting, which can compromise the apical seal.

Calcium-hydroxide-containing cements

Calcium-hydroxide-containing cements are presented in the form of a base paste and catalyst paste, which are mixed in equal amounts. They contain a resin similar to those used in the two-paste resin composites, to which calcium hydroxide is added as a filler in place of the

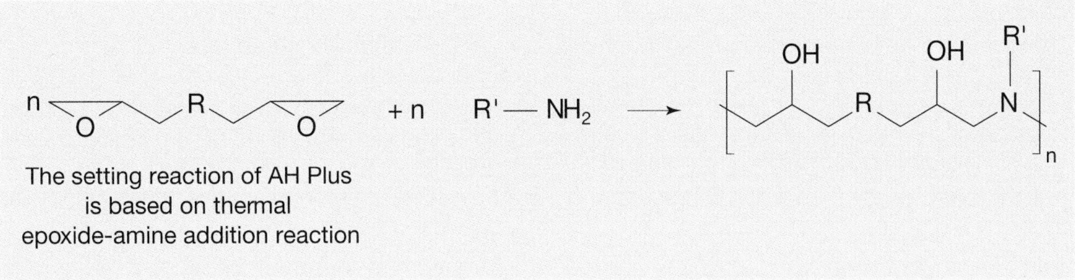

The setting reaction of AH Plus
is based on thermal
epoxide-amine addition reaction

Figure 2.6.5 The setting reaction of AH Plus

Table 2.6.6 Composition of Sealapex (Kerr Mf. Co., USA)

Base paste	%	Catalyst paste	%
Calcium hydroxide	46	Barium sulphate	39
Sulphonamide	38	Resin	33
Zinc oxide	12	Isobutyl salicylate	17
Zinc stearate	2	Colloidal silica	6
Colloidal silica	2	Titanium dioxide	4
		Iron oxide	<1

more usual glass fillers. The composition of one of these materials is presented in Table 2.6.6. As yet, little is known about the clinical performance of these materials. They have long working times and a high pH, which creates a highly alkaline environment where most bacteria will be killed. Biocompatibility is excellent with the formation of a cementum over the apical foramen. One drawback is their high solubility, which has raised concerns about possible coronal or apical micro-leakage after a time.

Glass–ionomer cements

The GICs consist of a fluoro-alumino-silicate glass, which is reacted with a polycarboxylic acid. Since GICs show low shrinkage on setting and possess the virtually unique ability to bond directly to dentine and enamel, these materials should make good root canal sealers. Surprisingly, it was not until the early 1990s that a GIC was developed specifically as a root canal sealant. The GICS used for restorative and lining purposes needed to be modified to deal with a range of problems. These included: too short a working time, difficulty in transporting the material to the root canal, adaptation to the root canal wall, lack of low film thickness, lack of radiopacity and questions about biocompatibility when in contact with the apical tissues. These problems have now been largely overcome by incorporating an X-ray contrasting agent and reducing the glass particle size to less than 25 µm. Some promising results have been obtained with GIC sealers, although working times still tend to be short and retreatment is a problem as the material sets very hard compared to the other root canal sealers.

Polydimethyl siloxanes

This root canal sealer is essentially a variant on the addition-cured polyvinylsiloxane impression materials, consisting of a polydimethylsiloxane, silicone oil, paraffin-base oil, a Pt catalyst and zirconium dioxide (see Chapter 2.7 for details of the setting chemistry). The delivery system ensures a homogeneous mix, free of air bubbles, and the rheology can be carefully controlled by the addition of the appropriate amount of filler. The small filler particle size ensures that this

material has excellent flow properties and can achieve a film thickness of 5 µm, which allows the sealer to flow into tiny crevices and tubules. As with the impression materials, the root canal sealer is insoluble and dimensionally stable, and has excellent biocompatibility. One concern is that this root canal sealer has neither the ability to bond to dentine, nor any antibacterial properties. It relies for its seal on the ability to adapt to the root canal wall and, according to the manufacturer, undergoes a slight expansion (0.2%) on setting. Further studies, especially clinical data, are needed to confirm the suitability of this product as a root canal sealer.

Mineral trioxide aggregate

The main features of MTA have already been described and are the same whether it is used for direct pulp capping or as a root canal sealant.

CLINICAL ASPECTS OF ROOT CANAL MATERIALS

Root-canal materials are in contact with living biological tissue that is not protected by any epithelial layer; therefore, their biocompatibility is of considerable importance. Their physical properties, relevant to the production of an apical seal, are also a major concern.

Biocompatibility

In general, it is assumed that for a material to be biologically acceptable, it must be as inert as possible. However, this is not always the case. In a sense, what is really desired is an interaction between the material and the biological environment that is beneficial to the biological environment and has no adverse effect on the material. This is very different from complete lack of interaction in the case of an inert material. The concern is over the form of the interaction.

When a sealer is placed at the apex of a root canal it will be in contact with vital tissue. It is important that the material does not elicit an inflammatory response in the tissues, as this may induce irritation, pain or tissue necrosis. All of these responses are likely to lead to the loss of the tooth, which is just the opposite of the intended outcome. A possibly beneficial response would be the formation of an intermediate layer of hard tissue that not only isolates the foreign material from the living tissue, but also helps to improve the quality of the apical seal.

A perennial problem in endodontic treatment is the likelihood of recurrent infection due to the presence of bacteria at the apex of the tooth. Thus, another feature one seeks in a root canal sealer is the ability to destroy bacteria.

As might be imagined, it is difficult to reconcile these two requirements, as they would require a high degree of selectivity in the biological response. In general, materials that show antibacterial properties also induce some inflammatory response in the local tissues, while those that do not elicit an inflammatory response are, at best, bacteriostatic.

If it is accepted that a perfect seal *cannot* be achieved, the materials used must have sufficient antibacterial activity to prevent bacteria from infiltrating the canal space and proliferating. However, the antibacterial property of a material should not be achieved at the expense of its biocompatibility.

Gutta percha is a highly biocompatible material, having such a low cytotoxicity that it is the cements that are used with it that will determine the tissue response.

The zinc oxide–eugenol-based cements are all inclined to induce some inflammatory reaction in the tissues, probably due to the presence of free eugenol. It is therefore important that measures are taken to ensure that the cement does not leak beyond the apex and into the vital tissues. Some formulations must be avoided because they contain paraformaldehyde, which may cause a severe inflammatory response, leading to tissue necrosis and bone resorption. Some cements have an incorporated steroid and, again, their use is contraindicated.

The resin systems should have comparatively excellent biocompatibility, as none of them contains the eugenol that contributes to the poor biocompatibility of the zinc oxide cements. Resins are known to be slightly toxic during the setting period but, once they have fully set, any inflammation rapidly recedes. The moderate cytotoxic response of freshly prepared AH26 may be associated with the release of formaldehyde, which is produced as a by-product of the setting process. Since AH26 takes some time to set, a certain degree of sensitivity may be associated with the use of this sealer. AH Plus has been shown to release only a tiny amount of formaldehyde (3.9 ppm), as compared with AH26 (1347 ppm). Nevertheless, AH26 has been shown to be cytotoxic, although this is much reduced after the material has set. In comparison, Diaket retains a degree of cytotoxicity even after it has set.

For the calcium-hydroxide-containing resins it is claimed that, in addition to the excellent biocompatibility, the material promotes cementum formation, similar to that observed for the pulp-capping agents based on calcium hydroxide.

Sealing properties

One of the difficulties in interpreting the information available on sealing properties is the lack of any standardized approach to the methods of measurement adopted, as this limits the value of the data available. This is particularly so for studies of the sealing properties, whether in vivo or in vitro, where so many methods have been used that direct comparison is unreliable, and only a general assessment is possible.

First, it is noticeable that there is no immediate distinction between the zinc oxide–eugenol cements and the resin-based materials. It would seem that some zinc oxide–eugenol cements are better than one or other resin system and that others are worse.

However, it should be appreciated that so much depends on the technique adopted that an acceptable result can most probably be obtained with any of them. As already noted, it is probably more important that an antibacterial seal is achieved than a physical seal, although both would be desirable. A physical seal by itself may not be good enough if the sealant does not provide an antibacterial barrier.

Physical properties

Since the results of endodontic treatment are so dependent on the operator, it is important to choose a material which has the handling characteristics that most suit the particular individual. The working and setting times and flows of the cements determine their handling

characteristics, while the film thickness, the solubility and the dimensional stability are important factors in determining their sealing ability.

Rickert's cement has a working time of some 15 minutes; it flows readily but is inclined to have a thick film width due to the gritty nature of the powder. Grossman's sealer has a working time of 1 hour and also shows good flow; its solubility is lower than that of Rickert's cement. Tubli-seal is a two-paste cement; it has a short working time (20 minutes), combined with good flow and a low film thickness.

The resin sealer Diaket has a very rapid set, and is sticky, viscous and difficult to manipulate. In comparison, AH Plus has a much longer working time, a better flow and lower film thickness. Once set, both of these materials are virtually insoluble.

The calcium-hydroxide-filled resins have good handling characteristics, but still require some clinical evaluation before they can be recommended for general use. The same applies to the glass–ionomer and the polyvinyl siloxane root canal sealer.

CLINICAL SIGNIFICANCE

Despite the introduction of a wide variety of root canal sealers, the preferred material among endodontists continues to be the zinc oxide–eugenol cement sealer.

SUMMARY

The ideal of a hermetic seal of the root apex has been abandoned in favour of an antibacterial seal for most of the root canal sealers. Perhaps only the GICs, with their intrinsic dentine-bonding capability, can possibly achieve a hermetic seal. For the present, the view is that an antibacterial seal can be achieved only by the combined use of gutta percha obturating points and root canal sealer cements. There are many cements to choose from and the paste–paste systems are the most popular.

Failure can be due to the presence of residual bacteria as a result of inadequate chemomechanical debridement, especially in inaccessible canals in multi-rooted teeth, and in unsealed lateral canals, or due to the coronal ingress of bacteria. With the currently available materials, it should be possible to obtain an adequate antibacterial seal.

POST AND CORE SYSTEMS

Extensive loss of tooth structure often requires endodontic treatment and, as a consequence, little may be left of the tooth crown. It is generally believed that, to rebuild such a tooth, there is a need for some form of reinforcement for the core. The most commonly used methods for reinforcing badly broken down and endodontically treated teeth are pin-retained cores or post and core systems (Figure 2.6.6). However, with regard to post and core systems, there has been passive acceptance of traditional concepts that have surprisingly little backing; more and more, the status quo is being challenged and some dentists are now asking if a post is really necessary. The factor that weakens the tooth is simply the extensive removal of tooth tissue. It is not a consequence of embrittlement of the dentine, as was once thought, since the root dentine does not significantly change in properties. The fractures often associated with endodontically treated teeth are simply a consequence of the removal of tooth tissue, weakening the tooth structure such that it is no longer able to withstand the forces exerted on it. Although one will often see the post and core system referred

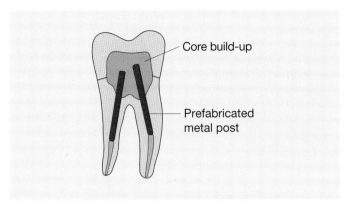

Figure 2.6.6 A post and core restored tooth

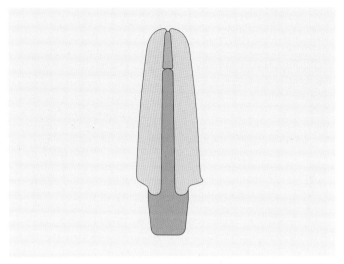

Figure 2.6.7 A cast post and core with ferrule, which is a lip of metal extending back over the preparation

to as a means of strengthening the tooth, this is possibly only the case when the post and core are effectively bonded to the tooth tissues such that the structural integrity of the tooth is improved. It is debatable how many, if any, of the current systems can claim to provide this benefit. Hence the function of a post and core system is not primarily to strengthen the tooth but to provide support for the retention of crown or other coronal superstructure, when a significant amount of coronal tooth structure has been lost. If there is sufficient remaining coronal tooth structure, then there really is no need for a post and core build-up. However, if most of the supragingival tooth structure is missing, then a post and a core becomes a prerequisite to crown preparation for anterior teeth; posteriorly, it may still be possible to use a pin-retained core.

The desirable features of a post and core system are that:

* the system provides maximum retention with minimal removal of tooth tissue
* the core provides a means of transferring stress from the restoration to the post and tooth
* the post is able to transfer the stresses to the remaining tooth structure without creating high stresses that may otherwise cause the tooth to fracture
* the post is retrievable in the case of failure
* the post and core system is aesthetically compatible with the restoration.

Types of post system

Posts are either prefabricated or cast. In the case of the prefabricated post, the core can be built up with one of a range of core materials (amalgam, composite, GIC, RMGIC). For the cast post, it is usual to use a prefabricated plastic blank, and the core can be incorporated with the blank such that the post and core are cast as a single unit. Whereas, at one time, a cast post and core would have been the system of choice, these days many dentists prefer some form of prefabricated post. The advantage is that the procedure is much quicker, simpler and cheaper than providing a cast system. The latter takes two appointments to complete and also requires the production of temporary restorations. However, cast post and core systems act as a single unit and can be cast with a ferrule (Figure 2.6.7), which supports the tooth against wedging forces and helps to prevent tooth fracture.

Prefabricated posts

The types of prefabricated posts available are:

* metal posts
* fibre-reinforced resin posts
* ceramic posts.

Metal posts

Metal prefabricated posts are made from stainless steel, nickel-chromium or titanium. The choice of these metals reflects the desire to use metals that have good corrosion resistance and a high yield strength. The posts come in a wide variety of designs, which include:

* non-threaded parallel-sided posts (e.g. Para-Post, Whaledent)
* non-threaded tapered posts (e.g. Endo-Post, Kerr)
* threaded parallel-sided posts (e.g. Kurer Anchor System, Teledyne)
* threaded tapered posts (e.g. Dentatus Screw Post, Dentatus).

It is impossible in a textbook such as this to cover in detail all the different designs of post systems that are available. Briefly, the post should be as long as possible without infringing on the apical 4–5 mm of the root canal seal. The post diameter should be as thin as possible to minimize removal of tooth tissue while also being sufficiently strong not to fracture itself. At the same time, the post should be stiff enough not to flex, as this will compromise the marginal seal. Increasing the post diameter will weaken the tooth and make it more liable to fracture. Retentive features, such as threads or surface roughening, can help but it should be noted that threads can give rise to local stress concentrations, which can contribute to tooth fracture. In this context, self-threading posts have excellent retention but are also associated with a high incidence of tooth fracture. Tapered posts are the least retentive; the greater the taper, the greater the possibility of root fracture due to a wedging effect.

Fibre-reinforced resin posts

Fibre-reinforced epoxy resin composite materials are increasingly finding a place in restorative dentistry and endodontics is no exception. The fibres are aligned in the long direction of the post, which provides strength and yet does not compromise the flexibility of the post. At present, there are two types of fibre-reinforced resin post system:

* carbon-fibre-reinforced posts (e.g. Composipost and Aestheti Post from RTD, Meylon, France; Carbonite from Harald Nordon SA, Montreux, Switzerland)
* glass-fibre-reinforced posts (e.g. Snowpost from Carbotech, Ganges, France; Parapost Fiber White from Coltene/Whaledent, New Jersey, USA; Aestheti Plus Post from RTD, Meylon, France; Glassix from Harald Nordon SA, Montreux, Switzerland).

The use of a resin matrix means that the post has the potential to be bonded to the remaining tooth structure and, in turn, the core can be bonded to the post. This, it is claimed, will improve the structural integrity of the tooth root and thus, unlike the metal posts, provide a stronger support structure for the crown with less chance of root fractures. This alters the requirements of the posts compared to metal posts, since the system acts as a single unit for supporting the crown. Whereas, in the case of metal posts, a high stiffness is important in preventing bending, as noted earlier, in the case of fibre-reinforced resin composite posts, the aim is to produce a restoration that, being bonded, acts as a homogeneous unit. The way to achieve this is to use a material with an elastic modulus similar to that of dentine. This would allow a more even stress distribution and should reduce the incidence of tooth fractures.

The carbon-fibre-reinforced posts are black, unless specifically coated to mask the black colour, as in the case of the Aestheti Post (RTD, Meylon, France). Glass-fibre-reinforced posts have the advantage that, being essentially white or white/translucent, they can produce superior aesthetic results when used in conjunction with all-ceramic restorations.

Ceramic posts

From the point of view of aesthetics, ceramic posts would seem to show considerable promise. Hence manufacturers have started recently to produce ceramic posts as an alternative to the white-fibre-reinforced posts. One of the materials that has become popular for such posts is zirconia because of its reputed high strength and toughness and its white appearance. Current systems include the Cosmopost (Ivoclar-Vivadent, Liechtenstein), the Biopost (Incermed, Lausanne, Switzerland) and the Cerapost (Brassler, Lemgo, Germany). However, the chemical inertness of zirconia is a potential problem with regard to retention and these systems must rely on mechanical means of retention. Dislodgement of the posts can occur due to rotation of the crown, resulting in torsional stresses. Zirconia posts have a lack of torsional resistance due to a lack of bonding, whereas the lack of torsional resistance in a fibre-reinforced post arises from the lack of stiffness of the post. As yet, information in these post systems is still very scarce.

CLINICAL SIGNIFICANCE

With the increasing use of all-ceramic restorations, it is likely that the demand for aesthetic post and core systems will increase significantly.

SUMMARY

Relative to the metal posts, both the fibre-reinforced and ceramic posts are new additions for the treatment of badly broken-down teeth. Considerably more knowledge and experience, both in vitro and in vivo, of the use of these materials is required before they can be accepted as readily as the metal post systems.

FURTHER READING

Anon (2000) New developments in fiber post systems. Am J Dent **13(special issue)**: 1B–24B

Asmussen E, Peutzfeldt A, Heitmann T (1999) Stiffness, elastic limit, and strength of newer types of endodontic posts. J Dent **27**: 275–278

Browne RM (1988) The *in vitro* assessment of the cytotoxicity of dental materials – does it have a role? Int Endod J **21**: 50–58

Camillera J, Montesin FE, Brady K et al (2005) The constitution of mineral trioxide aggregate. Dent Mater **21**: 297

Cox CF, Hafez AA (2001) Biocomposition and reaction of pulp tissues to restorative treatments. Dent Clin N Amer **45**: 31–48

Dammaschke T, Gerth HU, Züchner H et al (2005) Chemical and physical surface and bulk material characterization of white ProRoot MTA and two Portland cements. Dent Mater **21**: 731

Foreman PC, Barnes IE (1990) A review of calcium hydroxide. Int Endod J **23**: 283–297

Freedman GA (2001) Esthetic post-and-core treatment. Dent Clin N Amer **45(1)**: 103–116

Nair PNR, Duncan HF, Pitt Ford TR et al (2008) Histological, ultrastructural and quantitative investigations on the response of healthy human pulps to experimental capping with mineral trioxide aggregate: a randomized controlled trial. Int J Endod **41**: 128–150

Olsson H, Petersson K, Rohlin M (2006) Formation of hard tissue barrier after pulp capping in humans: a systematic review. Int Endod J **39**: 429–442

Orstavik D (1988) Antibacterial properties of endodontic materials. Int Endod J **21**: 161–169

Paque F, Sirtes G (2007) Apical sealing ability of Resilon/Epiphany versus gutta-percha/ AH Plus: immediate and 16-months leakage. Int Endod Journal **40**: 722–729

Pitt-Ford TR, Rowe AHR (1989) A new root canal sealer based on calcium hydroxide. J Endod **15**: 286–289

Stanley HR (1998) Criteria for standardizing and increasing credibility of direct pulp capping studies. Am J Dent **11**: Spec No: S17–34

Tobias RS (1988) Antibacterial properties of dental restorative materials – a review. Int Endod J **21**: 155–160

Watts A, Paterson RC, Cohen BD et al (1994) Pulp response to a novel adhesive calcium hydroxide based cement. Eur J Prosthodont Rest Dent **3**: 27–32

Impression materials

INTRODUCTION

Impression materials are used to produce a detailed replica of the teeth and the tissues of the oral cavity. From this replica, or impression, a model can be made that is used in the construction of full dentures, partial dentures, crowns, bridges and inlays.

Over the years, a wide variety of impression materials and associated techniques have been developed, all striving to achieve the optimum in desirable characteristics. The impression materials can be classified in terms of rigid and elastic impression materials (Table 2.7.1).

The rigid impression materials cannot engage undercuts that may be present on the teeth or the bone. Consequently, their use is restricted to edentulous patients without bony undercuts.

The elastic impression materials are subdivided into *hydrocolloid* and *elastomeric* impression materials. Both are able to engage undercuts and may be used in edentulous, partially dentate and fully dentate patients. The choice will depend on the particular requirements of each individual case.

The choice of impression material may also be affected by the technique to be adopted, with a major consideration being the selection of a stock tray or special tray. These trays are needed to support the impression material (especially when it is still fluid), so that it can be carried to the patient, inserted in the mouth, and removed once it is set. The trays also provide support when the model is poured from the impression.

The variety of applications of and techniques used with the impression materials are presented in Table 2.7.2. The choice of impression tray is determined, to some extent, by the viscosity of the impression material.

An impression material that is very fluid when it is first mixed cannot be used with a stock tray, and a close-fitting special tray needs to be produced. This can be done either by constructing an acrylic special tray from a preliminary model, or by using a high-viscosity material, which is placed in a stock tray; once this has set, a special tray is produced. Some impression materials are not available in a sufficiently high-viscosity version for use in a stock tray, and these include zinc oxide–eugenol, polyether and polysulphide elastomers. Others, such as impression compound (compo), plaster of Paris,

alginate and the silicones are available in formulations that *can* be used with a stock tray. Although compo can be used in a stock tray, the impression obtained does not reproduce surface details adequately unless a zinc oxide–eugenol wash is used with it. Similarly, alginates, when used in a stock tray, do not always give the required degree of accuracy and are then better used in a special tray.

CLINICAL SIGNIFICANCE

The choice of impression material and the type of tray to use will depend on the accuracy and the reproduction of the surface detail that is required.

REQUIREMENTS OF AN IMPRESSION MATERIAL

Some of the requirements of an impression material have already been touched on in the above discussion and now need to be defined more explicitly. The important characteristics of impression materials can be identified from the point of view of the patient or the dentist (Table 2.7.3).

Accurate reproduction of surface detail

The accuracy of reproduction of the surface detail depends on the viscosity of the mix and the ability of the impression material to adapt closely to both the soft and the hard tissues. A low viscosity is therefore desirable, but it should not be so low that the material is not easily contained within the impression tray.

Some materials are hydrophobic (water-repellent) and will be repelled by moisture on the surface. If this should happen in a critical area, then important surface detail may be lost as a blow hole is formed on the impression surface due to trapped air. A dry field is essential for such materials. If this is not feasible, an alternative material must be used that is compatible with moisture and saliva.

There are instances in which the patient will have mobile soft tissues. This occurs particularly with edentulous patients, who can present with a flabby ridge. If the impression material is very stiff, it may displace such tissues and produce a distorted impression. When this is reproduced in the prosthesis, the soft tissues will need to adapt to the prosthesis rather than the other way round; this will cause discomfort to the patient. Such impression materials are classed as being muco-compressive.

Ideally, the impression material to be used should be sufficiently fluid on placement to prevent displacement of the soft tissues, with such materials being considered to be mucostatic.

Dimensional accuracy and stability

These are dependent on the factors outlined below.

Type of tray

If the tray is prone to distortion, then the resultant model poured from such a tray will also be distorted. Hence, highly flexible trays should be avoided. A good bond between the tray and the impression material is very important. If the impression material comes away from the tray, this will again distort the impression. Manufacturers of impression materials will supply a suitable adhesive for their material to ensure a good bond. It is important that the manufacturer's instructions are followed to the letter; otherwise failure of the adhesive bond

may result. Additional retention may be achieved by the use of perforated trays.

Shrinkage of the impression material

Whether the impression material sets by a chemical reaction or some change in physical state, both usually result in some shrinkage of the impression material. Provided the impression material is firmly adhered to the tray, this increases the space previously occupied by the hard or soft tissues. In the case of a simple crown preparation, the result is a die which is slightly larger than the original tooth preparation (Figure 2.7.1). If the contraction of the impression material is excessive, this will result in a loosely fitting crown. Should the impression material expand on setting, then the opposite problem of a tightly fitting crown would result, with too little space for the cement that is needed to hold it in place.

In addition to the changes in dimensions on setting, there is also a slight thermal contraction of the impression material as it cools from mouth to room temperature. The coefficient of thermal expansion of both the tray and the impression material needs to be small. Ideally, an impression material should show a very small contraction (<0.5%), as this will result in the production of a crown that is slightly larger than the situation that it is designed for. This will provide the necessary space for the cement that is to be used.

Permanent set

When an impression is taken of a dentate patient, there will be undercuts due to the bulbous shapes of the tooth crowns. In this case, the impression material must be sufficiently flexible to allow removal from the undercut regions without causing distortion; rigid impression materials would therefore be unsuitable. The elastic impression materials must then be used, but, as most are actually viscoelastic materials (see Chapter 1.6), there is a possibility of some permanent deformation.

Storage stability

There is usually a significant delay between the taking of an impression and its arrival in the dental laboratory where the model is poured. It is important that the impression material neither shrinks nor expands nor distorts during this time period.

Impression technique

In the case of silicone impression materials in particular, there are a number of impression techniques that can be employed. It is

Table 2.7.1 Categorization of impression materials
Rigid
Plaster
Compo/zinc oxide–eugenol
Elastic
Hydrocolloid
Agar (reversible)
Alginate (irreversible)
Elastomeric
Polysulphide
Polyether
Silicone (condensation-cured)
Silicone (addition-cured)

Table 2.7.2 Indirect impression techniques

Application	Choice of material	Impression technique	Choice of viscosity	Type of tray
Full dentures	Plaster of Paris	Single stage	–	Stock/special
	Zinc oxide–eugenol	Single stage	–	Special
	Compo/zinc oxide–eugenol	Two stage	–	Stock
	Alginate	Single stage	–	Stock/special
Partial dentures	Alginate	Single	–	Stock/special
	Elastomers	Single	Medium	Special
Crowns, bridges and inlays	Compo	Copper ring	–	–
	Elastomer	Single	Medium	Special tray
		Twin mix	Heavy/light Putty/wash	Special tray Stock tray
		Two stage	Heavy/light Putty/wash	Special tray Stock tray

Table 2.7.3 Requirements of an impression material	
The patient	**The dentist**
Neutral taste and odour	Easily mixed
Short setting time	Short working time
Small tray	Easily removed
Easily removed	Good-quality impression
Non-toxic	Low-cost materials
	Easily disinfected

Table 2.7.4 Coefficient of expansion of waxes			
Source	**Name**	**Temperature range (°C)**	**Coefficient of expansion (ppm/°C)**
Mineral	Paraffin	20–28	307
		28–34	1631
Plant	Carnauba	22–52	156
Insect	Beeswax	22–41	344
		41–50	1048

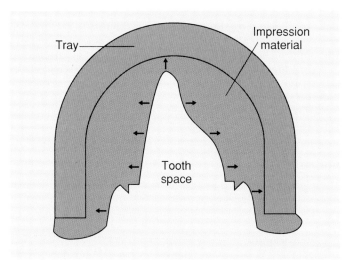

Figure 2.7.1 Shrinkage of the impression material towards the tray resulting in the production of a model which is slightly larger than the original preparation

important that the appropriate technique is used for each material. This will be dealt with later, in the discussion of the silicone impression materials.

CLINICAL SIGNIFICANCE

Impression materials have to comply with a very wide range of requirements and it is perhaps not surprising that there are so many on the market.

RIGID IMPRESSION MATERIALS

Impression compound (compo)

Impression compound is a thermoplastic material with a glass transition temperature of about 55–60°C. Above its glass transition temperature it becomes soft and will take up a new form. On cooling to mouth temperature, it hardens and can be removed, retaining an impression of the oral cavity. Thus, no chemical reaction is involved in the use of this material.

Composition

The composition of impression compounds tends to vary from product to product and is usually a trade secret. They consist of a combination of resins and waxes, plasticizers and fillers, each having a specific function:

- *Resins and waxes.* Resins are amorphous organic substances that are insoluble in water. Typical naturally occurring resins used in impression compound are shellac, dammar, rosin or sandarac. Some recent products use synthetic resins (e.g. coumerone indene) to give greater control and consistency of the composition. Waxes are straight-chain hydrocarbons of the general formula $CH_3(CH_2)_n CH_3$, where n is between 15 and 42. They are characteristically tasteless, odourless, colourless and greasy to the touch. Waxes used in impression compound include beeswax and colophony.
- *Plasticizers.* The waxes and resin, if used on their own, would tend to produce a brittle material with a tendency towards tackiness. The brittleness is overcome by the addition of plasticizers, such as gutta percha and now, more commonly, stearic acid.
- *Fillers.* To overcome the tackiness, control the degree of flow and minimize shrinkage due to thermal contraction, a filler is added. Commonly used fillers are calcium carbonate and limestone. The fillers also improve the rigidity of this impression material.

Properties

Impression compound is muco-compressive, as it is the most viscous of the impression materials used. This can present particular problems in those patients who have a flabby mandibular ridge.

Compo is rigid once cooled and therefore cannot be used to record undercuts. It has a high viscosity, so reproduction of surface detail is not very good. However, the reproduction can be improved by reheating the surface of the impression material after taking the first impression and then reseating it in the patient's mouth. Even then, the surface detail is not as good as can be achieved with virtually all of the other impression materials. It is therefore better to use compo as a simple and quick means of producing a special tray, and then use a wash of zinc oxide–eugenol to provide the surface detail.

The coefficient of thermal expansion of resins and waxes is very high, as indicated in Table 2.7.4, and are highly non-linear within the temperature range of dental interest (Figure 2.7.2). Shrinkage is in the order of 1.5%, and is due to the thermal contraction from mouth to room temperature.

The material has poor dimensional stability and the model must be poured as soon as possible after the impression is taken; this should take place within 1 hour.

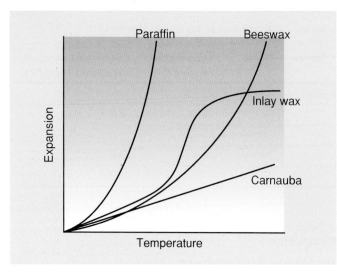

Figure 2.7.2 Thermal expansion of waxes

The thermal conductivity of impression compound is very low, meaning that, on softening, the outside will always soften first. This can give the impression that the material is ready for use when the inside might still be quite hard. Differential expansion gives rise to internal strains, which relieve themselves in due course by distortion of the impression. Thus, the material must be placed in the water bath to allow sufficient time for it to achieve a uniform temperature. Even then, internal strains will inevitably build up during cooling, and will eventually give rise to distortion, which is why the model must be poured as soon as possible.

Application

Its main application is for recording preliminary impressions of edentulous arches. This gives a model on which a special tray can be constructed, and which can subsequently be used with a low-viscosity impression material (such as zinc oxide–eugenol) for recording the fine surface detail (see below). The material is used relatively little these days, as other impression materials are preferred.

Zinc oxide–eugenol paste

Whereas there are many zinc oxide–eugenol products that are presented as powder–liquid systems, the impression material is in the form of two pastes. There is typically a *base paste* consisting of zinc oxide, olive oil, linseed oil, zinc acetate and a trace of water, and a *reactor paste*, consisting of eugenol and fillers, such as kaolin and talc.

Zinc oxide and eugenol are the reactive components that take part in the setting reaction (see Chapter 2.4). The water initiates the setting reaction, and the zinc acetate is present to speed up the setting process. The oils and fillers are inert substances, which allow the material to be used in a paste–paste formulation, and help to provide the appropriate handling characteristics.

Properties

The liquid is very fluid, i.e. mucostatic, and, being a water-based system, readily adapts to the soft tissues. It therefore provides a detailed reproduction of the soft tissues without causing displacement

of the soft tissues, but is rigid once set and is thus unable to record undercuts. This limits its application to the edentulous mouth, where it is used with a special tray.

It has the advantage of being dimensionally stable and shows little shrinkage on setting. However, as it is used with a special tray, the tray may impose limitations on the dimensional stability of the whole impression.

Although the material is non-toxic, eugenol can cause a burning sensation in the patient's mouth and leave a persistent taste that the patient may find unpleasant. The paste tends to adhere to skin, so the skin around the lips should be protected with petroleum jelly.

Impression plaster

Presentation and composition

Impression plaster consists of a powder to which water is added to produce a smooth paste. The composition of the powder is similar to that of the model materials discussed in more detail in Chapter 3.1, as is the setting process. The impression material consists typically of calcium sulphate β-hemihydrate $(CaSO_4)_2 \cdot H_2O$, potassium sulphate to reduce the expansion, borax to reduce the rate of setting, and starch to help disintegration of the impression on separation from the plaster/stone model.

Properties

The impression plaster is easy to mix, but great care must be taken to avoid trapping air bubbles, as these will give rise to surface inaccuracies. The material has well-controlled working and setting characteristics, which are governed by the relative amounts of borax and potassium sulphate.

The amount of potassium sulphate is generally more than would be found in model plaster, as for impressions the expansion must be kept to a minimum. Since the potassium sulphate also acts as an accelerator of the set, borax is needed to counteract it. The working time is of the order of 2–3 minutes, as is the setting time.

The mixed material has a very low viscosity, and so is mucostatic. It is hydrophilic and thus adapts readily to the soft tissues, recording their surface detail with great accuracy. The material is best used in a special tray, made of acrylic or shellac, to a thickness of 1.0–1.5 mm. Alternatively, it can be used as a wash with a compo special tray.

The dimensional stability of impression plaster is very good, so a time delay in pouring the model is of no consequence, although extremes of temperature should be avoided. A separating medium (usually a solution of sodium alginate) must be used between the model plaster and the impression plaster.

The material is rigid once set and thus unable to record undercuts. This limits its application to the edentulous patient.

From the patient's point of view it is not an unpleasant material, although it tends to leave a sensation of dryness in the mouth for some time after the impression has been taken.

ELASTIC IMPRESSION MATERIALS

The first elastic dental impression material was the hydrocolloid, which was introduced to dentistry in 1925. Since then, many elastomeric impression materials have become available, as indicated on the following time line:

Figure 2.7.3 The structure of a polysaccharide

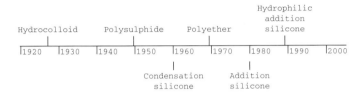

Colloids

The word colloid is derived from the word *kola*, meaning glue, and *oid*, meaning like. Thus a colloid has a glue-like physical character.

The colloidal state represents a highly dispersed phase of fine particles within another phase, somewhere between a solution and a suspension:

- A solution is a homogeneous mixture consisting of a single phase.
- A suspension is a mixture of two distinct phases.
- A colloid is a heterogeneous mixture of two phases, where the two phases are not readily differentiated.

The difference between a colloid and a suspension is that in a colloid the dispersed phase is not readily detectable microscopically. Examples of colloids in dental use are:

- colloidal silica in resin
- droplets of oil in the water supply to handpieces
- fillers in impression materials.

The size of the finely dispersed phase cannot easily be defined accurately, but it is slightly greater than the simple molecular size, usually in the range of 1–500 nm.

The colloid can exist in the form of a viscous liquid, known as a *sol*, or a solid, described as a *gel*. If the particles are suspended in water, then the suspension is called a *hydrocolloid*, with the liquid being a *hydrosol* and the solid a *hydrogel*. In the case of the hydrogel, there is an entanglement network of solid particles with the liquid trapped in the interstices. The solid particles are in the form of fibrils or chains of molecules.

The hydrocolloid impression materials come in two forms:

- reversible, e.g. agar
- irreversible, e.g. alginate.

Agar

Agar is a galactose sulphate, which forms a colloid with water. It liquefies between 71 °C and 100 °C and sets to gel again between 30 °C and 50 °C. It is a long-chain molecule, with a molecular weight of approximately 150 000. The structure of this polysaccharide is shown in Figure 2.7.3. The hydroxyl (OH) groups undergo hydrogen bonding, leading to the formation of a helical structure.

When heated, this hydrogen bond is broken, the helix is uncoiled and the gel is turned into a viscous fluid. This process is therefore reversible in the manner shown below:

$$\text{gel} \xrightarrow[\text{heating}]{} \text{sol} \xrightarrow[\text{cooling}]{} \text{gel}$$

These materials are analogous to thermoplastics and have the advantage that they can be used repeatedly.

The agar is heated in a water bath until it becomes fluid. It is placed in a special metal tray through which water can be passed when it is placed in the patient's mouth. The water cools the agar, whereupon it resolidifies as a gel, having taken up the shape of the oral tissues.

Composition

The composition and purpose of the various ingredients of a typical agar impression material are as shown in Table 2.7.5. As can be seen from the composition, only a small amount of agar is needed to form a gel.

Presentation and application

The material is provided in tube-like sachets for loading the tray, or in a syringe for easy adaptation to the teeth. The agar content of the syringe-applied material is lower than that of the tray material, so it is more fluid and easy to eject from the syringe and inject around the teeth.

When immersed in a temperature-controlled water bath, the material turns into a viscous liquid after approximately 8–12 minutes, and can be left for several hours. It is important that the material is not overheated, as this will cause breakdown of the polymer.

The water bath usually consists of three compartments, each held at a different temperature. One compartment contains water near its boiling point and is used for liquefying the agar. A second compartment is kept at 63–66 °C for storing the agar. The third compartment is kept at 46 °C and is used for tempering the agar after it is placed in the special water-cooled tray. This compartment is necessary to ensure that the agar is cooled to a temperature that the patient finds acceptable, and that will not burn the tissues. Due to the relatively small amount used, the syringe-applied material does not require tempering and can be kept in the storage compartment.

The contents of the tube are squeezed into an impression tray and placed in the tempering bath. Once the agar has cooled sufficiently, which takes about 2 minutes, the tray is placed in the patient's mouth. The water supply is connected only at this stage.

141

Table 2.7.5 Composition of an agar impression material

Component	Amount (%)	Purpose
Agar	12.5	Dispersed phase
Borax	0.2	Strengthens gel
Potassium sulphate	1.7	Accelerator for model
Alkyl benzoate	0.1	Prevents mould
Dyes and flavouring	Trace	Appearance and taste
Water	85.5	Continuous phase

The temperature of the water for the water-cooled tray should be around 13°C, so as to be comfortable for the patient; if it is too cold, the resultant thermal shock can cause considerable pain and discomfort. The water is allowed to circulate through the tray and after about 5 minutes the agar will have solidified. The tray can now be removed from the patient's mouth and an accurate reproduction of the tissues obtained.

Should the material not be used, for whatever reason, it can be used again at a later date. The time required to reliquefy the material may be somewhat longer and can add up to 4 minutes to the process. Each time the material is heated, it will cause some breakdown of the polymer structure and the agar will become noticeably stiffer. Thus, it should not be reheated more than four times.

Properties

As it is a highly fluid liquid when placed in the mouth and adapts readily to the contours of the hard and soft tissues because of its hydrophilic nature, this material provides very accurate reproduction of surface detail. In addition, the material closest to the water-cooled tray gels first, while the material in contact with the tissues stays liquid longest and can compensate for any inaccuracies due to shrinkage or unintentional movement of the tray.

The model should be poured from the impression immediately, and should this not be possible, the impression material should be kept at a relative humidity of 100% by wrapping it in a wet towel. In any case, the model needs to be poured within 1 hour as the material suffers from two potential problems:

1. Syneresis. This is a process whereby water is forced out on to the surface of the impression as the gel molecules are drawn closer together, with the main driving force being the relief of internal stresses. The water evaporates from the surface and causes the impression material to shrink.
2. Imbibition. This is the uptake of water that occurs if the material has become dry, possibly due to inadequate storage technique. Distortion of the impression will result if this occurs, as the internal stresses that are always present are relieved during this process.

The material can readily be removed from undercuts, but great care must be exercised as it tears very easily and does not bond to the stock tray. Although the tray is perforated, there is always the possibility that some separation occurs when dealing with an oral anatomy that has severe undercuts.

The material is highly viscoelastic, so it is important that the tray is removed by a rapid snap action so that a near-elastic response results. This applies equally to many of the other polymer-based impression materials. It is necessary to have a reasonable thickness of the impression material to limit the extent of the deformation arising on the removal from an undercut.

The borax in the material, which is present to control the pH, has the adverse effect of reacting with the model material and thus slowing down its setting behaviour; this can result in a soft surface to the model. Potassium sulphate is added in order to avoid this.

The material is non-toxic and is non-irritant to the patient, provided the recommended procedure is followed carefully. It is relatively cheap, and is used in some laboratories for making duplicate models, as it can be recycled up to four times.

There are some disadvantages with the agar impression materials, in that one needs special equipment such as water-cooled trays and a temperature-controlled bath, and there is an initial cost in providing this equipment. Also, the water-cooled tray is very bulky, which may cause some discomfort to the patient. Whilst the material can, in principle, be recycled, in these days of cross-infection concerns this is no longer viable. Also, great care must be exercised that the water baths are not contaminated. For these reasons, this impression material is now relatively little used.

Alginates

The alginates are based on alginic acid, which is derived from a marine plant. The structure of alginic acid is quite complex and is shown in Figure 2.7.4. Some of the hydrogen molecules on the carboxyl groups are replaced by sodium, thus forming a water-soluble salt, with a molecular weight of 20000 to 200000. The setting process in this material is by the creation of cross-links between the polymer chains of the sodium alginate. The composition of a typical alginate impression material is presented in Table 2.7.6.

Setting process

When mixed with water, a chemical reaction occurs that cross-links the polymer chain, forming a three-dimensional network structure. As these cross-links cannot be broken once formed, this is an irreversible process, such that the material can only be used once:

$$\text{sol} \xrightarrow{\text{chemical reaction}} \text{gel}$$

Setting reaction

Calcium sulphate dihydrate provides the Ca ions for the cross-linking reaction that converts the sol to a gel. The calcium ions are released from calcium sulphate dihydrate, which is partially soluble in the water:

$$(CaSO_4)\cdot 2H_2O \rightarrow 2Ca^{2+} + 2SO_4^{2-} + H_2O$$

The cross-linking mechanism is shown in Figure 2.7.5 and can be described by the general reaction:

$$Na_nAlg + n/2\, CaSO_4 \rightarrow n/2\, Na_2SO_4 + Ca_{n/2}Alg$$

$$\underset{\text{alginate}}{\text{sodium}} + \underset{\text{dihydrate}}{\underset{\text{sulphate}}{\text{calcium}}} \rightarrow \underset{\text{sulphate}}{\text{sodium}} + \underset{\text{gel}}{\underset{\text{alginate}}{\text{calcium}}}$$

The working and setting times are determined by the rate of release of calcium ions and their availability for cross-linking. Rapid dissolution of the calcium sulphate would give the material an inadequate working time, so, to overcome this, sodium phosphate is added to regulate the initial burst of calcium ions. The sodium phosphate acts as a retarder, and the amount included can be varied to produce regular and fast-setting versions of this impression material. Sodium ions are produced by the following reaction:

$$Na_3PO_4 \rightarrow 3Na^+ + PO_4^{3-}$$

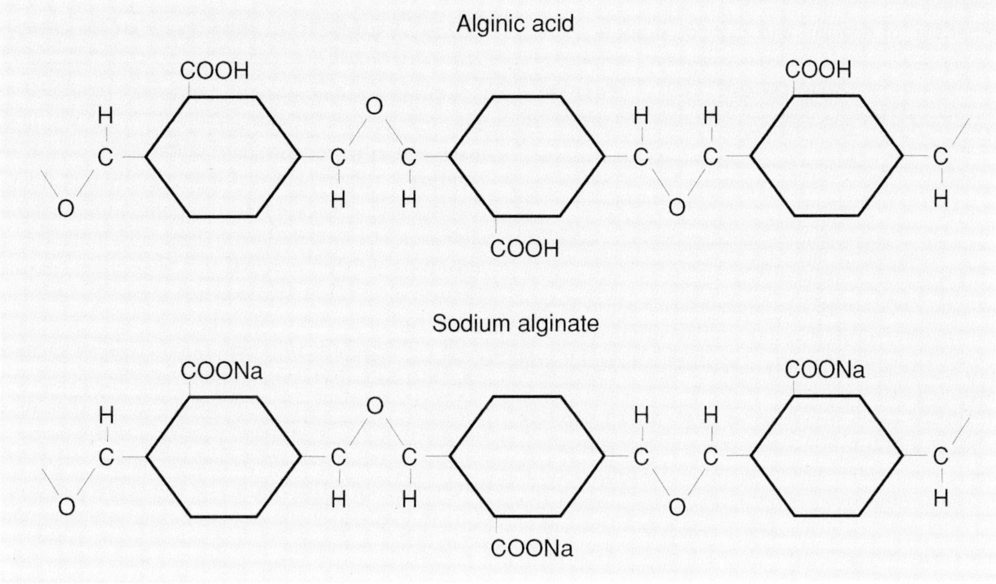

Alginic acid

Sodium alginate

Figure 2.7.4 Structure of sodium alginate with hydrogen ions in alginic acid replaced by sodium ions

Figure 2.7.5 Cross-linking reaction of sodium alginate in the presence of calcium ions

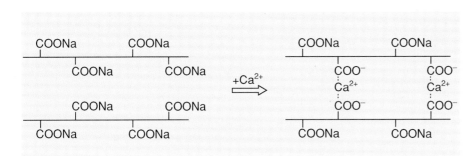

Table 2.7.6 Composition of an alginate impression material

Component	Amount (%)	Purpose
Sodium alginate	18	Hydrogel former
Calcium sulphate dihydrate	14	Provides calcium ions
Sodium phosphate	2	Controls working time
Potassium sulphate	10	Setting of model
Fillers (diatomaceous earth)	56	Controls consistency
Sodium silicofluoride	4	Controls pH

The calcium ions will react preferentially with the phosphate ions to form an insoluble calcium phosphate:

$$3Ca^{2+} + 2PO_4^{3-} \rightarrow Ca_3(PO_4)_2$$

Thus, the calcium ions that are released initially from the calcium sulphate dihydrate are not available for cross-linking as they react with the phosphate ions. Only when sufficient calcium ions have been released to react with all the sodium phosphate that has been added, will the subsequently released calcium ions be free to form cross-links.

There is a considerable pH change on setting, from a pH of 11 to one of about 7. This change in pH has been utilized in some formulations by the incorporation of pH indicators to allow a visual perception of the working and setting process.

Properties

These materials are provided as dust-free powders that overcome any potential irritation due to fine dust particles entering the atmosphere and being inhaled. The powder should be mixed thoroughly before use to eliminate the segregation of the components that may occur during storage, and to incorporate the surface layer, which is often contaminated with moisture picked up from the atmosphere. The container must be resealed as soon as the required amount of powder has been removed. The correct proportioning of the powder and water is important, and the manufacturers supply a suitable measuring spoon. Mixing is most easily done in a rubber bowl with a spatula of the type used for mixing plaster and stone.

This material has a well-controlled working time, but it does vary from product to product. One can affect the working and setting times by using warm water, but it is preferable to choose a product with working and setting times suited to your individual needs and use water at a temperature between 18°C and 24°C. Typical values for a regular- and fast-setting alginate impression material are shown in Table 2.7.7. The clinical setting time can be detected by the loss of tackiness of the surface. The impression should be left in place for 2–3 minutes after the tackiness has gone from the surface.

143

Table 2.7.7 A comparison of regular- and fast-set alginate

	Regular-set	Fast-set
Mixing time (minutes)	1	0.75
Working time (minutes)	3–4.5	1.25–2
Setting time (minutes)	1–4.5	1–2

The surface reproduction with these materials is not as good as that with agar or elastomers, and thus they are not recommended for crown and bridge work. However, they are very popular for full and partial denture work.

Alginates suffer from the same problems as agar in that they are susceptible to syneresis and imbibition, giving poor dimensional stability. As with the agar, the model should be poured within 1 hour and kept wet in the meantime by placing a wet towel around the impression.

Like agar, alginate is highly viscoelastic and a snap-removal technique needs to be employed in order to obtain an elastic response. The amount of compression strain the material may experience on removal from undercuts can be as high as 10%. The permanent deformation in such circumstances may be of the order of 1.5%, which is just about acceptable for the sort of applications in which these materials are used. The permanent deformation is somewhat higher than for agar impression materials, where, under the same conditions, this would be of the order of 1%.

The permanent deformation can be minimized by ensuring that there are no deep undercuts, as the deeper the undercut, the greater the amount of compression strain. Using a snap removal will ensure that the time for which the material is under compression is as short as possible; this is an advantage because the longer the material is under compression, the higher the amount of permanent deformation due to the viscoelastic nature of the alginates. Some recovery of the deformation will occur once the impression is removed and the compressive load taken off. However, although longer recovery times result in lower permanent sets, this advantage must be offset against the dimensional instability of the material.

Alginate impression materials have a lower tear strength than agar.

CLINICAL SIGNIFICANCE

Although increasing the loading rate – for example, by using a snap-removal technique – will raise the tear strength slightly, alginates cannot be used for crown and bridge work as excessive tearing will result on removal.

The impression must be rinsed after removal from the patient's mouth to remove any saliva, as this will interfere with the setting of the gypsum model. Any surface water should be removed prior to pouring the model, as residual water will dilute the model material and result in a soft surface, which is easily damaged.

The alginate should not be left on the model for too long as it becomes difficult to separate if allowed to dry out. This would result in a poor surface finish, as bits of the alginate are left on the surface of the model.

Patient acceptability is not a problem with this impression material. The material is cheap but does have a limited shelf life, probably related to water contamination.

ELASTOMERIC IMPRESSION MATERIALS

The impression materials discussed so far are not good enough generally for taking accurate impressions of the dentate patient. The alginates are inherently weak materials and provide a poor reproduction of surface detail; agar is dimensionally unstable and only suitable if laboratory facilities are close at hand; and the rigid impression materials cannot be removed from deep undercuts. Thus, there is still a need for an impression material that is accurate, shows a large recoverable deformation, and has adequate long-term dimensional stability. These goals can all be met with the elastomeric impression materials.

The elastomeric impression materials are characterized as polymers that are used at a temperature above their glass transition temperature, Tg. Such materials become more and more fluid as their temperature is raised above their glass-transition temperature.

The viscosities of the polymers that are used for impression materials are governed primarily by the molecular weight of the polymer (i.e. the length of the polymer chains) and by the presence of additives, such as fillers.

Thus, we have a material that is fluid at room temperature, but that can be turned into a solid by binding the long-chain molecules together.

This process of binding the chains to form a three-dimensional network is known as cross-linking (as described in Chapter 1.5) and forms the basis of the liquid-to-solid transition of all the elastomeric impression materials.

There are, essentially, three main groups of elastomeric impression materials:

- polysulphides
- polyethers
- silicones.

First, the chemistry of these impression materials will be described and then their relative merits will be considered.

Polysulphides

The polysulphide polymer shown below has a molecular weight of 2000–4000, with terminal and pendant mercaptan groups (–SH) (Figure 2.7.6). The subscripts x and y in Figure 2.7.6 denote different numbers of repeating units. These materials are also known as thiokol rubbers as they are derived from thiols, which are the sulphur analogues of alcohols (e.g. ethanethiol, CH_3CH_2SH, rather than ethanol, CH_3CH_2OH).

The mercaptan groups are oxidized by an accelerator to bring about both chain lengthening and cross-linking, as shown in Figure 2.7.7. This reaction causes a rapid increase in the molecular weight of the polymer, which causes the paste to be converted into a rubber. Water is a by-product of the reaction.

The polymerization reaction is exothermic, with a temperature rise of 3–4 °C being typical, although this does depend on the amount of polysulphide used.

Presentation

Polysulphides are presented as a base paste (containing polysulphide and an inert filler, such as titanium dioxide TiO_2 as 0.3 μm particles) and an activator paste (containing lead dioxide, which gives the distinctive brown colour, sulphur and dibutyl or dioctyl phthalate).

Polyethers

An interesting feature of the polyether-based impression materials is that they were developed specifically with the dental profession in

Figure 2.7.6 A typical polysulphide

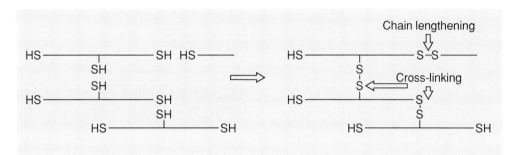

Figure 2.7.7 Cross-linking and chain lengthening of a polysulphide impression material

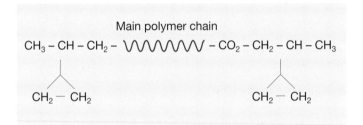

Figure 2.7.8 Structure of a polyether

mind. They were introduced in the late 1960s. A simplified version of the polymer structure is shown in Figure 2.7.8.

The polymer is cured by a reaction with imine end groups. The setting reaction is shown in Figure 2.7.9. There is no by-product associated with this reaction, which is one reason why this material has good dimensional stability. However, it *is* inclined to absorb water on storage and must therefore be kept in a dry environment; certainly, the polymer should never be placed in the same bag as an alginate impression.

Presentation

The polyethers come as two-paste systems: a base paste (consisting of polyether, a plasticizer such as glycoether or phthalate, and colloidal silica as an inert filler) and an activator paste (consisting of an aromatic sulphonate ester, a plasticizer and an inert filler).

Silicones

There are two important groups of silicone impression materials. One group is known as the *condensation-cured silicones* and the other as the *addition-cured silicones*. Both are based on the polydimethyl siloxane

polymer but have different end-groups, giving rise to different curing mechanisms.

Condensation-cured silicones

These materials are based on a polydimethyl siloxane polymer with hydroxyl terminal groups, as shown in Figure 2.7.10. Crosslinking is achieved by the use of a tetraethyl silicate (TES), such that as many as three polymer chains can be linked together, as shown in Figure 2.7.11. Three functional groups are needed to form a cross-linking network, as a functionality of two only gives rise to chain lengthening. The by-product of this reaction is an alcohol (R-OH).

CLINICAL SIGNIFICANCE

The release of an alcohol from condensation-cured silicones compromises the storage stability.

Presentation

The material comes as a base paste, containing silicone fluid and a filler, and an activator paste of tetra-ethyl silicate (the cross-linking agent). It is important for the amount of activator paste used to be carefully controlled. Insufficient TES gives rise to an incomplete cure, leaving a material with poor mechanical characteristics, such as high permanent set. Conversely, an excess of TES also gives an incomplete cure, leaving many unreacted ethyl end-groups.

Addition-cured silicones

These materials are similar to the condensation-cured silicones in that they are also based on a polydimethyl siloxane polymer. However, in this case, the terminal groups are vinyls, as shown in Figure 2.7.12. The setting reaction is via a platinum catalyst and a silanol, as depicted

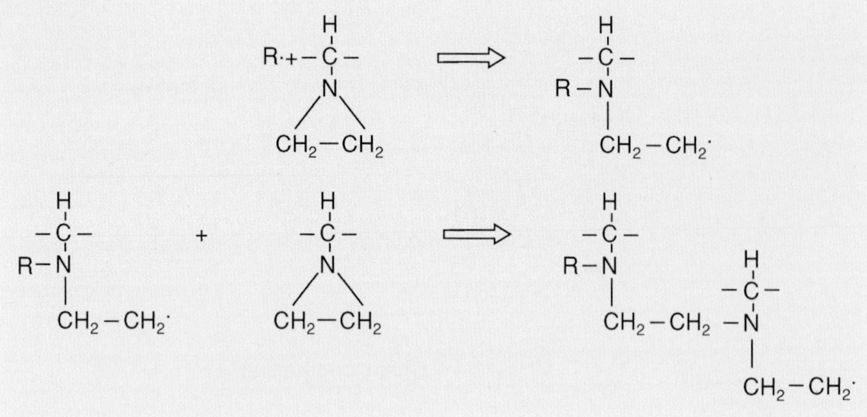

Figure 2.7.9 Cross-linking reaction via the imine pendant groups of a polyether

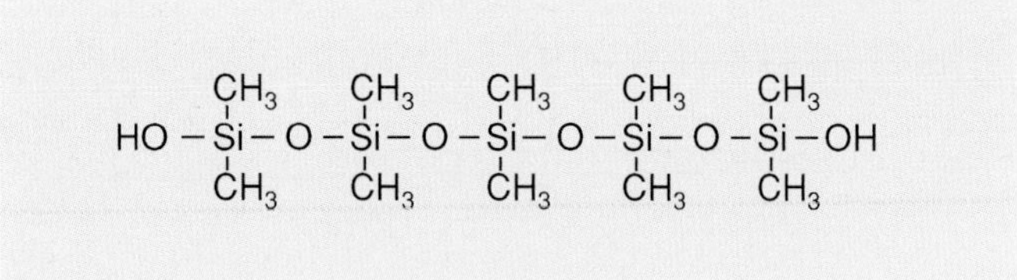

Figure 2.7.10 Hydroxyl-terminated polydimethyl siloxane

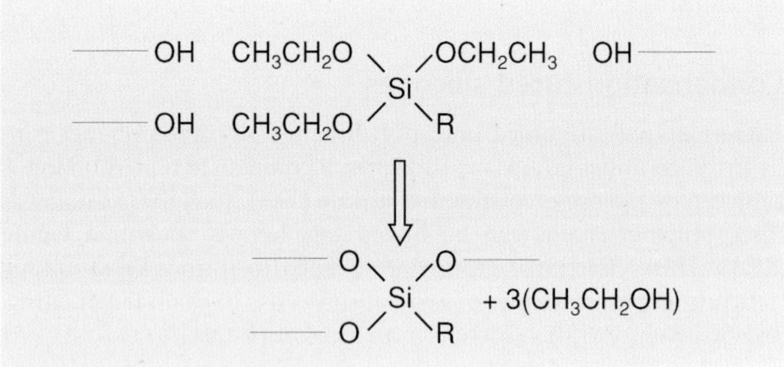

Figure 2.7.11 Cross-linking reaction for a condensation-cured silicone impression material

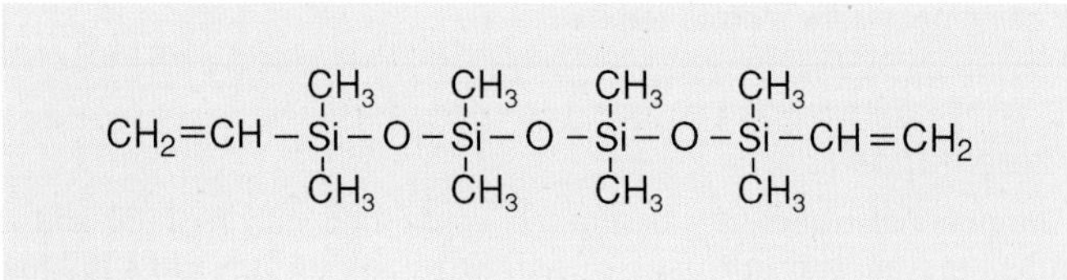

Figure 2.7.12 Polydimethyl siloxane with vinyl end-groups

in Figure 2.7.13. An important feature of this setting reaction is the fact that there is no by-product.

Presentation

The addition-cured silicones present as a base paste (of polyvinyl siloxane, silanol and a filler) and a catalyst paste (of polyvinyl siloxane, platinum catalyst and a filler).

RELATIVE MERITS OF THE ELASTOMERIC IMPRESSION MATERIALS

Handling characteristics

The setting process of the polysulphide impression material is highly susceptible to changes in environmental conditions, such as temperature and humidity variation, and unless these are carefully controlled, the working and setting times can be very erratic. Typically, the working time and setting times are 6 and 13 minutes respectively, which are quite long compared to some of the other impression materials, which have setting times in the region of 4–5 minutes. A high ambient temperature combined with high humidity can give rise to very much shorter working and setting times, and the converse is also true.

The condensation-cured silicones, too, can suffer from erratic setting behaviour, not only due to the possibility of a non-uniform mixing procedure, but also because the TES is susceptible to hydrolysis. If TES becomes contaminated with moisture, it can become inactive, which could result in some embarrassing moments.

The setting behaviour of the polyether and addition-cured silicone impression materials is more consistent. However, it has been noticed that there is an inhibition of the setting of addition-cured silicone putties when the mixer is wearing latex gloves.

The mixing of the low-viscosity addition-cured silicones has been made considerably easier with the introduction of gun delivery systems. These avoid both the potential for incomplete mixing and the introduction of air bubbles.

The elastomeric impression materials are available in a range of viscosities depending on the amount of filler that is incorporated, and include a light-bodied (wash), medium-bodied and heavy-bodied viscosity, and a putty.

The light-bodied materials are used in the double mix (single-step, two-phase) impression technique in combination with a high-filler-loaded, high-viscosity material (heavy-bodied) in a customized tray. The other use is in the putty/wash (single- or two-step, two-phase) impression technique, where it is used in combination with a very highly filled putty in a stock tray.

The medium-bodied material can be used as a single-material, single-step impression technique using a customized tray, or in combination with a light-bodied material in a single-step two-phase technique, again in a customized tray.

Polysulphides

The viscosity of the base paste depends on the amount of filler present, and heavy-, medium- and light-bodied impression paste forms are

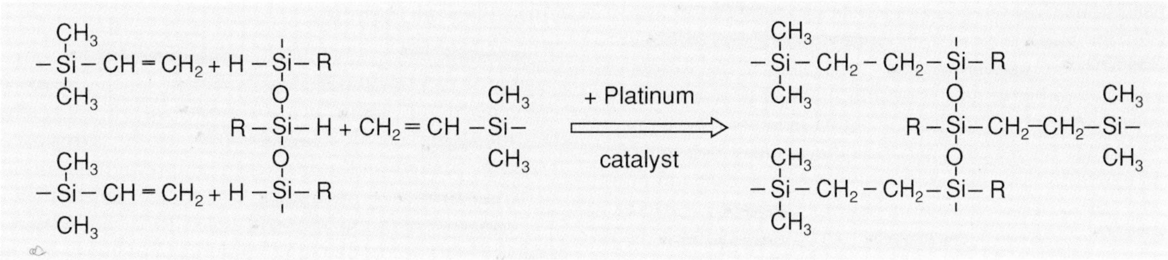

Figure 2.7.13 Cross-linking reaction for an addition-cured silicone impression material

available. Note that there is no putty version of this impression material, so it must be used with a special tray, using either the medium-bodied material by itself or a combination of the heavy- and light-bodied materials.

Polyethers

These materials are available only in a single viscosity and can be used in a special tray using a single viscosity mix. However, a thinner *is* available to produce a low-viscosity wash.

Condensation-cured silicones

A wide range of viscosities are available, varying from a putty to a heavy-, a medium- and a light-bodied material. There are also some extra-fine materials of very low viscosity available. Thus, these materials can be used in a wide variety of impression techniques. The difference in viscosity between the activator and base paste can present a problem in that it is difficult to obtain a uniform mix unless a good technique is employed.

Addition-cured silicones

As with the condensation-cured silicones, the material is available in a wide range of viscosities, varying from a putty to a heavy-, a medium- and a light-bodied material. Thus, these materials can also be used in a wide range of impression techniques. They have the advantage over the condensation-cured silicones in that the base paste and the catalyst paste for a given grade of material have the same consistencies, which make them relatively easy to mix.

If a stock tray is to be used for a single-step impression technique, then there are some addition-cured silicone impression materials, which do not have a tendency to flow when stationary (i.e. when loaded into the tray) but will flow readily under pressure. These are the monophase impression materials.

Mechanical properties

Stiffness

The stiffness of the impression material once it has set can be a major consideration in the ease with which it is removed from undercuts. Polysulphide impression materials are the most flexible and the relative stiffness of the set materials can be ranked as follows:

$$PS < CCS < ACS < PE$$

when comparing similar viscosity materials. However, in the case of addition-cured silicones, problems have been experienced with the extremely stiff putties, where removal can be very difficult if the putty has been allowed to flow into large interdental spaces. Newer versions of the putties have been introduced which have a lower stiffness once set, the so-called *soft putties*.

Permanent set

Ideally, when the impression is removed from an undercut, the deformation that results should be totally and immediately recoverable. All of the elastomeric impression materials are viscoelastic in behaviour, so it is important that they are removed from the mouth with a sharp tug. This will ensure that the impression material is strained for only a short time and that a near-elastic response will be obtained. If the impression is removed slowly, the material will be given the opportunity to flow and not all of the induced strain may be relieved.

The silicones are particularly good at showing virtually no permanent deformation, while the polysulphides have a relatively high degree of viscous flow. The impression materials can be ranked as follows:

$$PS > PE > CCS > ACS$$

with the polysulphides most prone to permanent deformation, and the addition-cured silicones least prone.

Tear strength

The tear strength of the impression material is also important when an impression is taken of the dentate patient. The polysulphides have the highest tear strength, followed a long way down by the polyethers and finally the silicones.

A high tear strength is, nevertheless, not necessarily a good thing, as too high a tear strength may give rise to difficulties in removing the impression from the mouth in cases where the impression material has flowed into the interdental spaces. Also, a considerable amount of deformation may occur for materials with a high tear strength before the impression material tears, and this deformation may not be totally recoverable.

Thus, the tear strength should be sufficient to prevent catastrophic failure, but not so high as to result in excessive deformation or difficulty in removal of the impression.

Reproduction of surface detail

All of the elastomeric impression materials are able to reproduce the details of the surface very accurately when a low-viscosity material is employed. The ability to reproduce the surface detail is directly related to the viscosity of the impression material: the lower the viscosity, the better the reproduction. In fact, the reproduction is generally so good that the stone dies are unable to reproduce it.

Factors which give rise to inadequacies in the surface reproduction are generally related to poor technique. For example, great care must be exercised during the mixing of the two pastes to minimize the presence of air bubbles. Air bubbles are not a problem when they are within the bulk of the impression material, but they will present difficulties when close to or at the surface, as detail will be lost. Another problem that may manifest itself is the occurrence of areas where the impression material has not set properly and retains a tacky feel. This is usually due to improper mixing resulting in a non-homogeneous mix.

All of the elastomeric impression materials are hydrophobic and, if the surface of the tooth has become contaminated with saliva, the impression material is unable to wet it – this can give rise to loss of surface detail. The ability of an impression material to wet a surface can be determined from contact angle measurements. The contact angles for water on the set materials have been measured, and are 49.3°, 82.1° and 98.2° for a polyether, polysulphide and an addition-cured silicone, respectively. This shows that the silicones are particularly problematic, and that the polyethers are the easiest to work with from this point of view.

A number of so-called hydrophilic addition-cured silicones are available. A surfactant has been added to these materials to alter the hydrophobicity of the surface and so reduce the contact angle to be closer to that of the polyether impression materials.

Dimensional stability and accuracy

It is important that the model of the oral cavity is an accurate three-dimensional replica, since all laboratory work will be based on this model. Besides the problems of distortion, there are also the dangers of expansion and contraction of the impression.

With the advent of the addition-cured silicones and the polyethers, impression materials are most probably as accurate as they will ever need to be. Recently, attention has been paid to improving their handling characteristics; the dimensional stability of the addition-cured silicones can sometimes turn out to be somewhat of an embarrassment, as discussed below.

Other factors

Factors which contribute to the production of an inaccurate model have already been discussed, but some deserve further comment in relation to specific impression materials.

Setting shrinkage and thermal contraction

In general, the setting shrinkage of the elastomeric impression materials is very low. The cross-linking process results in considerably less shrinkage than is usually associated with polymerization, as it merely involves a process of linking the pre-existing polymer chains to each other. Polyether and addition-cured silicones have the lowest setting shrinkage, followed by the polysulphides. The condensation-cured silicones have the highest degree of contraction due to setting shrinkage. Thus, the impression materials can be ranked as follows in terms of their setting shrinkage:

$$PE = ACS < PS < CCS$$

The thermal contraction is important as the impression is cooled from mouth temperature to room temperature. The polyethers have the highest thermal contraction (320 ppm/°C), followed by the polysulphides (270 ppm/°C) and then the silicones (200 ppm/°C). These can be ranked as follows:

$$CCS = ACS < PS < PE$$

Of course, both the setting shrinkage and the thermal contraction are affected by the amount of filler present, in that the higher the filler loading, the smaller the contraction.

CLINICAL SIGNIFICANCE

The amount of light-bodied material used should always be kept to a minimum.

Dimensional stability

The polysulphides are inclined to contract on storage, especially if they are kept in a low humidity environment, as the by-product of the setting reaction is water. Thus, the model will always be slightly larger than the tooth, leaving adequate space for the luting agent. Models should be poured very soon after the impression has been taken.

The polyethers are very stable on storage, unless they are placed in a high-humidity environment when they will absorb water and expand. If this occurs, the resultant model is going to be smaller than the original tooth and a crown produced on such a model will not fit under any circumstances. As this impression material absorbs water readily from alginate impression materials, the two should never be placed in direct contact.

CLINICAL SIGNIFICANCE

The condensation-cured silicones show a considerable contraction with time. This has been ascribed to the loss of the alcohol by-product. So, as with the polysulphides, models should be prepared as soon as possible after allowing for elastic recovery: that is, between 30 minutes and 1 hour after taking the impression.

The addition-cured silicones are extremely stable once set and show virtually no dimensional change on storage. Thus these materials are particularly good to use in situations where duplicate stone dies are needed.

Impression technique

The polysulphide and condensation-cured silicones display a small measure of shrinkage, such that the model poured from the impression is invariably slightly larger than the tooth.

The amount of space thus created for the luting agent will depend on the time that has elapsed between taking the impression and making the model. For the polyether impression material and the addition-cured silicones, the shrinkage is so small that there is very little space for the luting agent. The high dimensional stability of the addition-cured silicones can cause problems if the wrong impression technique is used.

The wide variety of presentations of the silicone impression materials provides an opportunity to use various impression-taking techniques. The most popular are putty/wash procedures, which allow the use of a stock tray.

The consequences for the size of the model produced from the three impression techniques are shown graphically in Figure 2.7.14.

Twin-mix technique

In this technique, the low-viscosity wash is mixed and placed in a syringe and, while the impression material is placed around those teeth for which an accurate impression is needed, the putty is mixed and placed in the stock tray. The loaded tray is then inserted in the patient's mouth, and the two impression materials allowed to set simultaneously. There will be some deformation of the impression material on removal, most of which is recovered immediately by a recoil action.

CLINICAL SIGNIFICANCE

The permanent set is a measure of the ability for elastic recovery; the larger the permanent set, the greater is the potential for distortion on removal of the impression from the mouth.

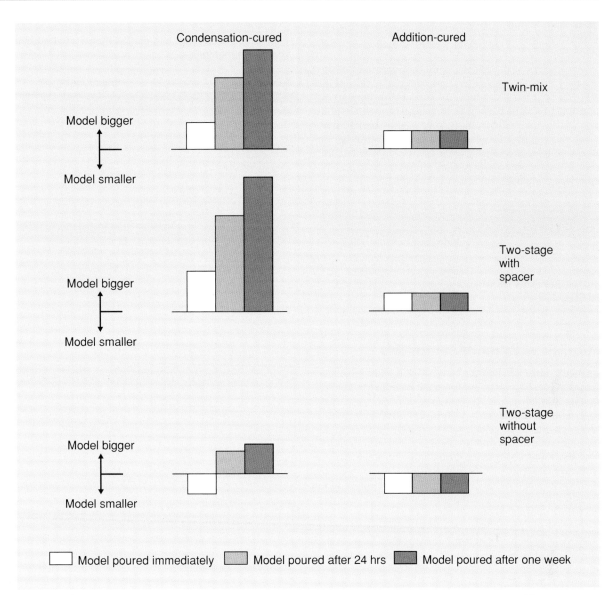

Figure 2.7.14 Dimensional changes for an addition-cured and a condensation-cured silicone impression material following different impression-taking techniques

If the model is poured virtually immediately, little or no shrinkage (due to cooling and storage contraction) will have taken place and the resultant model will be only slightly bigger than the tooth. Due to storage contraction (in the case of the condensation-cured silicone), the longer the delay before pouring the model, the larger the model will be. As the addition-cured silicones are extremely stable on storage, the model will be of the same size no matter when it is poured.

The potential problems with this technique are related to the removal of the addition-cured silicones. Although there are now some softer putties, removal can be difficult if the putty has flowed into the interdental spaces; the larger these are, the more difficult it will be to remove the impression. Another problem that may arise is that the putty may displace the wash in areas where surface accuracy is desirable.

Two-stage with spacer technique

This technique effectively involves the production of a special tray by using the putty first. A primary impression is taken either directly from the oral surfaces or sometimes with a thin cellophane sheet laid over

the putty. In the former situation, the poor-quality impression of the teeth is then cut out, creating a channel for the wash material. After this, a second impression is produced using the low-viscosity wash, which provides the necessary surface detail.

Generally, more of the wash material is required in this technique than in the twin-mix approach, and this means that there is more setting shrinkage as the wash has a much lower filler content. This is especially the case with the condensation-cured silicones, which also show more shrinkage on storage.

The addition-cured silicones are relatively unaffected by such problems. The setting shrinkage is compensated for to some degree, as the putty will have already set. When this method is used with the addition-cured silicones, it avoids the need to remove a stiff putty material from undercuts.

Two-stage without spacer technique

In this technique, the first impression is taken with the putty. Subsequently, the wash is placed around the teeth and in the tray containing the set putty, and is reseated in the mouth. The process of reseating in itself can be quite problematic. As a certain amount of space is required by the wash, there will be some compression of the putty to accommodate this.

The excellent recovery of the silicone impression materials means that, immediately after the material has set and is removed from the mouth, there will be a recoil action as the pressure on the putty is relieved. If a model is poured virtually immediately, then for both impression materials the model is likely to be slightly smaller than the tooth. For the condensation-cured silicones, the shrinkage on storage will ensure that, after a delay of 24 hours, this situation will have reversed. However, the addition-cured silicones are so dimensionally stable that the model will always be too small.

CLINICAL SIGNIFICANCE

The two-stage without spacer technique is inappropriate for addition-cured silicones because the primary impression would be extremely difficult to remove from undercuts, once it has set, due to the high stiffness of the putty.

Compatibility with model materials

The compatibility with the model materials does not present a problem for any of the elastomeric impression materials. However, for the silicone impression materials, the hydrophobicity can make them susceptible to poor wetting by the aqueous slurries of the gypsum-based products used to pour models or dies, which can lead to air bubbles and voids. Whilst this problem has been addressed to some degree by the inclusion of surfactants in the impression material, it has not completely disappeared. One way in which the occurrence of air bubbles and voids can possibly be minimized is by the application of a surfactant to the surface of the impression after it has been disinfected and before pouring the model.

One limitation of the polysulphide impression material is that it cannot be electroplated with copper to produce reinforced dies, as the polysulphide reacts with the electrolyte. The alternative process of silver plating is not readily available because of the dangers associated with the silver cyanide used in the plating process. The susceptibility of the polyether impression materials to absorb water may give rise to some distortion during the plating process.

The condensation- and addition-cured silicones can be plated with either copper or silver. The only problem here is that the surface has to be made conductive, and it is difficult to apply a graphite coating because of the low surface tension of the silicones.

Acceptability

The polysulphides have an unpleasant odour due to the mercapto groups. (Small amounts of thiols are added to natural gas to make it easier to detect and thiols are excreted by the skunk to ward off predators.) The polysulphides are also difficult to clean off clothing if spilled. The polyether and silicone impression materials are highly acceptable and very clean to handle.

Cost

The elastomers are considerably more expensive than the hydrocolloids and the rigid impression materials, with the addition-cured silicones being more expensive still.

The relative merits of the elastomeric impression materials are summarized in Table 2.7.8.

Table 2.7.8 Advantages and disadvantages of elastomeric impression materials

Advantages	Disadvantages
Polysulphides	
Good wettability	High permanent deformation
Good surface detail	Unpleasant taste and odour
Easy to remove	Must pour within 1 hour
High tear strength	Long setting time
	Care needed when disinfecting
Condensation-cured silicones	
Good surface detail (dry surfaces)	Hydrophobic
Good dimensional accuracy	Shrinks on storage
Low permanent deformation	Must pour within 1 hour
Wide range of viscosities	Low tear strength
Easy to disinfect	
Highly acceptable to patient	
Polyethers	
Hydrophilic	High permanent deformation
Good surface detail	Swells in disinfectants or moist environments
Good dimensional accuracy	Difficult to remove
Good resistance to deformation	Low tear strength
Highly acceptable to patient	Care needed when disinfecting
Addition-cured silicones	
Good surface detail (dry surfaces)	Hydrophobic (unless surfactant added)
Good dimensional accuracy	Low tear strength
Good storage stability	
Low permanent deformation	
Wide range of viscosities	
Easy to disinfect	
Highly acceptable to patient	

DISINFECTION OF IMPRESSION MATERIALS

The dental team is constantly exposed to microorganisms, which can cause infections such as the common cold, pneumonia, tuberculosis, herpes and hepatitis. Particularly since the advent of AIDS (the acquired immunodeficiency syndrome), there has been an increased awareness of the potential pathways for cross-infection when handling impression materials. Cross-infection may occur from the patient to the dentist, to the dental surgery assistant and eventually to the laboratory technician. Thus the whole dental team is at risk.

Most dental laboratories will not accept impressions unless there is a guarantee from the dentist that they have been disinfected. This has presented the dentist with a serious problem, as the taking of accurate impressions is a difficult procedure at the best of times. All the care and attention paid to the taking of a good-quality impression could be totally undermined if the impression should distort during the disinfecting procedure.

It is up to the dentist to choose the most appropriate impression material and the associated disinfection procedure.

Disinfectants

Since sterilization of impressions is not possible because of the high temperature and time needed, disinfection is the method of choice. The most effective means of disinfecting impressions is to immerse them in disinfectant solution for up to 30 minutes. When disinfection of impressions cannot be carried out by immersion, a disinfectant spray may be used. There are a variety of solutions, which may be used for spray or immersion disinfection of impression materials. These fall into the following main groups:

- *Chlorine solutions.* These tend to be harmful to skin, eyes etc., and they bleach clothing, have an unpleasant odour and are highly corrosive to metals.
- *Aldehyde solutions.* These give off a suffocating odour and are irritating to the skin and eyes. Commercial products tend to be made from glutaraldehyde-based solutions rather than formaldehyde-based solutions. Glutaraldehyde 2% solutions are the preferred disinfectants.
- *Iodine solutions* (Iodophors 1%).
- *Phenols.*

Effects of disinfectants on the accuracy of impression materials

The effects of disinfectants on the accuracy and dimensional stability of impression materials have been extensively studied and a summary is provided below of the current knowledge relating to the various classes of impression materials.

Reversible hydrocolloids

Agar impression materials can be immersed in sodium hypochlorite solutions, iodophors or glutaraldehyde with phenolic buffer. It is important that the manufacturers' instructions are carefully followed with regard to dilution and immersion time. The immersion time should, on no account, exceed 30 minutes. Another potential hazard with agar is associated with the danger of cross-contamination from the conditioning baths.

Irreversible hydrocolloids

A highly significant dimensional change occurs for alginate impression materials when immersed for more than 15 minutes in glutaraldehyde, formaldehyde or sodium hypochlorite, while those sprayed and left in contact with phenol derivatives for 30 minutes resulted in casts which also demonstrated statistically and clinically significant dimensional changes. Sodium hypochlorite will also cause partial dissolution of alginates. Immersion for up to 15 minutes in neutral glutaraldehyde or iodophor appears to result in an acceptable dimensional change. However, alginate impressions soaked in aldehyde agents for as little as 2 minutes have been shown to produce casts of inferior surface quality.

Thus, irreversible hydrocolloid (alginate) impression materials distort when immersed and should be disinfected by spraying and placing in a sealed plastic bag for the manufacturer's recommended time.

Internal disinfection (replacing water with disinfectant before impression-taking) is another possibility for alginates, since it allows immediate pouring of the impression after removal from the oral cavity. Although it appears highly effective, it still does not overcome the problem of how to disinfect the impression tray.

Polysulphides

Studies using a wide range of disinfectants and periods of immersion varying from 10 to 30 minutes indicate that no adverse effects are observed with polysulphide impression materials and that spray disinfectants are also acceptable.

Polyethers

Polyether impression materials are known to expand when exposed to moisture. It is not surprising then that immersion in a variety of disinfectants caused excessive swelling after 10 minutes. Dimensional changes become highly significant after 4 hours' immersion in 10% aqueous succinic aldehyde, but are acceptable after 10 minutes' immersion. Spray disinfectants are acceptable. Hence the recommendation for polyether impression materials is to use a spray disinfectant or immersion in products with a short disinfection time (less than 10 minutes), such as chlorine compounds.

Condensation-cured silicones

Although condensation-cured silicones are chemically unaffected by prolonged immersion in a wide variety of disinfectants, the limiting factor with this impression material is its inherent dimensional instability.

Addition-cured silicones

Many studies have been undertaken of the effects of disinfectants on the dimensional stability of addition-cured silicones. They conclude that no adverse effects result from even an extended exposure (up to 18 hours) of addition-cured silicones to all varieties of disinfectant. The only drawback appears to be a reduced wettability of the model material on the set impression for the hydrophilic silicone impression materials.

Disinfection procedure

Impressions should be rinsed in water immediately on removal from the patient's mouth to remove any obvious signs of saliva, blood and debris. Disinfection of the impression should be carried out before the model is cast or the impression is sent to an outside laboratory. It is the responsibility of the dentist to ensure that impressions are received by the dental laboratory without carrying contaminants. As can be seen from the above, the disinfection procedure to be adopted depends on the type of impression material and the disinfectant used. It must be appreciated that the objective of the procedure is to disinfect and not to sterilize, the latter requiring extended immersion for an unacceptable period; in any case, it is not warranted.

The British Dental Association Advisory Service (Advice Sheet A12) makes the comment that certain types of impression material can be disinfected with glutaraldehyde, but also note that there is, as yet, no universally applicable method for disinfecting all types of impression materials. They go on to recommend that disposable trays should be used and that technicians should wear gloves when handling impression materials and pouring models.

The American Dental Association suggests immersion for 30 minutes in a glutaraldehyde-based disinfectant for polysulphide, condensation- and addition-cured silicone impression materials and a chlorine compound spray disinfectant for irreversible hydrocolloid and polyether impression materials. However, it is important in each case that the manufacturers' recommendations are adhered to and that appropriate disinfection procedures are used to suit each type of impression material.

From the information available to date, the only impression materials that can be disinfected with virtually no adverse effects are the addition-cured silicones.

To summarize, the various disinfection procedures are as follows:

- *Alginates*: spray with disinfectant and place in a sealed plastic bag for the manufacturer's recommended time.
- *Polysulphides and silicones*: immerse in a disinfectant for the manufacturer's recommended time (preferably <30 minutes)
- *Polyethers*: spray with disinfectant or immerse in products with a short disinfection time (<10 minutes).

FAILURES OF IMPRESSION-TAKING

As the quality of the prosthesis is directly dependent on the quality of the impression, it is important that a poor-quality impression is identified readily and is not passed to the dental laboratory for processing.

In many instances, the need for retakes can be avoided by being aware of the kinds of problem that might arise and how these may be avoided. The main failures are associated with poor reproduction of surface detail and poor fit of the prosthesis.

Poor reproduction of surface detail

Factors that give rise to poor reproduction of surface detail are:

- *Rough or uneven surface on impression*. This may be due to incomplete setting (usually associated with premature removal), improper mixing or the presence of surface contaminants. A set that is too rapid will also give a poor surface reproduction and may be due to the wrong temperature, humidity or mix.
- *Bubbles*. These usually arise if the material is allowed to set too quickly or if bubbles have been introduced during the mixing process.
- *Irregular-shaped voids*. These will appear due to moisture or debris on the surface.

Poor fit of prosthesis

Factors that give rise to poor fit are:

- *Distortion*. The use of excessively flexible trays will result in distortion of the impression as the tray is distorted during seating. If the working time of the impression material is exceeded, the material will not flow properly and there is a temptation to use more pressure when taking the impression, causing distortion of the tray and permanent set of the impression material. Movement of the tray while the impression material is setting will also cause distortion. Adhesive failure between the tray and the impression material can occur if there is insufficient adhesive, if the wrong adhesive is used, or if insufficient time is allowed for the adhesive to become effective. An inappropriate disinfecting procedure will also give rise to distortion.
- *Castings too big or too small*. Although it would be difficult to distinguish between prostheses that fit poorly due to being the wrong size or being distorted, the most common causes of the wrong-sized castings are: the use of inappropriate impression techniques, pouring the model at the wrong time, or the

impression having been stored under unsuitable conditions of temperature and humidity.

DIGITAL IMPRESSIONING

Intraoral digital impression systems are rapidly coming to the forefront of dentistry. The first serious application of the intraoral impressioning system was developed for the chair-side computer-aided design–computer-aided manufacture (CAD–CAM) system from Sirona (CEREC™). In order to be able to produce a CAD–CAM-processed restoration at the chair side, it is necessary to have a digital image of the oral anatomy. The imaging system is based around an infrared (840 nm) or blue light-emitting diode (LED; 470 nm) scanner. A process known as triangulation is used to determine the position of the laser dot. In most cases, a laser stripe, instead of a single laser dot, is swept across the object to speed up the acquisition process. One drawback is that the surfaces of the teeth need to be covered with a white powder to aid the data collection. Once the intraoral data have been captured, they can be used to produce a milled definitive restoration in a single visit. The advantage is that the digital impression can be reviewed on screen for accuracy and it is easy to ensure that the margins of the prepared teeth are readily identified.

However, CEREC™ is a fully integrated system and not all dentists are able or willing to devote the extra time and effort needed to learn the various stages of designing, milling and characterization of the restorations. A number of manufacturers, including 3M/ESPE (LAVA COS™) and Cadent (iTero™), have invested heavily in free-standing chair-side intraoral scanners. The LAVA COS™ system, for example, captures three-dimensional data in a video sequence that is able to record approximately 20 three-dimensional data sets per second, or close to 2400 data sets per arch, for an accurate and high-speed scan. The most impressive achievement is the ability of the system to model those data in real time at the chair side, which is due to the increased processing power of the latest computers. This has made it possible to display on the monitor the three-dimensional image that is being taken in the mouth as it is being captured. As with the CEREC™ system, the dentist can confidently and immediately assess whether enough information has been captured for a completed digital impression. These free-standing intraoral scanners are intended to capture the digital data, which are then transferred to a facility that can either proceed directly to the manufacture of the restoration or convert the data into a highly accurate model; this, in turn, can be sent to the laboratory of the dentist's choice for more conventional processing.

The potential benefits of these systems are enormous, as they replace the tray and putty method of impressing patients with a highly detailed digital scan of the tooth preparation area. This approach has a number of benefits, as it:

- eliminates the imprecision synonymous with conventional impressions
- improves patient interaction
- improves patient comfort, as no bulky tray is needed and there is no waiting while the impression material sets
- improves communication between the dental laboratory and the dentist
- increases productivity
- reduces the need for retakes.

At present, the systems are only able to take accurate impressions of the hard tissues, so that the type of restoration that can be made from digital impressions from the various systems include inlays, onlays, crowns, fixed bridges and mouthguards, occlusal guards and orthodontic appliances.

FURTHER READING

Birnbaum NS, Aaronson HB (2008) Dental impressions using 3D digital scanners: virtual becomes reality. Compend Contin Educ Dent **29(8)**: 498–505

CDMIE (1996) Infection control recommendations for the dental office and the dental laboratory. ADA Council on Scientific Affairs and ADA Council on Dental Practice. J Am Dent Assoc **127**: 672–680

Jagger DC, Al Jabra O, Harrison A et al (2004) The effect of a range of disinfectants on the dimensional accuracy of some impression materials. Eur J Prosthodont Rest Dent **12**: 154

Jamani KD, Harrington E, Wilson HJ (1989) Rigidity of impression materials. J Oral Rehab **16**: 241–248

Johnson GH, Chellis KD, Gordon GE et al (1998) Dimensional stability and detail reproduction of irreversible hydrocolloid and elastomeric impressions disinfected by immersion. J Prosthet Dent **79**: 446–453

Kess RS, Combe EC, Sparks BS (2000) Effect of surface treatments on the wettability of vinyl polysiloxane impression materials. J Prosthet Dent **83**: 98

McCabe JF, Storer R (1980) Elastomeric impression materials. The measurement of some properties relevant to clinical practice. Brit Dent J **149**: 73–79

Millstein P, Maya A, Segura C (1998) Determining the accuracy of stock and custom tray impression/casts. J Oral Rehab **25**: 645–648

Pamenius M, Ohlsen NG (1987) The clinical relevance of mechanical properties of elastomers. Dent Mater **3**: 270

Pratten DH, Craig RG (1989) Wettability of a hydrophilic addition silicone impression material. J Prosthet Dent **61**: 197–201

Rosen M, Touyz LZG, Becker PJ (1989) The effect of latex gloves on setting time of vinyl polysiloxane putty impression materials. Brit Dent J **166**: 374–375

Rubel BS (2007) Impression materials: a comparative review of impression materials most commonly used in restorative dentistry. Dent Clin North Am **51(3)**: 629–642

Chapter | 2.8 |

Nanotechnology in dental materials

INTRODUCTION

Nanotechnology is concerned with the development and application of matter at the scale of nanometres, or 10^{-9} m. By convention, a nanomaterial is any material which includes components or features with at least one dimension less than 100 nm. The term is sometimes 'stretched' to cover those materials with features of several hundred nanometres, perhaps to cash in on the current vogue for all things 'nano'! To use features at this scale offers a wide range of advantages and opportunities to the materials engineer, and for this reason nanotechnology continues to have a profound effect on many areas of science, technology, medicine and consumer products.

In this chapter we will discuss the impact of nanotechnology on dental biomaterials. This is a rapidly developing field and what we present here is something of a snapshot of the state of play in late 2012. Doubtless some of the innovations that are in their infancy now will become commonplace in the dental surgery in years to come, while others will prove to be ineffective, or too expensive, or too challenging in scale-up to become widespread.

NANOFILLED DENTAL COMPOSITES

Dental composites (Chapter 2.2) are composed predominantly of silica filler particles embedded in a polymer matrix. The size of the filler particles has a profound effect on the properties of the material. To an extent, smaller is better – the composite can be better polished and the translucency and aesthetics controlled if the filler particles are small. The earliest composites, which had large filler particles, suffered from rough and therefore dull, plaque-retentive surfaces. However, reduce the particle size too far and you are likely to run into trouble with wettability. Since specific surface area increases with decreasing particle diameter, there comes a point for a given filler loading where there is insufficient resin to wet the filler particle surfaces and the composite becomes porous, crumbly and dry. This places a limit on the total filler surface area that can be incorporated into a composite, which is a function of both particle size and total loading.

Nevertheless, nanoscale filler particles have found application in dental composites, in combination with larger filler particles. In fact this is nothing new; 'nanofilled' composites, composites which contain nanoparticle fillers, were on the market long before the term 'nanoparticle' was applied to dental biomaterials! The 'microfilled' composites developed in the 1970s contained filler particles as small as 40 nm [1], and modern 'hybrid' composites contain filler particles of the size that would be defined as nanoparticles now we have a name to put to them.

So, one could easily be cynical about the array of 'nanocomposites' that adorn the catalogues of the dental materials suppliers; dentists have been using products that could be described as exactly that for decades. That would be a hasty judgement, however. Nanocomposite development is certainly a very active area of research and there are some promising early indications. To be a true nanomaterial, a nanocomposite should contain structural features where at least one dimension is less than 100 nm, although the term is sometimes used, both in the scientific literature and in marketing material, to apply to those materials where the features are anything below 1 μm, or those where nanoparticles are arranged in clusters that might themselves form more of a microscale object. It would be beneficial to the dental community if a globally accepted definition of a dental nanocomposite could be developed, and this might quite reasonably insist on a scale of <100 nm. In the absence of such an accepted definition, we will discuss nanocomposites with these and with larger features as well.

It can be difficult to form a thorough and balanced picture of the properties of nanofilled composites since any one study may evaluate only a few materials and the results cannot necessarily be extrapolated to apply in a wider context. In some published studies, the nanofilled composites are compared to non-nanofilled materials that also exhibit other differences in composition or structure, making a genuine evaluation of the effect of the nanofillers impossible. Thus one must interpret research findings with caution and scrutinize studies and claims with a critical eye.

A recent large study compared 72 different commercial brands and models of composite and compomer, of which 7 were classed by the authors as 'nanohybrid'. It appears that the source of the classification was in the marketing material supplied by the manufacturer rather than a more rigorous criterion such as fraction of filler with diameter below, say, 100 nm, and this is a limitation of the study. It appears from this comparison that the materials classified as nanohybrids exhibited a moderate flexural strength and modulus of elasticity but a high tensile and compressive strength in comparison to other composite classifications [2].

Nanoscale fillers may, of course, be composed of materials other than silica. Nanoparticles of calcium phosphate have been incorporated into experimental composites, and the preliminary indications are that the wear rates of these and conventional composites were comparable while the mechanical properties of the nanocomposites were somewhat superior and a sustained release of calcium and phosphate was observed, which may potentially foster remineralization in the surrounding tissue [3,4]. The calcium and phosphate release was able to elevate the pH in an artificial plaque model, while a conventional composite was not [5]. The same team has investigated calcium fluoride nanofillers which appear to confer fluoride release on the nanocomposite materials and might conceivably offer remineralization benefits [6]. Given that secondary or recurrent caries around the restoration is a common reason for the failure and replacement of composites, this could represent a significant step forward. These are interesting nanocomposites developed by respected researchers and will be watched with anticipation, although they are not yet independently tested or commercially available.

Of course, roughly spherical particles are not the only option for nanoscale fillers. There has been recent interest in developing nanoscale fibres to reinforce dental composites; fibre-reinforced materials are already used extensively and to great effect in civil and aerospace engineering. Composites containing zirconia–silica and zirconia–yttria–silica nanofibres (albeit rather large ones with diameters in the 100–300 nm range) [7] substituted for the regular glass filler had significantly higher flexural strength, flexural modulus and energy at breakage than the same composites with only the silica fillers, and some compositions had increased fracture toughness as well. However, these improvements were at the expense of the degree of conversion of monomer to polymer in the material [8]. Composites containing modest substitutions (5–10%) of hydroxyapatite nanofibres, again with diameters around 100 nm, also exhibited increased flexural strength compared to those containing only silica fillers, but these composites also showed elevated water sorption and solubility [9,10]. The contrast between fibre-like and spherical nanofillers was investigated in a study utilizing smaller hydroxyapatite nanofibres, with diameters of around 50 nm, and comparing these with roughly spherical hydroxyapatite nanoparticles. The nanofibre-reinforced composite was found to have superior flexural strength and fracture toughness when comparing composites with the same mass fraction of substituted spherical nanofillers [11]. This is thought to be because the nanofibres act as crack deflectors and crack bridges as well as being more easily wetted by the resin, and less likely to aggregate, than the spherical nanoparticles. The highly nanofibre-filled composites did, however, display a rather high porosity. Thus there are some interesting developments in this area, but also a number of significant drawbacks which will need to be addressed if these formulations are ever to reach the chairside.

NANOFILLED GLASS–IONOMER CEMENTS AND RELATED MATERIALS

Nanoscale filler particles have been incorporated into glass–ionomer cements (GICs) and their resin-modified counterparts. For the fundamental chemistry and properties of GICs the reader should consult Chapter 2.3. The reader will recall that one of the significant properties of GICs is that they release fluoride, although there remains some controversy regarding the clinical outcome of this. The primary focus so far on nano-GICs has been the impact of the nanofiller on fluoride release and uptake characteristics. Two independent studies have indicated that a resin-modified GIC containing nanoscale *silica* fillers as well as conventional (size and composition) fillers exhibited similar fluoride release and recharge behaviour to a regular resin-modified GIC [12,13]. Enhanced fluoride release has been achieved by adding nanoparticulate fillers to resin-modified GICs, not of the conventional silica–alumina–calcium fluoride glass but of fluorapatite or fluorhydroxyapatite, although this was only measured up to 70 days after preparation so it is not clear how long this would be sustained and whether it could be recharged as with conventional fluoride release from GICs [14], or indeed whether it would make any difference to caries in the area surrounding the restoration.

As regards other properties of nanofilled GICs, the data are rather scattered, with only a few properties tested for any one composition, and there is less of a feel for what these fillers might be able to offer this class of material than there is for composites.

Hydroxyapatite and fluorapatite nanofillers have been added to a commercial GIC and have been shown to increase the compressive, tensile and flexural strength [15] and enhance the bond strength to dentine [16]; other physical, chemical or biological properties were not investigated. Titania (titanium dioxide) nanoparticles have been added to GICs with the primary intention of conferring an alternative, or additional, antimicrobial efficacy on the material, since titania exhibits antimicrobial properties when activated by exposure to light of wavelength 380 nm. GICs containing 3% titania nanofillers reduced growth of *Streptococcus mutans* and also improved some mechanical properties such as fracture toughness and flexural and compressive strength; higher concentrations of nanofillers were also efficacious against the streptococci but resulted in a deterioration of mechanical properties and a reduction in setting time [17]. Of course with these materials one would have to consider what intensity of UV light was necessary to activate the antimicrobial function of the titania – the patient is unlikely to want to spend most of their day with their mouth wide open, gathering the sun's rays, and is certainly going to resist the suggestion of placing a UV light source in their mouth for therapeutic purposes. Perhaps if the patient had a class V restoration in the anterior region of the mouth this could be used as a motivation for them to put on a broad smile on their way out of the dentist's surgery.

OTHER NANOFILLED MATERIALS

Nanoscale fillers have been incorporated into many other dental materials, with rather mixed results.

Nanoparticles of montmorillonite (a clay-forming mineral) have been incorporated into poly(methyl methacrylate) (PMMA), a denture base material (Chapter 3.2), and appear to have a good biocompatibility profile as investigated using laboratory and animal tests [18]. The inclusion of these nanoparticles confers a reduction in the polymerization shrinkage of the material [19] so may offer advantages in processing and fit. One might well expect that such inclusions would influence the mechanical and physical properties but this has yet to be established. PMMA has also been modified by addition of nanoscale (4–6 nm) particles of industrial diamond, and it was found that 0.1 wt% substitution of these nanoparticles made the material tougher and more resistant to impact, although higher substitutions caused these properties to deteriorate [20]. This team also noted a change in the colour of the nanofilled PMMA which may represent a limitation to this application.

A modified mineral trioxide aggregate (MTA), used for endodontic applications (Chapter 2.6), has been developed containing nanofillers

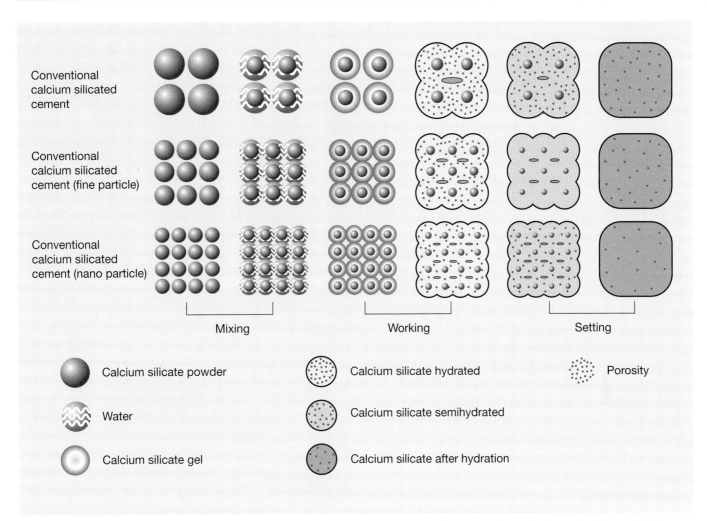

Figure 2.8.1 A schematic showing the setting of calcium silicate cements with different particle size. Note the reduced porosity with nanofilled cement. *Courtesy of Professor Mohammed Ali Saghiri, Azad University, Iran, with thanks*

(US patent http://www.google.com/patents/US20120012030). It seems that the nanofilled material exhibited increased hardness and a shorter setting time compared to a similar material with larger particle size, as well as a reduced porosity (Figure 2.8.1) [21]. The researchers noted that the nanofilled material exhibited a dimensional change on setting which they feared could lead to the material becoming dislodged, but a later comparison of the force needed to push a root filling of the nanofilled MTA out of position with that of conventional MTA materials suggested that the reverse was true and the adhesion of the nano-MTA was superior [22]. Only time will tell whether these properties offer significant clinical benefit, but the initial investigations are quite promising.

Silica nanofillers have been incorporated into polyvinylsiloxane impression materials (Chapter 2.7), and it was found that by carefully adjusting the ratio of nano- to traditionally sized silica fillers, properties such as the viscosity, tensile strength and working and setting time could be adjusted [23]. A good deal more research will be needed, though, before these materials are fully characterized.

As discussed in Chapter 3.6, zirconia is finding increasing application in dentistry, including in indirect restorations which are then veneered with a more translucent ceramic. These have been very welcome developments but the restorations are sometimes hampered by difficulty in machining the restoration without chipping the veneering ceramic. Using small zirconia particles in the processing phase can result in an increase in the strength of the finished material,

but it is of paramount importance to ensure that the particles are well distributed rather than present in clumps and agglomerates, and this has confounded some attempts to use nanoscale zirconia. This has recently been achieved using diatomite (a porous silicate) coated with nanoparticles of zirconia, and the resultant materials had a higher flexural strength and a decreased porosity, although disappointingly there was no improvement in fracture toughness [24].

Thus nanofilled dental materials offer some tantalizing improvements in some properties, particularly the physical and mechanical, but these improvements are sometimes at the expense of other properties. There is room for a good deal of development in this field and this will surely come over the next few years, particularly as manufacturers become more acutely aware of the research being conducted in the academic environment.

CLINICAL EVALUATION OF NANOFILLED MATERIALS

Owing to the relatively recent development of most of these materials, there is not yet a great deal of clinical data available.

There is one report of non-carious cervical lesions filled using a nanofilled composite, a nanofilled and a traditional RMGIC, observing the restorations at baseline and 6 and 12 months' recall [25]. The main conclusions of this study were that the nanofilled RMGIC exhibited more marginal staining and discoloration than the other materials. However, the materials were not matched for other properties and were of three different categories, so it is not possible to conclude that it was the nanofillers that were responsible for this difference or if it is simply a facet of the composition and structure of this particular RMGIC.

Another clinical study compared 49 class I and II restorations in 32 patients using a nanohybrid, a microfilled hybrid and a conventional hybrid composite [26]. This suffers from the same problem as the study described above, in that the materials were not matched for other properties and there is an incomplete data set describing the size, distribution and relative proportions of the different filler particles. This study has the benefit that restorations were assessed at regular intervals over 5 years, giving a longer view of the materials' performance. Although the three materials performed very similarly overall, there was a slight but statistically significant reduction in wear for the nanofilled hybrid.

One further clinical study compared 68 class II restorations in 30 patients over a 6-year period using a nanohybrid and conventional hybrid material [27]. Suffering from the same confounding factors as the previous two studies, this study found no significant difference between the two materials in terms of a range of clinical criteria such as marginal integrity and development of defects. A study comparing *indirect* restorations created using a nanofilled composite and an ormocer could again detect no differences related to material choice at a 36-month recall [28].

Such clinical data can be confounded by the pace of development of dental biomaterials, which is so rapid that, once sufficient data has been gathered to describe the clinical efficacy of a given material, the material is virtually out of date and new generations of material have superseded it. We must of course continue to strive to establish the efficacy of nanofilled materials in a clinical environment but the reader should be aware that there is inevitably a degree of delay and consequent redundancy in some of this data.

SURFACE ENGINEERING OF DENTAL IMPLANTS

Dental implants are fabricated from titanium or, more rarely, titanium alloys such as Ti–6Al–4V where the titanium is alloyed with 6% aluminium and 4% vanadium. Titanium and its alloys exhibit the unusual property of osseointegration, whereby the interaction of the bone-forming cells, osteoblasts, with the implant surface results in a stable, strong, resilient interface that can withstand the rigours of chewing, eating and talking for a lifetime. Although osseointegration can happen with a smooth titanium surface, it is widely accepted that using an implant surface with moderate roughness accelerates and assists the process.

In years gone by the primary focus has been on the micrometre scale roughness, or microroughness, of implant surfaces. Implants have been developed with many different microrough surface finishes, such as those shown in Figure 2.8.2. Many interesting observations have been made, including that osteoblasts and other cells respond to the specific pattern and separation of features on the surface and will align themselves in grooves or pits of an appropriate size. More recently, the concept of nanoroughness has been developed and the response of osteoblasts to nanoscale features has become a topic of interest to researchers in the field of implantology. It is difficult to quantify the effect of nanoroughness on osseointegration since the methods used to alter the nanoroughness of an experimental fixture often simultaneously change the microroughness and/or the surface

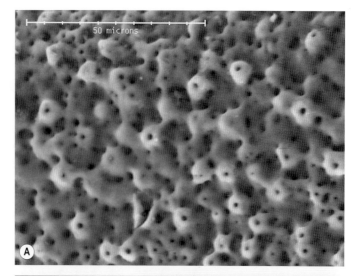

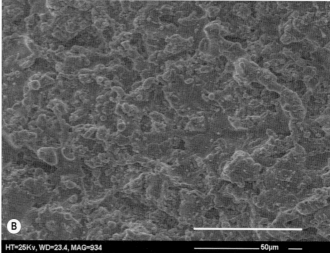

Figure 2.8.2 Scanning electron micrographs showing the surfaces of two commercial dental implants: (a) anodically oxidized; (b) plasma sprayed. Scale bar = 50 μm

chemistry of the titanium, meaning that if the implant generates a different response one does not know whether it was the change in nanoroughness or in one of the other factors which caused it [29]. Very careful study design is necessary if we are to separate out the effects of nanoroughness and random and ordered nanoscale features from other factors such as microroughness and surface chemistry. The best that can be said at present is that a number of commercially available implants have shown enhanced osseointegration compared with their predecessors from the same manufacturers, and one factor that the new models have in common is increased nanoroughness [29]. This is tantalizing but only further investigations will give a conclusive answer on the importance of nanoroughness and nanoscale features in implant technology.

There is, however, good motivation for pursuing this line of enquiry, and it comes from recent results in cell biology and protein chemistry. Cells have fundamental structural components that are of the order of tens and hundreds of nanometres, and it is therefore perhaps not surprising that many material–cell interactions are governed by features of comparable sizes (Figure 2.8.3) [30]. Tissues, including the tissues of the oral cavity, also have important structural features of the order of nanometres; Figure 2.8.4 shows the micro- and nanoscale features characteristic of human enamel. Remember that a biomaterial

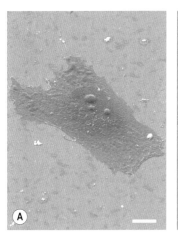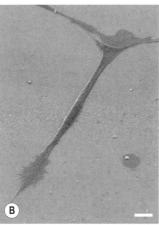

Figure 2.8.3 Scanning electron micrographs images show osteoblast cells grown on 15-nm high nano-dot Ti surface (a) are polygonal, while they become more elongated when grown on 100-nm high nano-pillar Ti surface indicating a less favourable interaction (b). Scale bar: 10 μm.
Courtesy of Dr Terje Sjostrom and Dr Bo Su, University of Bristol, with thanks

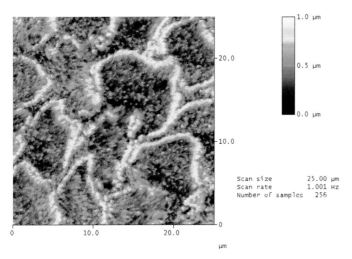

Figure 2.8.4 Atomic force microscopy image showing the exquisitely fine crystallite arrangement characteristic of human enamel. The specimen has been acid etched to reveal the crystallite alignment. Vertical scale 1.0 μm, horizontal scale 50 μm

is replacing a body tissue such as a bone; biomaterials with surface features similar to the natural tissue might profitably cash in on millennia of evolution by providing a very similar substrate for the body cells to interact with. For this reason a number of research teams are attempting to mimic the nanoscale roughness and features of extracellular matrix which coats many surfaces within the body, while maintaining consistent surface chemistry so that the specific effect of the nanotopography is elucidated. Fibroblasts [31] and endothelial cells [32] respond differently according to the size of surface features; 13 nm domains favour the development of a mature cytoskeleton over 35 or 95 nm features. Endothelial cells also adhere more readily to surfaces that are nanorough rather than microrough [33], and adhesion is particularly promoted by surfaces with *vertical* features in the range 5–19 nm than with lower or higher values; horizontal features size appears to be less important than vertical [34]. Interestingly, this was directly correlated with increased collagen and fibronectin adhesion to surfaces with these features suggesting that the successful adhesion of proteins is what causes the increased adhesion of the cells [34]. Osteoblasts are also rather fussy when it comes to surface

features, with more favourable behaviour (cell number, formation of focal adhesions and microfilaments, reduction in apoptosis) on surfaces exhibiting features of around 50 nm than those with features of 10, 100 or 200 nm [35].

The interaction of large molecules such as proteins does appear to be largely controlled by nanodomains on materials, both in terms of the morphology and chemical functionality of the surfaces. Collagen, which has a molecular length of around 300 nm, will preferentially align along 30–90 nm wide chemically labelled domains on a substrate [36]. Adsorption of fibrinogen increases as the nanoroughness of a tantalum surface is increased, over and above what one would expect simply from the associated increase in surface area, and this has been attributed to certain nanoroughnesses being particularly suited to the specific conformation of the protein [37]. A related study using bovine serum albumin confirmed that nanoscale features can elicit structural changes in the protein on adsorption, which in turn can lead to changes in functionality [38].

Thus it can confidently be said that human body cells of importance to the field of dental biomaterials in general, and implantology in particular, are profoundly affected by features on the biomaterial surface of the order of nanometres. There remains much work to be done, but one can imagine that such nanopatterning might be used to good effect in modulating the interaction of dental implants with proteins and cells.

Tailoring the nanoscale topography of dental implant surfaces is not the only way in which nanotechnology is being exploited in implant science. There have also been attempts to graft or otherwise attach nanoparticles, nanofibres and nanocoatings to implants with a view to conferring favourable properties on them. Calcium phosphates are of particular interest owing to their chemical similarity to bone. Titanium surfaces coated with hydroxyapatite nanoparticles in combination with polymer and collagen microfibres exhibited improved wettability and increased mesenchymal stem cell adhesion, proliferation and differentiation [39]. Titanium implants coated with calcium phosphate nanoparticles exhibited a greater bone–implant contact compared to uncoated implants in an animal model, although this was the only one of a number of factors which showed a difference between the two implants [40]. Titanium implants with a slightly different calcium phosphate nanoparticle surface coating resulted in the same clinical outcomes as non-coated implants in another animal model [41]. Thus the data are yet to convince, but there may be some progress made in this area in years to come.

Of course, any careful sculpting, texturing or coating of the surface would have to withstand the implant placement procedure, so it will be necessary to check that these intricate and subtle surfaces are still intact after the implant has been vigorously screwed into place in the bone of the maxilla or mandible. There is also the matter of other, less desirable, cells interacting with nanotextured surfaces. Oral bacteria adhere more readily to roughened surfaces (Figure 2.8.5) and the impact of nanoroughness on biofilm accumulation is not yet known.

ANTIMICROBIAL NANOPARTICLES IN DENTAL MATERIALS

Nanoparticles are finding increasing application in the field of antimicrobial and antifungal biomedical materials. The majority of studies are on the application of silver nanoparticles, which exhibit a broad spectrum of efficacy against bacteria and yeasts.

We have already described the application of calcium phosphate nanoparticles in resin-based composites as agents which might mediate remineralization of demineralized tooth tissue. The same research team has incorporated silver nanoparticles into the same

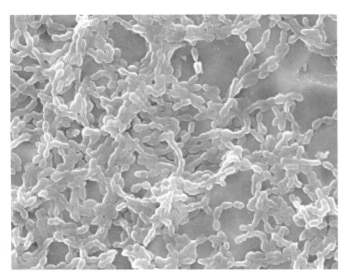

Figure 2.8.5 The characteristic chains of *Streptococcus gordonii*, a primary oral colonizer, on a section of anodized titanium exhibiting micro- and nanoroughness. Observe how the bacteria are often aligned into the lower-lying regions where they are protected from shear forces. Scanning electron micrograph; scale bar 10 μm

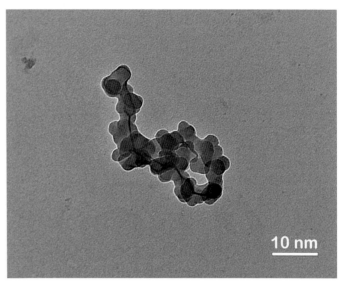

Figure 2.8.6 Sulphur nanoparticles which exhibit antifungal properties against two common yeasts. Image contributed by Professor Arunava Goswami and his team at the Indian Statistical Institute, with thanks from the authors

composites, and has shown that, in a laboratory model, this reduces the proliferation of plaque bacteria on the composite surface by around 75% [42,43].

Silver nanoparticles have been incorporated into denture base materials. A fungicidal effect (against *Candida albicans*, a common oral yeast) was observed in one study, although only at rather high nanoparticle doping levels of 20% or greater, and this extent of doping resulted in problems with colour stability which have yet to be resolved [44]. The exact mechanism is unclear; there is some disagreement as to whether, and how much, silver is released from the material once polymerized [44,45]. Another study found no fungicidal effect of silver nanoparticle-doped denture bases, suggesting that perhaps it is only when silver is free to migrate that it can be efficacious against Candida [46]. Denture soft linings have also been modified by addition of silver nanoparticles [47], and the nanofunctional materials do show some reduction in colonization by Candida, but the inclusion of even modest quantities of silver nanoparticles results in a change in the colour and appearance of the soft lining material [48] which will have to be overcome if they are to find clinical application.

Dental implants have also been functionalized with silver nanoparticles. Of course, a confluent layer of silver could also be applied to an implant thus conferring antimicrobial function, but the problem with this approach is first that you then are reliant on the junction between titanium (dioxide) and silver for strength of the interface, and second that you have obscured the titanium dioxide surface which is necessary for osseointegration. The use of nanoparticles circumvents these problems since it is possible to have a dispersed antimicrobial phase on the implant surface but retain plenty of exposed titanium dioxide for the osteoblasts to interact with.

The nanoparticles must be made to adhere to the implant surface somehow; unlike with polymers or cements, they cannot be usefully embedded within the titanium. This can be achieved using a ~1 μm layer of a hydrogel [49] or a coating of soda lime glass [50] from which ionic silver is gradually leached, but of course this raises the problem of obscuring the titanium dioxide. Silver nanoparticles embedded in the hydrogel layer did inhibit growth of *Staphylococcus aureus*, *Pseudomonas aeruginosa* and *Escherichia coli*, but also had adverse effects on osteoblast-like cells [49]. Silver nanoparticles on a soda lime glass coating inhibited growth of *Streptococcus oralis*, but their effect on osteoblasts was not investigated [50]. Clearly this approach needs

careful attention with regard to osseointegration and potential toxicity if it is to progress towards the clinic. An alternative approach is to use something to embed the silver nanoparticles that itself has a positive effect on osseointegration; one team has recently reported a composite implant coating of silver nanoparticles and fibroblast growth factor which shows promise [51].

Silver nanoparticles have been incorporated into dentine bonding systems, and have been shown in the laboratory to reduce the growth of a plaque biofilm without compromising bond strength or affecting the formation of resin tags [52]. The effect is enhanced further when the silver nanoparticles are added in combination with another antimicrobial agent, quaternary ammonium [53].

These and other nanoparticles based on metals and metal oxides, such as platinum and copper, are showing considerable promise as antimicrobial agents in dentistry and elsewhere. They are not, however, without their drawbacks, and safety concerns have certainly been raised (for a further discussion of the safety of dental nanomaterials see below). Non-metal based antimicrobial nanoparticles are also being developed. These have yet to find much application in dental materials, but research in other specialist fields may well translate to dentistry in the future. For instance, polymer nanoparticles can be loaded with antibiotics or antivirals for more sustained and/or targeted delivery than systemic or topical applications [54–58]. Inorganic elemental nanoparticles have also been tested and found to display some potentially useful antimicrobial attributes, such as sulphur nanoparticles of diameter <10 nm (Figure 2.8.6) which displayed significant fungicidal properties [59]. Small molecules such as antimicrobial peptides are increasingly popular, and are often encased, for ease of delivery, in structures such as nanoparticles or nanotubes [60]. Finally, small organic antimicrobial nanoparticles are in development (Figure 2.8.7) and may find application in various dental biomaterials.

NANOSTRUCTURED SCAFFOLDS IN TISSUE ENGINEERING

Tissue engineering is an immense research field and, owing to the scale of structural components of cells and tissues, nanotechnology is

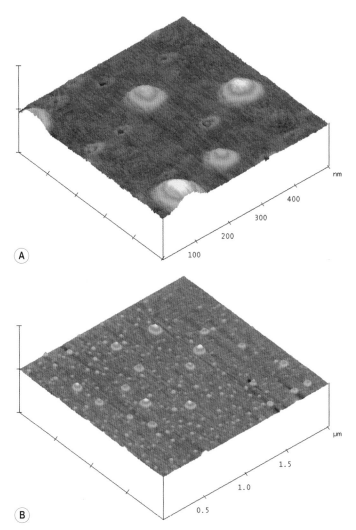

Figure 2.8.7 Organic antimicrobial nanoparticles for applications in dental biomaterials developed in the Oral Nanoscience research group at the University of Bristol. Atomic force microscopy image where false colour is used to indicate height, so the green area is the substrate and the blue–yellow objects are the nanoparticles, which are 4–8 nm in height. (a) Horizontal scale 500 nm, vertical scale 10 nm; (b) horizontal scale 2 μm, vertical scale 30 nm

An ambitious approach is to use a scaffold to engineer the pulp and create new pulp tissue and dentine [62]. The scaffold can be constructed from a wide range of materials such as a nanofibre hydrogel [63] or a polymer [64]. The scaffold is not just an inert structure on and around which the cells grow; recent developments allow for a bioactive and exquisitely tailored structure, carefully designed to elicit a favourable cell response. Some of these lines of enquiry might ultimately lead to an injectable material that could radically change endodontic treatment planning [62].

A recent report describes the use of silica and hydroxyapatite nanoparticles as a strategy to remineralize severely demineralized dentine (Figure 2.8.8) [65]. The nanoparticles were used to infiltrate the collagen network of the demineralized dentine and it was proposed that this could be used as a scaffold for the deposition of new mineral. The hydroxyapatite occurring naturally within and among the dentine collagen lattice can be lost due to caries or acid erosion, and the replacement of this mineral with the same or very similar structure and mechanical and physical properties is something of a holy grail of modern dentistry.

These approaches are still some way from finding clinical application but are without doubt a very exciting area and may provide a whole new approach to managing dental tissue restoration in the medium-term future.

SAFETY OF DENTAL NANOMATERIALS

There has been much concern, even hype, in the press and in popular fiction about the potential health risks of all things 'nano'. In some cases this is probably well founded; in others there is certainly a degree of scaremongering. It should be noted that some of the more dramatic instances of toxic or other deleterious effects observed in laboratories and reported in the media are the result of extraordinarily high doses that are unlikely to have any bearing in the real world.

One might ask why toxicology of dental nanomaterials is a concern at all, when most of the nanoscale components we have discussed are fabricated from rather prosaic materials that are already in widespread use in dental and other biomaterials. Silver is a noble metal; titanium exhibits passivation and is thus moderately inert when coated with its customary layer of titanium dioxide; calcium phosphates are the materials of which teeth and bones are made; silica is in every dental composite placed over the past 40 years.

In one sense, the very property that makes nanomaterials so attractive to the biomedical materials engineer is also the property which renders them potentially hazardous: their size. Cells and proteins respond to features of a comparable size to the cell structures and proteins themselves. However, because nanoparticles are of a comparable size to cells, and in some cases a good deal smaller, they can sometimes cross cell membranes and even enter cell nuclei, disrupt cell and tissue structure and function and thus interfere with normal processes, when a larger, micrometre plus size particle of an identical composition would have no opportunity for doing so. Furthermore, any consideration of the toxicity of a material must be in the context of the dose; the surface area of nanoparticles is many orders of magnitude greater than the same mass of the same material in microparticle form, and thus any ion release from that material is likely to be very much greater when presented as a nanomaterial. Thus even the most innocuous material, in classical terms, must be reconsidered when presented to the body in 'nano' form.

When considering the potential toxicity of dental nanomaterials one is concerned predominantly with two aspects: first, are the nanoparticles, nanofibres or other nanoscale objects released into the body, and if so where do they go and what do they do when they get there;

inevitably a lynchpin of this whole area of science. The interface between tissue engineering and dental materials is a very exciting field.

One area which has received a good deal of attention in the biomedical materials research community is the use of scaffolds for bone tissue engineering and regeneration [61]. Bone grafting from either the patient or a donor has been carried out for decades but is not without its problems, and these form a powerful driver for the development of methods to create bone de novo rather than transplant it from another source. This has been achieved by creating scaffolds which are gradually resorbed or remodelled in the body and promote a process of osteogenesis, or bone formation. Since bone itself is structured at the macro-, micro- and nanoscale, it is no surprise that scaffolds benefit from nanoscale engineering as well. It is by no means clear exactly how nanoscale topographic features modulate the behaviour of the osteoblasts, or bone-forming cells, only that this is probably a significant factor in the response to a given scaffold. Progress in this area could have a profound impact on treatment strategies in oral and maxillofacial surgery.

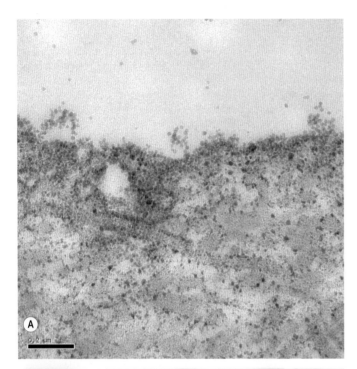

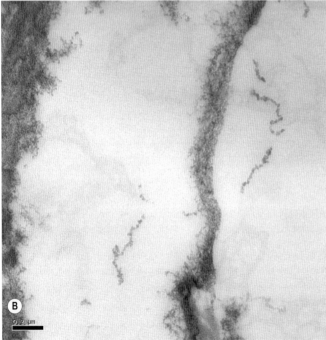

Figure 2.8.8 Demineralized dentine infiltrated with silica (a) and hydroxyapatite (b) nanoparticles. *Image courtesy of Dr Alex Besinis, University of Sheffield*

and, second, do the nanoparticles etc., dissolve, degrade or otherwise disintegrate and release their components into the body, and if so what effect does this have, locally and systemically? One of the few reports to address this directly used radioactive labelling to investigate what becomes of the hydroxyapatite nanoparticles after nanoparticle-coated implants are placed in animals – in this case, rats [66]. There was a measurable release of calcium from the implants which appeared to be cleared by the rats' normal metabolic processes rather than accumulating in any organs, which is encouraging.

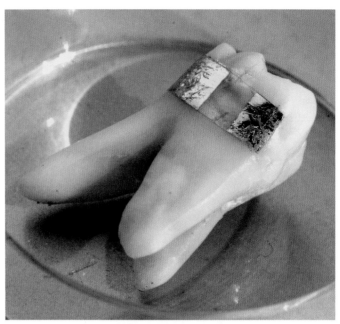

Figure 2.8.9 Graphene sensor deposited on a human tooth. The authors are indebted to Professor Mike McAlpine and his team at Princeton University for this image

Of course, in some cases the degrading of the nanoparticle is exactly what is intended; the composite resins described above which contain calcium phosphate nanoparticles and nanofibres have been cleverly designed specifically so that the calcium phosphate dissolves under caries-like conditions, releasing calcium and phosphate ions just when they are most needed [67]. Silver nanoparticles are thought to exert their antimicrobial effects through the gradual release of silver ions.

The extremely rapid pace of development of nanofunctional bio-materials is such that the methodology for assessing the safety and biocompatibility of these materials is still playing catch-up. It seems, however, that at the current time there is no convincing reason for the dental community, or indeed the public, to harbour concerns about any commercially available dental nanomaterials.

THE WEIRD AND THE WONDERFUL

Nanotechnology seems to fire the imagination of some very creative and talented researchers. One exciting recent development might have been inspired by the awarding of the 2010 Nobel Prize for Physics to a team from the University of Manchester, UK, for the discovery and investigation of graphene. Graphene is a single layer of carbon atoms joined together in a honeycomb structure. It has been rather charm-ingly described as atomic-scale chicken wire. It has a number of extraordinary properties including strength 200 times greater than steel and remarkable thermal and semiconducting qualities.

It has been suggested that graphene could be used as an exquisitely sensitive sensing device. This has recently been applied to dentistry. A graphene sheet has been deposited on the surface of an extracted human tooth with a view to developing a system for remote detection of respiration and the presence of plaque bacteria (Figure 2.8.9) [68]. While this technology is very much in the developmental stage, it could open up some interesting opportunities for remote and non-invasive monitoring of oral health.

Quantum dots are tiny particles of materials, often semiconductors, with particular and unusual electronic and optical properties. They have been studied and developed extensively in physics and engineering laboratories around the world, but have only recently found a potential application in dentistry. This is because quantum dots exhibit fluorescence that can be controlled by careful control of the precise size of the dots. Of course, tooth enamel also exhibits fluorescence, and this is notoriously difficult to recreate in a direct restorative dental biomaterial. In a recent report, quantum dots consisting of a core-shell structure of cadmium selenide innermost and zinc sulphide outermost with a range of diameters of 1.9–5.2 nm (Figure 2.8.10) were incorporated into a commercial composite and, by careful tuning of the dot diameter, the researchers were able to produce fluorescence spectra similar to those of natural teeth, opening up the possibility of creating more natural-looking restorations [69].

Nanorobots, tiny mobile devices that can travel through the human body acting as targeted delivery vehicles, repair modules or other clever agents, might be thought to be the stuff of fiction but in fact are the subject of intensive research [70,71]. One can imagine that these might find application in dentistry for the delivery of drugs or other compounds and the repair of damaged oral tissues.

Many times have scientists been caught out by claims of 'in five years we are confident that…' and so claims of imminent invasions by swarms of nanorobots into dentistry and medicine might perhaps be viewed with scepticism, but the developments in dental nanomaterials over the coming years and decades will certainly be worthy of scrutiny.

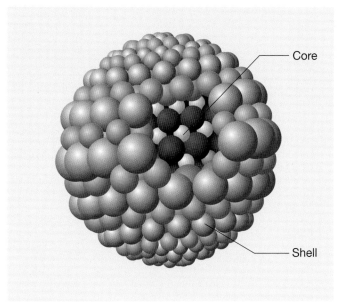

Figure 2.8.10 Quantum dot used in resin-based composites by Professor Egberto Munin and his team at the Universidade Camilo Castelo Branco, Brazil, to mimic the fluorescence spectrum of natural tooth tissue. The core material is cadmium selenide and the shell is zinc sulphide.
Figure courtesy of Prof Munin, with thanks

REFERENCES

1. Lutz F, Phillips RW (1983) A classification and evaluation of composite resin systems. J Prosthet Dent 50: 480–488

2. Ilie N, Hickel R (2009) Investigations on mechanical behaviour of dental composites. Clin Oral Investig 13: 427–438

3. Xu HH, Moreau JL, Sun L, Chow LC (2011) Nanocomposite containing amorphous calcium phosphate nanoparticles for caries inhibition. Dent Mater 27: 762–769

4. Moreau JL, Weir MD, Giuseppetti AA, Chow LC, Antonucci JM, Xu HH (2012) Long-term mechanical durability of dental nanocomposites containing amorphous calcium phosphate nanoparticles. J Biomed Mater Res B Appl Biomater 100: 1264–1273

5. Moreau JL, Sun L, Chow LC, Xu HH (2011) Mechanical and acid neutralizing properties and bacteria inhibition of amorphous calcium phosphate dental nanocomposite. J Biomed Mater Res B Appl Biomater 98: 80–88

6. Weir MD, Moreau JL, Levine ED, Strassler HE, Chow LC, Xu HH (2012) Nanocomposite containing CaF(2) nanoparticles: thermal cycling, wear and long-term water-aging. Dent Mater 28: 642–652

7. Xu X, Guo G, Fan Y (2010) Fabrication and characterization of dense zirconia and zirconia-silica ceramic nanofibers. J Nanosci Nanotechnol 10: 5672–5679

8. Guo G, Fan Y, Zhang JF, Hagan JL, Xu X (2012) Novel dental composites reinforced with zirconia-silica ceramic nanofibers. Dent Mater 28: 360–368

9. Chen L, Yu Q, Wang Y, Li H (2011) BisGMA/TEGDMA dental composite containing high aspect-ratio hydroxyapatite nanofibers. Dent Mater 27: 1187–1195

10. Chen L, Xu C, Wang Y, Shi J, Yu Q, Li H (2012) BisGMA/TEGDMA dental nanocomposites containing glyoxylic acid-modified high-aspect ratio hydroxyapatite nanofibers with enhanced dispersion. Biomed Mater 7: 045014

11. Zhang H, Darvell BW (2012) Mechanical properties of hydroxyapatite whisker-reinforced bis-GMA-based resin composites. Dent Mater 28: 824–830

12. Mitra SB, Oxman JD, Falsafi A, Ton TT (2011) Fluoride release and recharge behavior of a nano-filled resin-modified glass ionomer compared with that of other fluoride releasing materials. Am J Dent 24: 372–378

13. Neelakantan P, John S, Anand S, Sureshbabu N, Subbarao C (2011) Fluoride release from a new glass-ionomer cement. Oper Dent 36: 80–85

14. Lin J, Zhu J, Gu X, Wen W, Li Q, Fischer-Brandies H et al (2011) Effects of incorporation of nano-fluorapatite or nano-fluorohydroxyapatite on a resin-modified glass ionomer cement. Acta Biomater 7: 1346–1353

15. Moshaverinia A, Ansari S, Movasaghi Z, Billington RW, Darr JA, Rehman IU (2008) Modification of conventional glass-ionomer cements with N-vinylpyrrolidone containing polyacids, nano-hydroxy and fluoroapatite to improve mechanical properties. Dent Mater 24: 1381–1390

16. Moshaverinia A, Ansari S, Moshaverinia M, Roohpour N, Darr JA, Rehman I (2008) Effects of incorporation of hydroxyapatite and fluoroapatite nanobioceramics into conventional glass ionomer cements (GIC). Acta Biomater 4: 432–440

17. Elsaka SE, Hamouda IM, Swain MV (2011) Titanium dioxide nanoparticles addition to a conventional glass-ionomer restorative: influence on physical and antibacterial properties. J Dent 39: 589–598

18. Zheng J, Su Q, Wang C et al (2011) Synthesis and biological evaluation of PMMA/MMT nanocomposite as denture base material. J Mater Sci Mater Med 22: 1063–1071

19. Salahuddin N, Shehata M (2001) Polymethylmethacrylate-montmorillonite composites: preparation, characterization and properties. Polymer 42: 8379–8385

20. Protopapa P, Kontonasaki E, Bikiaris D, Paraskevopoulos KM, Koidis P (2011) Reinforcement of a PMMA resin for fixed interim prostheses with nanodiamonds. Dent Mater J **30**: 222–231

21. Saghiri MA, Asgar K, Lotfi M, Garcia-Godoy F (2012) Nanomodification of mineral trioxide aggregate for enhanced physiochemical properties. Int Endod J **45**: 979–988

22. Saghiri MA, Garcia-Godoy F, Gutmann JL, Lotfi M, Asatorian A, Ahmadi H (2012) Push-out bond strength of a nano-modified mineral trioxide aggregate. Dent Traumatol doi: 10.1111/j.1600-9657.2012.01176.x. [Epub ahead of print]

23. Choi JH, Kim MK, Woo HG, Song HJ, Park YJ (2011) Modulation of physical properties of polyvinylsiloxane impression materials by filler type combination. J Nanosci Nanotechnol **11**: 1547–1550

24. Lu X, Xia Y, Liu M et al (2012) Improved performance of diatomite-based dental nanocomposite ceramics using layer-by-layer assembly. Int J Nanomedicine **7**: 2153–2164

25. Perdigao J, Dutra-Correa M, Saraceni S, Ciaramicoli M, Kiyan V (2012) Randomized clinical trial of two resin-modified glass ionomer materials: 1-year results. Oper Dent [Epub ahead of print]

26. Palaniappan S, Elsen L, Lijnen I, Peumans M, Van Meerbeek B, Lambrechts P (2012) Nanohybrid and microfilled hybrid versus conventional hybrid composite restorations: 5-year clinical wear performance. Clin Oral Investig **16**: 181–190

27. Kramer N, Garcia-Godoy F, Reinelt C, Feilzer AJ, Frankenberger R (2011) Nanohybrid vs. fine hybrid composite in extended Class II cavities after six years. Dent Mater **27**: 455–464

28. Dukic W, Dukic OL, Milardovic S, Delija B (2010) Clinical evaluation of indirect composite restorations at baseline and 36 months after placement. Oper Dent **35**: 156–164

29. Wennerberg A, Albrektsson T (2009) On implant surfaces: a review of current knowledge and opinions. Int J Oral Maxillofac Implants **25**: 63–74

30. Variola F, Brunski JB, Orsini G, Tambasco de Oliveira P, Wazen R, Nanci A (2011) Nanoscale surface modifications of medically relevant metals: state-of-the art and perspectives. Nanoscale **3**: 335–353

31. Dalby MJ, Riehle MO, Johnstone HJ, Affrossman S, Curtis AS (2002) Polymer-demixed nanotopography: control of fibroblast spreading and proliferation. Tissue Eng **8**: 1099–1108

32. Dalby MJ, Riehle MO, Johnstone H, Affrossman S, Curtis AS (2002) In vitro reaction of endothelial cells to polymer demixed nanotopography. Biomaterials **23**: 2945–2954

33. Miller DC, Thapa A, Haberstroh KM, Webster TJ (2004) Endothelial and vascular smooth muscle cell function on poly(lactic-co-glycolic acid) with nano-structured surface features. Biomaterials **25**: 53–61

34. Carpenter J, Khang D, Webster TJ (2008) Nanometer polymer surface features: the influence on surface energy, protein adsorption and endothelial cell adhesion. Nanotechnology **19**: 505103

35. Pan HA, Hung YC, Chiou JC, Tai SM, Chen HH, Steven Huang G (2012) Nanosurface design of dental implants for improved cell growth and function. Nanotechnology **23**: 335703

36. Denis FA, Pallandre A, Nysten B, Jonas AM, Dupont-Gillain CC (2005) Alignment and assembly of adsorbed collagen molecules induced by anisotropic chemical nanopatterns. Small **1**: 984–991

37. Rechendorff K, Hovgaard MB, Foss M, Zhdanov VP, Besenbacher F (2006) Enhancement of protein adsorption induced by surface roughness. Langmuir **22**: 10885–10888

38. Dolatshahi-Pirouz A, Rechendorff K, Hovgaard MB, Foss M, Chevallier J, Besenbacher F (2008) Bovine serum albumin adsorption on nano-rough platinum surfaces studied by QCM-D. Colloids Surf B Biointerfaces **66**: 53–59

39. Ravichandran R, Ng C, Liao S et al (2012) Biomimetic surface modification of titanium surfaces for early cell capture by advanced electrospinning. Biomed Mater **7**: 015001

40. Artzi Z, Nemcovsky CE, Tal HE et al (2011) Clinical and histomorphometric observations around dual acid-etched and calcium phosphate nanometer deposited-surface implants. Int J Oral Maxillofac Implants **26**: 893–901

41. Schouten C, Meijer GJ, van den Beucken JJ et al (2010) In vivo bone response and mechanical evaluation of electrosprayed CaP nanoparticle coatings using the iliac crest of goats as an implantation model. Acta Biomater **6**: 2227–2236

42. Cheng L, Weir MD, Xu HH et al (2012) Effect of amorphous calcium phosphate and silver nanocomposites on dental plaque microcosm biofilms. J Biomed Mater Res B Appl Biomater **100**: 1378–1386

43. Cheng L, Weir MD, Xu HH et al (2012) Antibacterial amorphous calcium phosphate nanocomposites with a quaternary ammonium dimethacrylate and silver nanoparticles. Dent Mater **28**: 561–572

44. Nam KY, Lee CH, Lee CJ (2012) Antifungal and physical characteristics of modified denture base acrylic incorporated with silver nanoparticles. Gerodontology **29**: e413–419

45. Monteiro DR, Gorup LF, Takamiya AS, de Camargo ER, Filho AC, Barbosa DB (2012) Silver distribution and release from an antimicrobial denture base resin containing silver colloidal nanoparticles. J Prosthodont **21**: 7–15

46. Wady AF, Machado AL, Zucolotto V, Zamperini CA, Berni E, Vergani CE (2012) Evaluation of Candida albicans adhesion and biofilm formation on a denture base acrylic resin containing silver nanoparticles. J Appl Microbiol **112**: 1163–1172

47. Chladek G, Barszczewska-Rybarek I, Lukaszczyk J (2012) Developing the procedure of modifying the denture soft liner by silver nanoparticles. Acta Bioeng Biomech **14**: 23–29

48. Chladek G, Mertas A, Barszczewska-Rybarek I et al (2011) Antifungal activity of denture soft lining material modified by silver nanoparticles – a pilot study. Int J Mol Sci **12**: 4735–4744

49. De Giglio E, Cafagna D, Cometa S et al (2012) An innovative, easily fabricated, silver nanoparticle-based titanium implant coating: development and analytical characterization. Anal Bioanal Chem [Epub ahead of print]

50. Cabal B, Cafini F, Esteban-Tejeda L et al (2012) Inhibitory effect on in vitro Streptococcus oralis biofilm of a soda-lime glass containing silver nanoparticles coating on titanium alloy. PLoS One **7**: e42393

51. Ma Q, Mei S, Ji K, Zhang Y, Chu PK (2011) Immobilization of Ag nanoparticles/FGF-2 on a modified titanium implant surface and improved human gingival fibroblasts behavior. J Biomed Mater Res A **98**: 274–286

52. Zhang K, Melo MA, Cheng L, Weir MD, Bai Y, Xu HH (2012) Effect of quaternary ammonium and silver nanoparticle-containing adhesives on dentin bond strength and dental plaque microcosm biofilms. Dent Mater **28**: 842–852

53. Cheng L, Zhang K, Melo MA, Weir MD, Zhou X, Xu HH (2012) Anti-biofilm dentin primer with quaternary ammonium and silver nanoparticles. J Dent Res **91**: 598–604

54. Abdelghany SM, Quinn DJ, Ingram RJ et al (2012) Gentamicin-loaded nanoparticles show improved antimicrobial effects towards Pseudomonas aeruginosa infection. Int J Nanomedicine **7**: 4053–4063

55. Misra R, Sahoo SK (2012) Antibacterial activity of doxycycline-loaded nanoparticles. Methods Enzymol **509**: 61–85

56. Cavalli R, Donalisio M, Bisazza A et al (2012) Enhanced antiviral activity of acyclovir loaded into nanoparticles. Methods Enzymol **509**: 1–19

57. Surolia R, Pachauri M, Ghosh PC (2012) Preparation and characterization of monensin loaded PLGA nanoparticles: in vitro anti-malarial activity against Plasmodium falciparum. J Biomed Nanotechnol **8**: 172–181

58. Wang JJ, Zeng ZW, Xiao RZ et al (2011) Recent advances of chitosan nanoparticles as drug carriers. Int J Nanomedicine **6**: 765–774

59. Roy Choudhury S, Goswami A (2012) Supramolecular reactive sulphur nanoparticles: a novel and efficient antimicrobial agent. J Appl Microbiol doi: 10.1111/j.1365-2672.2012.05422.x. [Epub ahead of print]

60. Urban P, Valle-Delgado JJ, Moles E, Marques J, Diez C, Fernandez-Busquets X (2012) Nanotools for the delivery of antimicrobial peptides. Curr Drug Targets **13**: 1158–1172

61. Saiz E, Zimmermann EA, Lee JS, Wegst UG, Tomsia AP (2012) Perspectives on the role of nanotechnology in bone tissue engineering. Dent Mater [Epub ahead of print]

62. Galler KM, D'Souza RN, Hartgerink JD, Schmalz G (2011) Scaffolds for dental pulp tissue engineering. Adv Dent Res **23**: 333–339

63. Chan B, Wong RW, Rabie B (2011) In vivo production of mineralised tissue pieces for clinical use: a qualitative pilot study using human dental pulp cell. Int J Oral Maxillofac Surg **40**: 612–620

64. El-Backly RM, Massoud AG, El-Badry AM, Sherif RA, Marei MK (2008) Regeneration of dentine/pulp-like tissue using a dental pulp stem cell/poly(lactic-co-glycolic) acid scaffold construct in New Zealand white rabbits. Aust Endod J **34**: 52–67

65. Besinis A, van Noort R, Martin N (2012) Infiltration of demineralized dentin with silica and hydroxyapatite nanoparticles. Dent Mater **28**: 1012–1023

66. Wennerberg A, Jimbo R, Allard S, Skarnemark G, Andersson M (2011) In vivo stability of hydroxyapatite nanoparticles coated on titanium implant surfaces. Int J Oral Maxillofac Implants **26**: 1161–1166

67. Xu HH, Weir MD, Sun L (2009) Calcium and phosphate ion releasing composite: effect of pH on release and mechanical properties. Dent Mater **25**: 535–542

68. Mannoor MS, Tao H, Clayton JD et al (2012) Graphene-based wireless bacteria detection on tooth enamel. Nat Commun **3**: 763

69. Alves LP, Pilla V, Murgo DO, Munin E (2010) Core-shell quantum dots tailor the fluorescence of dental resin composites. J Dent **38**: 149–152

70. Patel GM, Patel GC, Patel RB, Patel JK, Patel M (2006) Nanorobot: a versatile tool in nanomedicine. J Drug Target **14**: 63–67

71. Cavalcanti A, Shirinzadeh B, Freitas Jr RA, Kretly LC (2007) Medical nanorobot architecture based on nanobioelectronics. Recent Pat Nanotechnol **1**: 1–10

Section | 3 |

Laboratory and related dental materials

The materials described in this section are used mostly by the dental technician to construct prostheses, although there is a considerable overlap, such as in the chapter on cementation. Information on the detailed aspects of the construction of prostheses has been avoided, as this is the prerogative of the dental technician. However, responsibility for the choice of materials to be placed in the patient's mouth remains with the dental practitioner and this requires a knowledge of what is available. While the clinician may not be engaged in the various stages of construction of a prosthesis, a thorough knowledge of the characteristics of the materials used and an appreciation of the processes involved is of paramount importance if the correct choice of materials is to be made for a particular clinical situation. Additionally, the clinician will find that awareness of the various materials and procedures involved in the construction of a prosthesis greatly aids communication with the dental technician and avoids possible misunderstanding.

Chapter | 3.1 |

Models, dies and refractories

INTRODUCTION

Materials that are derived from gypsum are used in a variety of dental applications. They include:

- models and dies
- impression materials
- moulds
- refractory investments.

A *model* is a replica of the fitting surfaces of the oral cavity; it is poured from an impression of the oral anatomy, and is then used to construct an appliance, such as a full or a partial denture. A *mould* is used for the construction of a denture. *Dies* are replicas of individual teeth, and are generally used in the construction of crowns and bridges. A *refractory investment* is a high-temperature-resistant material that uses gypsum or phosphates as a binder and is used as a mould material for lost wax casting of dental casting alloys and a mould or support structure for the construction of ceramic restorations such as veneers, crowns and inlays using sintering or hot pressing. In this chapter we will focus on the chemistry and properties of these materials.

MODELS AND DIES

The basic ingredient for models and dies is gypsum, more commonly known as plaster of Paris.

Chemistry of gypsum

Composition

Gypsum is calcium sulphate dihydrate, $CaSO_4 \cdot 2H_2O$. When this substance is calcined – that is, heated to a temperature sufficiently high to drive off some of the water – it is converted into calcium sulphate hemihydrate $(CaSO_4)_2 \cdot H_2O$, and at higher temperatures the anhydrite is formed as shown below:

Gypsum	$CaSO_4 \cdot 2H_2O$
↓ Up to 130°C	
Hemihydrate	$(CaSO_4)_2 \cdot H_2O$
↓ Up to 200°C	
Anhydrite	$CaSO_4$

The production of calcium sulphate hemihydrate can be undertaken in one of three ways, producing versions of gypsum with different properties and hence different applications. These are plaster, dental stone and densite (improved stone). It should be noted that the three versions are chemically identical, differing only in form and structural detail.

Plaster

Calcium sulphate dihydrate is heated in an open vessel. Water is driven off, the dihydrate is converted into hemihydrate, known as calcined calcium sulphate or β-hemihydrate. The resultant material consists of large irregular porous particles and these particles do not pack together very tightly. The powder needs to be mixed with a large amount of water to obtain a mix satisfactory for dental use, as much of the water is absorbed into the pores between the particles. The usual mix is 50 mL of water to 100 g of powder.

Dental stone

If the dihydrate is heated in an autoclave, the hemihydrate that is produced consists of small, regular-shaped particles which are relatively non-porous. This autoclaved calcium sulphate is known as α-hemihydrate. Due to the non-porous and regular structure of the particles, they can be packed more tightly together using less water. The mix is 20 mL water to 100 g of powder.

Densite (improved stone)

In the production of this form of calcium sulphate hemihydrate, the dihydrate is boiled in the presence of calcium chloride and magnesium chloride. These two chlorides act as deflocculants, helping to separate the individual particles that would otherwise tend to agglomerate. The hemihydrate particles that are produced are yet more compact and smoother than those of the dental stone. The densite is mixed in the ratio of 100 g of powder to 20 mL of water.

Applications

Plaster is used as a general purpose material, mainly for bases and models, as it is cheap and easy to use and shape. The setting expansion (see below) is not of great importance for these applications. A similar composition is used for plaster impression material (see Chapter 2.7) and for gypsum-bonded refractory investments, although for these applications the working and setting times and the setting expansion are carefully controlled by the incorporation of various additives (see below).

The dental stone is used for models of the mouth, while the denser, improved stone is used for individual tooth models, called dies. The latter are used for the shaping of wax patterns from which castings are produced.

Setting process

Heating the hydrate to drive off some of the water produces a substance which is effectively dehydrated. As a consequence of this, the hemihydrate is able to react with water and revert back to calcium sulphate dihydrate as follows:

$$(CaSO_4)_2 \cdot H_2O + 3H_2O \rightarrow 2CaSO_4 \cdot 2H_2O$$

The setting process for gypsum products is believed to occur in the following sequence:

1. Some calcium sulphate hemihydrate dissolves in the water.
2. The dissolved calcium sulphate hemihydrate reacts with the water and forms calcium sulphate dihydrate.
3. The solubility of calcium sulphate dihydrate is very low and a supersaturated solution is formed.
4. This supersaturated solution is unstable and calcium sulphate dihydrate precipitates out as stable crystals.
5. As the stable calcium sulphate dihydrate crystals precipitate out of the solution, more calcium sulphate hemihydrate is dissolved and this continues until all the hemihydrate has dissolved.

Working and setting times

The material must be mixed and poured before it reaches the end of its working time. The working times vary from product to product, and are chosen to suit the particular application.

For impression plaster, the working time is only 2–3 minutes, whereas it approaches 8 minutes for a gypsum-bonded refractory investment. Short working times give rise to short setting times, as both are controlled by the speed of the reaction. Hence, for an impression plaster, the setting time is typically 2–3 minutes, whereas the setting time can vary from 20–45 minutes for gypsum-bonded refractory investments.

The model materials have working times similar to those of impression plaster but their setting times are somewhat longer. For plaster the setting time is 5–10 minutes, while for stone it can be up to 20 minutes.

The handling characteristics are controlled by the inclusion of various additives. Additives which speed up the setting process are gypsum (<20%), potassium sulphate and sodium chloride (<20%). These act as nucleating sites for the growth of dihydrate crystals. Those that slow down the setting rate are sodium chloride (>20%),

potassium citrate and borax, which interfere with dihydrate crystal formation. These additives also affect the dimensional change on setting, as discussed later.

The manipulation of the powder–liquid system will also affect the setting characteristics. The operator can change the powder-to-liquid ratio, and, by adding more water, the setting time is extended, because it takes longer for the solution to become saturated and thus for the dihydrate crystals to begin to precipitate out. Increasing the spatulation time will result in a reduction of the setting time, as it has the effect of breaking up the crystals as they form, hence increasing the number of sites for crystallization.

> ### CLINICAL SIGNIFICANCE
>
> Longer spatulation times will tend to reduce the setting time and increase the setting expansion.

An increase in temperature has only a minimal effect, since the increased rate of dissolution of the hemihydrate is offset by the higher solubility of the calcium sulphate dihydrate in the water.

Dimensional changes on setting

On setting, the crystals that are formed are spherulitic in appearance (Figure 3.1.1), not unlike snowflakes. These crystals impinge on one another as they grow, and try to push each other apart. The result of this action is that there is a dimensional expansion on setting. The material in fact does shrink, in the sense that its molar volume is less by 7.1 vol. %, as shown in Table 3.1.1. However, large, empty spaces form between the crystals, leading to a high porosity. It is this that accounts for the observed dimensional expansion of 0.6 vol. %.

This ability to expand on setting is a very important feature of this material, and it is the factor that makes it so useful for a large number of dental applications. In particular, models and dies are best produced slightly larger than the oral anatomy. This is to ensure that crowns, bridges and dentures are not too tight a fit when placed in the mouth. The expansion is also made use of in investments, as it helps to compensate for the shrinkage of metallic casting on cooling from the melting temperature.

Although it is desirable generally that models produced from plaster or stone are slightly on the big side, the unchecked expansion of this material would be excessive.

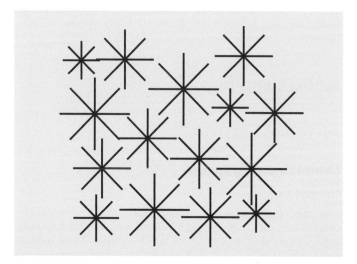

Figure 3.1.1 Spherulitic structure of calcium sulphate dihydrate

Table 3.1.1 Change in molar volume that occurs as calcium sulphate hemihydrate is rehydrated

	$(CaSO_4)_2 \cdot H_2O$	+ $3H_2O$	$\rightarrow$ $2CaSO_4 \cdot 2H_2O$
Molecular weight	290	54	344
Density	2.75	1.0	2.32
Molar volume	105	54	148

Change in volume = (148–159)/159 = −7.1%

Table 3.1.2 Setting expansions of some gypsum products

Plaster	0.20–0.30%
Stone	0.08–0.10%
Densite	0.05–0.07%

Table 3.1.3 Compressive strengths of some gypsum products

Plaster	12 MPa
Stone	30 MPa
Densite	38 MPa

CLINICAL SIGNIFICANCE

There are various additives in gypsum products that are used to control the degree of expansion, which in the case of plaster is 0.2–0.3 vol. % and for stones and dies is in the region of 0.05–0.10 vol. %.

CLINICAL SIGNIFICANCE

The low setting expansion of stone and densite makes these materials ideal for the production of dies and models for both metal and ceramic work.

Sodium chloride

Sodium chloride provides additional sites for crystal formation. The higher density of crystals limits the growth of the crystals and hence reduces their ability to push each other apart. This results in a reduction of the observed expansion. The increased number of sites for nucleation of the dihydrate crystals has the effect of increasing the rate of setting of the material. The hemihydrate also dissolves more rapidly, which again increases the rate of reaction.

If present in high concentrations (>20%), the sodium chloride will deposit on to the surface of the crystal and prevent further growth. This reduces the reaction rate, rather than increasing it.

Potassium sulphate

Potassium sulphate (K_2SO_4) reacts with the water and calcium sulphate hemihydrate to produce $K_2(CaSO_4)_2 \cdot H_2O$. This compound crystallizes very rapidly and encourages the growth of more crystals. This has the effect of reducing the overall expansion and accelerating the setting reaction. When present as a 2% solution in water, it will reduce the setting time from approximately 10 minutes to 4 minutes.

Calcium sulphate dihydrate

The addition of a small amount of calcium sulphate dihydrate will provide additional sites for nucleation and act as an accelerator; it will reduce both the working and the setting times.

Borax

The addition of borax ($Na_2B_4O_7 \cdot 10H_2O$) is important because it counteracts the increased rate of setting due to the inclusion of the above additives. It is a *retarder* of the setting process. The addition of borax leads to the formation of calcium tetraborate, which deposits on the dihydrate crystals and prevents further growth.

Potassium citrate

Potassium citrate acts as a retarder, and is sometimes added in addition to borax.

Thus, by carefully regulating the amount of the above additives, gypsum-based products can be produced with the correct degree of expansion and the correct working and setting times appropriate for various applications. The typical setting expansions for gypsum products are as shown in Table 3.1.2.

Hygroscopic expansion

The setting expansion can be increased substantially by immersing the material in water whilst it is setting. When it is in air, the surface tension of the free water tends to draw the crystals together, and this limits the ability of the crystals to grow.

However, when the crystals are immersed in water they can grow more freely, resulting in a greater degree of expansion. This process is called *hygroscopic expansion*, and is sometimes used with gypsum-bonded refractory investments for the casting of alloys that have a high coefficient of thermal expansion or a high contraction on solidification.

Properties

Dimensional stability

Once the material has set, there is little or no dimensional change. The storage stability is excellent, although the material *is* slightly soluble in water. For this reason, washing the surface with hot water should be avoided.

Compressive strength

The compressive strength is the mechanical property most commonly used for assessing the strength of gypsum products. These values are typically as shown in Table 3.1.3.

The compressive strength is affected considerably by the powder-to-liquid ratio that is used. It is clear from the above data that the reduction in the amount of water that is required to produce an acceptable mix gives a significant improvement in the compressive strength. Thus, the compressive strength of the set product is affected by straying from the recommended powder-to-liquid ratio. The use of an excessive amount of water has the advantage that a smooth mix, which can be readily poured, is obtained. The air that is incorporated during the mixing process is more readily removed from such a mix for stone and densite by vibration, but the compressive strength after setting will be inferior. On the other hand, using less water than is recommended results in a thick mix from which incorporated air is more difficult to remove, leading to an increased porosity and a significantly reduced strength. There is also a danger that insufficient water will be present for the full reaction to take place.

Thus, using less water has the potential of increasing the compressive strength, but inferior properties are obtained if too little is used.

There is a marked difference in the wet and dry strength of plaster products. In general, the dry strength is about twice the wet strength.

Tensile strength

The wet tensile strength of plaster is very low (approximately 2 MPa). This is due to the porosity and brittle nature of the material, which has the disadvantage that teeth and margins on the model can be easily damaged if handled roughly. Dental stone has a tensile strength about twice that of plaster, and is therefore preferred for the production of crown and bridge models and dies.

Hardness and abrasion resistance

The surface hardness of gypsum products is very low, so the material is highly susceptible to scratching and loss through abrasion. The epoxy resins are explored as alternative die materials since these exhibit much better detail reproduction, abrasion resistance and transverse strength than the gypsum materials, but are subject to polymerization shrinkage.

CLINICAL SIGNIFICANCE

The contraction of epoxy resins during setting can compromise the fit of castings unless this is taken into account in the processing.

Reproduction of surface detail

In the American National Standards Institute/American Dental Association specification no. 19, compatibility of impression materials with dental stones is assessed by the presence of a 20-μm-wide line reproduced on an unmodified calcium sulphate dihydrate cast. As the surface of gypsum products is slightly porous, minute surface details that are less than 20 μm are not readily reproduced. However, macroscopic surface details are very accurately reproduced, although air bubbles (trapped between the plaster and the impression, for example) can contribute to the loss of surface details.

When a mould is being waxed up for casting, the die has to be kept moist. Since the gypsum is, to some degree, soluble in water, some surface loss of material will occur and therefore repeated drying and wetting should be avoided.

CLINICAL SIGNIFICANCE

Whenever a die needs to be rewetted, this should be done with a saturated solution of calcium sulphate dihydrate in water.

Summary

The advantages and disadvantages of the use of plaster for the production of models can be summarized as shown in Table 3.1.4.

Table 3.1.4 Advantages and disadvantages of plaster for model making

Advantages	Disadvantages
Dimensionally accurate and stable	Low tensile strength, brittle Poor abrasion resistance
Cheap	Poor surface detail
Good colour contrast	Poor wetting of rubber impression materials

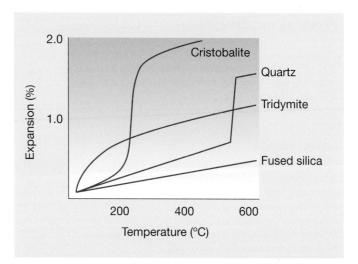

Figure 3.1.2 Thermal expansion behaviour of three silica allotropes

REFRACTORIES

As mentioned previously, refractories are materials that can withstand high temperatures of up to 1500°C. They are used to construct moulds used in the lost wax casting technique for the fabrication of metal restorations and the hot pressing of ceramic restorations, and are also used as a base in the sintering process for the production of ceramic restorations such as veneers, crowns and inlays.

In 1929, Coleman and Weinstein invented a gypsum-bonded cristobalite investment to replace the plaster of Paris, eliminating most of the shrinkage and distortion problems that had plagued the production of gold castings up to that point. Cristobalite is one of the three allotropic forms of silica, the others being quartz and tridymite, and it has thermal expansion qualities that make it especially suitable as an investment material for gold casting (Figure 3.1.2). The term investment originated from the solid mould process, in which a material like plaster of Paris is poured or 'invested' into a container that holds the wax pattern that is identical to the gold casting to be produced. After the plaster has set, the mould is heated up to a temperature of 900–1000°C, so that the wax pattern is burnt out and a high degree of thermal expansion is achieved, leaving a hollow cavity into which the molten metal is poured. However, the addition of cristobalite to plaster of Paris to create a gypsum-bonded investment did not immediately produce perfect gold alloy castings, and it was not until the 1940s that cristobalite investment materials were formulated that compensated for all of the distortions encountered in the original lost wax technique.

Refractories for lost wax casting of dental alloys

The basic principles of lost wax casting are described in Chapter 3.3. The most important feature of a dental refractory investment is the amount it will expand on heating without distorting or disintegrating. The concept is that the mould cavity will expand by an amount sufficient to compensate for the shrinkage of the wax pattern due to the change in temperature at which the wax pattern is prepared and subsequently invested, and the shrinkage of the metal as it cools down from its casting temperature.

wax shrinkage + metal shrinkage =
setting expansion + hygroscopic expansion + thermal expansion

The aim is to produce a restoration that will be a perfect fit. Naturally, the degree of expansion required from the refractory investment depends on the contraction behaviour of the metal used to manufacture a restoration. For example, the effective contraction of dental gold alloys on cooling from the casting temperature (1100–1300°C) to room temperature is in the range of 1.25 to 1.80%, and the mould has to be heated to a temperature of 900–1000°C to provide adequate expansion of the mould space. This contrasts with the casting of titanium, where the mould is heat-soaked at a temperature of 900°C but then has to be cooled to 350°C because above this temperature the molten titanium will react with the mould materials. Yet the mould still has to compensate for a thermal contraction of titanium of 1.6%.

The amount of expansion of the refractory investment is governed by a combination of the setting expansion derived from the binder and the thermal expansion/contraction of the binder and filler.

The type of refractory and its properties depend on the particular application, but there are currently two types of refractory materials that are still widely used: namely, gypsum-bonded and phosphate-bonded refractories. The gypsum-bonded investments are used primarily for casting with low-melting-temperature gold alloys, while the phosphate-bonded investments are used with base metal alloys and with high-melting-temperature gold and precious metal alloys, and for the casting, hot pressing and sintering of dental glasses and glass–ceramics.

Gypsum-bonded refractory investments

Gypsum-bonded dental refractory investments are used primarily in conjunction with relatively low-melting-temperature gold alloys and silver/palladium alloys, which are typically melted in the range of 1100–1300°C. Gypsum-bonded dental refractory investments consist of some 70% silica, typically a mixture of quartz and cristobalite, and 30% binder (calcium sulphate hemihydrate).

The setting expansion is governed by the composition of the binder and will clearly be a function of the relative amounts of plaster and stone and all the other ingredients that are incorporated to control the expansion and the setting time, as explained in detail above when considering models and dies. The setting expansion can be enhanced by placing the mould in water or adding water to the surface of the mould during the intial setting process. The hygroscopic expansion that this gives rise to is caused by the capillary action of the water, which is attracted into the spaces between the dihydrate crystals as they form and pushes the crystals further apart. It is important to appreciate that, when hygroscopic expansion is used, the mould temperature at casting may need to be some 200°C lower. Along with the addition of sodium chloride and/or potassium sulphate, the setting expansion can vary from 0.25 to 0.80%. However, much of this is lost when the investment is heated, when the gypsum binder will shrink as it loses water and it converts from calcium sulphate dihydrate, through calcium sulphate hemihydrate to anhydrite (CaSO4).

The thermal expansion of most refractory materials would be insufficient to provide enough expansion to compensate for the contraction of a dental casting alloy. To overcome this problem, cristobalite is used as a major ingredient in dental refractory investments along with the binder. Cristobalite undergoes a rapid expansion at 220°C due to an inversion from cubic high cristobalite to tetragonal low cristobalite, resulting in a less dense crystal structure. At the same time, the room-temperature form of quartz, α-quartz, undergoes a reversible change in crystal structure at 573°C to form β-quartz, and this is accompanied by a linear expansion of 0.45%. The thermal expansion of a gypsum-bonded investment can be carefully controlled by selecting appropriate amounts of each ingredient and is typically in the range of 1.20 to 1.50%.

Phosphate-bonded refractory investments

Gypsum-bonded refractory investments are not suitable for use with many high-melting-temperature gold alloys used to construct metal–ceramic restorations and most base metal alloys such as Ni–Cr and Co–Cr alloys. For such alloys, which typically are cast at temperatures between 1400°C and 1550°C, a phosphate-bonded investment is required, since the gypsum-bonded investment would disintegrate on contact with the molten metal. Also, as a consequence of the high casting temperature, the thermal contaction for such alloys is typically around 2.0–2.3% and the gypsum-bonded investments are not able to compensate for this degree of contraction.

A phosphate-bonded investment consists of a powder containing ammonium diacid phosphate ($NH_4 \cdot H_2 \cdot PO_4$), calcined magnesia (MgO) and silica (quartz and cristobalite). The powder is mixed with a liquid consisting of water, colloidal silica, surfactant, defloculant, glycerine and defoaming agent. On mixing, a reaction takes place between the phosphate, magnesia and water as follows:

$$NH_4 \cdot H_2 \cdot PO_4 + MgO + 5H_2O \rightarrow Mg \cdot NH_4 \cdot PO_4 \cdot 6H_2O$$

The crystalline solid that forms as a result of this setting reaction binds the silica particles together. As with the plaster of Paris, the crystals push each other apart and this results in a small setting expansion, but again most of this is lost when the mould is heated. When the temperature reaches approximately 300°C, ammonia and water are released:

$$2(Mg \cdot NH_4 \cdot PO_4 \cdot 6H_2O) \rightarrow Mg_2 \cdot P_2O_7 + 2NH_3 + 13H_2O$$

On further heating, any remaining $NH_4 \cdot H_2 \cdot PO_4$ reacts with the colloidal silica to form a silicophosphate, which helps to increase the strength of the investment at high temperatures.

The release of ammonia on heating the refractory investment is a potential environmental hazard but there are now phosphate-bonded investments that do not relase ammonia. This has been achieved by substituting the ammonium diacid phosphate ($NH_4 \cdot H_2 \cdot PO_4$) with $Mg(H_2PO_4)_2$.

When considering the use of a phosphate-bonded refractory investment as a mould for hot pressing or support for the construction of ceramic restorations, there is, in fact, very little literature on the subject. During the laboratory construction stage of, for example, a veneer, careful consideration must be given to the dimensional changes that may take place within the variety of refractory and ceramic materials available. When the ceramic is fired on a refractory mould, it is important that there is no differential contraction, as this may cause distortion or even cracking of the restoration. Generally speaking, matched refractory investment and ceramic systems have a closely matched coefficient of thermal expansion (CTE), but huge discrepancies, by as much as a factor of 2, can arise with the injudicious selection of a refractory/ceramic combination. Some veneering ceramics, such as those based on a feldspathic glass, will have a CTE of 6–7 ppm/°C and the phosphate-bonded refractory investments can have a CTE of up to 13 ppm/°C.

CLINICAL SIGNIFICANCE

By carefully controlling the composition of the binder and the refractory investment, the setting and thermal expansion can be controlled and, in turn, it is possible to compensate for the contraction of the metal or the ceramic such that the restoration will have a clinically acceptable quality of fit on the tooth.

FURTHER READING

Chan TK, Darvell BW (2001) Effect of storage conditions on calcium sulphate hemihydrate-containing products. Dent Mater 17: 134

Derrien G, Le Menn G (1995) Evaluation of detail reproduction for three die materials by using scanning electron microscopy and two-dimensional profilometry. J Prosthet Dent 74: 1

Duke P, Moore BK, Haug SP (2000) Study of the physical properties of type IV gypsum, resin-containing, and epoxy die materials. J Prosthet Dent 83: 466

Eames WB, Edwares CR, Buck WH (1978) Scraping resistance of dental die materials: a comparison of brands. Oper Dent 3: 66

Fan PL, Powers JM, Reid BC (1981) Surface mechanical properties of stone, resin and metal dies. J Am Dent Assoc 103: 408

Paquette JM, Taniguchi T, White SN (2000) Dimensional accuracy of an epoxy resin die material using two setting methods. J Prosthet Dent 83: 301

Takashiba S, Zhang Z, Tamaki Y (2002) Experimental ammonia-free phosphate-bonded investments using Mg(H2PO4)2 solution. Dent Mater J 21(4): 322–331

Whyte MP, Brockhurst PJ (1996) The effect of steam sterilization on the properties of set dental gypsum models. Aust Dent J 41: 128

Wildgoose DG, Winstanley RB, van Noort R (1997) The laboratory construction and teaching of ceramic veneers: a survey. J Dent. 25(2): 119–123

Denture base resins

INTRODUCTION

There is an ageing population in the Western world and the projection is that, by 2025, more than 50% of the population will be over the age of 50. Despite developments in oral hygiene, it is likely that many of these people will require full or partial dentures to replace missing teeth. At present, some 32 million North Americans wear full or partial dentures and the number of dentures prescribed annually runs at 9 million full dentures and 4.5 million partial dentures. For these patients, it is important that they are provided with an attractive, highly functional denture, as this will have a very positive influence on their quality of life.

The construction of a denture involves many steps. The first step is taking an impression, which is then followed by the various laboratory stages. These include producing a model, setting the teeth, preparing a waxed model, investing in a denture flask and boiling out the wax, which then leaves a space to be filled by the denture base material.

Various materials have been used to construct dentures, including cellulose products, phenol-formaldehyde, vinyl resins and vulcanite. However, they have suffered from a variety of problems:

- Cellulose products suffered from warpage in the mouth, and from a taste of camphor due to its use as a plasticizer. This camphor leached out of the denture, causing blistering, staining and loss of colour within a few months.
- Phenol-formaldehyde (bakelite) proved to be too difficult to process and also lost its colour in the mouth.
- Vinyl resins were found to have a low resistance to fracture, and failures were common, possibly due to fatigue.
- Vulcanite was the first material to be used for the mass production of dentures, but its aesthetic qualities are not very good and it has now been replaced by acrylic resins.

Acrylic resin (poly methyl methacrylate) is now the material of choice; it has the required aesthetic quality, and is cheap and easy to process. Even so, it is not ideal in all respects. The ideal properties of a denture base material are shown in Table 3.2.1.

Acrylic resins are popular because they meet many of the criteria set out in Table 3.2.1. In particular, dentures made from acrylic resin are easy to process using inexpensive techniques, and are aesthetically pleasing. Besides its use in the construction of full dentures, the material is also used for a wide range of other applications such as the construction of customized trays for impression taking, the soft-tissue replication on cast metal frameworks, denture repairs, soft liners and denture teeth.

COMPOSITION AND STRUCTURE OF ACRYLIC RESIN

An acrylic resin denture is made by the process of free radical addition polymerization to form poly methyl methacrylate (PMMA). The monomer is methyl methacrylate (MMA):

$$
\begin{array}{ccc}
H & & Me \\
| & & | \\
C & = & C \\
| & & | \\
H & & C = O \\
& & | \\
& & O \\
& & | \\
& & Me
\end{array}
$$

where Me stands for CH_3. The conversion of the monomer into a polymer involves the normal sequence of activation, initiation, propagation and termination, as described in Chapter 1.5. The resins are available in either heat-cured or cold-cured forms.

Heat-cured resins

These materials consist of a powder and a liquid, which, on mixing and subsequent heating, form a rigid solid. The constituents of the powder and liquid are shown in Table 3.2.2.

The reasons for the particular formulation of a powder–liquid system are threefold:

- Processing is possible by the dough technique.
- Polymerization shrinkage is minimized.
- The heat of the reaction is reduced.

<table>
<tr><td>

Table 3.2.1 Criteria for an ideal denture base material

Natural appearance
High strength, stiffness, hardness and toughness
Dimensional stabililty
Absence of odour, taste or toxic products
Resistance to absorption of oral fluids
Good retention to polymers, porcelain and metals
Ease of repair
Good shelf life
Ease of manipulation
Low density
Accurate reproduction of surface detail
Resistance to bacterial growth
Good thermal conductivity
Radiopacity
Ease of cleaning
Inexpensiveness to use

</td></tr>
</table>

Table 3.2.2 Constituents of a heat-cured resin

Powder
Beads or granules of poly methyl methacrylate
Initiator – benzoyl peroxide
Pigments/dyes
Opacifiers – titanium/zinc oxides
Plasticizer – dibutyl phthalate
Synthetic fibres – nylon/acrylic

Liquid
Methyl methacrylate monomer
Inhibitor – hydroquinone
Cross-linking agent – ethylene glycol dimethacrylate

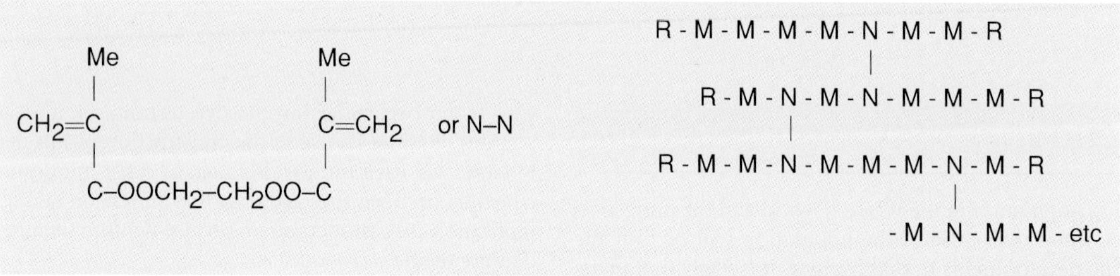

Figure 3.2.1 Diethylene glycol dimethacrylate (a) and its formation of cross-links (b)

The dough technique helps to make the processing of dentures a relatively straightforward process. A flask containing the teeth set in plaster is packed with the dough and then closed under pressure such that the excess dough is squeezed out. In addition, by adapting the dough to the model and trimming off any excess, cold-cure varieties of the acrylics are easily manipulated (when in the doughy stage) to produce special trays. Granules dissolve more readily in the monomer than beads and hence reduce the time taken to reach the doughy stage.

The polymerization shrinkage is reduced when compared to using a monomer because most of the material that is being used (i.e. the beads or granules) has already been polymerized.

The polymerization reaction is highly exothermic, as a considerable amount of heat energy (80 kJ/mol) is released in reducing the C=C to –C–C– bonds. Since a large proportion of the mixture is already in the form of a polymer, the potential for overheating is reduced. As the maximum temperature reached will be less, so the amount of thermal contraction will also be reduced.

The monomer is extremely volatile and highly flammable, so the container must be kept sealed at all times and must be kept away from naked flames. The container is a dark glass bottle, which extends the shelf life of the monomer by avoiding spontaneous polymerization from the action of light.

Hydroquinone also extends the shelf life of the monomer by reacting rapidly with any free radicals that may form spontaneously within the liquid and producing forms of stabilized free radicals that are not able to initiate the polymerization process.

Contamination with the polymer beads or granules must be avoided, as these carry the benzoyl peroxide on their surface and only a tiny amount of the polymer is needed to start the polymerization reaction.

The polymer powder is very stable and has a virtually indefinite shelf life.

A cross-linking agent, such as diethylene glycol dimethacrylate, is included in order to improve the mechanical properties (Figure 3.2.1a). These are incorporated at various points along the methyl methacrylate polymer chain and form cross-links with adjacent chains by virtue of their two double-bond sites (Figure 3.2.1b).

Thus, although the PMMA is a thermoplastic resin, the inclusion of the cross-linking agent prevents post-processing.

Cold-cure resins

The chemistry of these resins is identical to that of the heat-cured resins, except that the cure is initiated by a tertiary amine (e.g. dimethyl-P-toluidine or sulphinic acid) rather than heat.

This method of curing is not as efficient as the heat curing process, and tends to result in a lower-molecular-weight material. This has an adverse effect on the strength properties of the material and also raises the amount of uncured residual monomer in the resin. The colour stability is not as good as for the heat-cured material, and the cold-cured resins are more prone to yellowing.

The size of the polymer beads is somewhat smaller than in the heat-cured resin (which has a bead size of 150 μm) to ease dissolution in the monomer to produce a dough. The doughy stage has to be reached before the addition curing reaction begins to affect the viscosity of the mix and prevents the adaptation of the mix to the mould walls.

The lower molecular weight also results in a lowering of the glass transition temperature, with Tg being typically 75–80°C. Whilst one might think that this makes the material more inclined to warpage, this is not so. As no external heat source is used to cure the resin, there is less build-up of internal strain. Nevertheless, the material is highly susceptible to creep, and this can contribute significantly to the eventual distortion of the denture when in use.

Pour-and-cure resins

These are cold-cure resins that are sufficiently liquid when mixed that they can be poured into a mould made of a hydrocolloid. They give excellent reproduction of surface detail but are inferior to both the heat- and cold-cured acrylics in so many other respects that they are not much used.

Visible-light-cured resins

A visible-light-activated denture base resin was first introduced in the 1980s, on the premise that it did not contain methyl methacrylate, which is a known sensitizer. Thus the material was advocated for its biocompatibility, but also because of its low bacterial adherence, ease of fabrication and manipulation, patient acceptance, ability to bond to other denture resins and a lack of requirement for proportioning and mixing. The chemistry of these materials has more in common with a composite restorative material than with the denture base resins considered above (see Chapter 2.2). The material is composed of a matrix of urethane dimethacrylate that contains a small amount of colloidal silica to control the rheology. The filler consists of acrylic beads that become part of an interpenetrating polymer network structure when it is cured. Initially, its application was limited because of a lack of impact strength and high brittleness, but a superior product has now become available that is claimed to have superior properties (Eclipse™, Dentsply). It is widely used as a denture hard reline material, for the construction of customized impression trays and for the repair of fractured dentures.

ASPECTS OF MANIPULATION

Powder-to-liquid ratio

It is important to use the correct powder-to-liquid ratio (2.0/1.0 wt %; 1.6/1.0 vol. %). Too much powder could result in inadequate filling by the monomer of the free space between the powder particles, resulting in a weak material as a consequence of porosity in the final product. Too much monomer will produce excessive polymerization shrinkage and a loss of quality of fit to the denture-bearing surface.

The additives tend to settle out at the bottom of the container and it is important that the container is shaken before use to ensure an even distribution of the powder ingredients.

Control of colour

The colouring pigment is usually incorporated in the polymer powder, but in some cases it may simply be on the surface of the polymer beads and may be washed off by too rapid a contact of the monomer. In this case, the polymer should be added to the monomer slowly. Too little powder will produce too light a shade.

Mould lining

There is a danger that the resin may penetrate the relatively rough surface of the plaster mould and adhere to it. To prevent this, a separating medium must be employed. Nowadays, the separating medium

is usually a solution of sodium alginate, although some still recommend the use of tin foil.

Processing

There are two problems in particular to watch out for in the processing of acrylics for dentures: one is their porosity and the second is the presence of processing strains.

Porosity

The problem one is most likely to experience with acrylic resin dentures is the occurrence of porosity during the processing stage. There are two major causes of porosity: polymerization shrinkage-associated *contraction porosity*, and volatilization of the monomer, termed *gaseous porosity*.

Contraction porosity

Contraction porosity occurs because the monomer contracts by some 20% of its volume during processing. By using the powder–liquid system, this contraction is minimized and should be in the region of 5–8%. However, this is not translated into a high linear shrinkage, which, on the basis of the volumetric shrinkage, should be of the order of 1.5–2%, but is in fact somewhere in the region of 0.2–0.5%. It is believed that this is because the observed contraction is due in large part to the thermal contraction as a result of the change from curing temperature to room temperature, rather than due to the polymerization contraction. In order to activate the polymerization process, the temperature in the flask has to be raised to more than 60°C, such that the benzoyl peroxide breaks down and forms free radicals (see Chapter 1.5). Once the reaction has been initiated, it continues to generate heat of its own due to the exothermic reaction. This can push up the temperature of the acrylic to well above 100°C.

At the processing temperature, the resin is able to flow into the spaces created by the curing contraction. The driving force for this flow is provided by pressure that is exerted during the processing; packing a slight excess of denture base material into the mould ensures that the material is under pressure when the mould is closed. This pressure is maintained throughout the processing cycle.

The resin only becomes rigid once it gets below its glass transition temperature, at which point the curing contraction will have been completed. From this point on, it is the thermal contraction that contributes to the observed changes in dimensions of the denture base. Cold-cure resins should give a better fit for the denture, as the processing temperature is considerably lower (around 60°C, compared to 100°C for the heat-cured resin). However, the fit is normally compromised due to the increased likelihood of creep at the lower Tg.

It is therefore important that sufficient dough is packed in the mould to ensure that the material is constantly under pressure during processing. This will cause any voids present in the mix to collapse, and should also help to compensate for the curing contraction. Thus, the packing of the mould should only be carried out when the mix has reached the doughy stage, as, prior to this, the high flow causes a rapid loss of pressure.

If there is evidence of localized porosity, this may be due to poor mixing of the components or to packing the mould before the doughy stage is reached. The associated differential contraction can lead to distortion of the denture.

Gaseous porosity

As noted above, on polymerization, there is an exothermic reaction. This could cause the temperature of the resin to rise above 100°C, which is just above its boiling temperature. If this temperature is exceeded before the polymerization process is completed, gaseous monomer will be formed – which is the cause of gaseous porosity. The amount of heat generated depends on the volume of resin present, the proportion of monomer and the rapidity with which the external heat reaches the resin. The occurrence of gaseous porosity can be avoided by allowing the temperature to be raised in a slow and controlled fashion.

CLINICAL SIGNIFICANCE

Polymerization must be carried out *slowly* (to prevent gaseous porosity) and *under pressure* (to avoid contraction porosity), such that the temperature of the denture acrylic never exceeds 100°C.

Processing strains

The restriction imposed on the dimensional change of the resin will inevitably give rise to internal strains. If such strains were allowed to relax, the result would be warpage, crazing, or distortion of the denture base. Although many of the strains generated during the curing contraction can be relieved by the flow that occurs above the glass transition temperature, some strain that is due to thermal contraction will remain. The level of the internal strain can be minimized by using acrylic rather than porcelain teeth (so that there is no differential shrinkage on cooling) and by allowing the flask to cool slowly.

The relief of internal strain can produce tiny surface defects in the resin. These are known as *crazes*, and can be identified by a hazy or foggy appearance to the surface of the denture base. A craze is a localized region of high plastic deformation of the polymer, which may be filled with tiny voids. At this stage it is not yet a crack since, unlike a crack, the crazed region can still support stress. However, crazing can lead to brittle fracture of the polymer. As the voids in the crazed region grow, these become separated only by thin fibrils of polymer until eventually the fibrils fail and a crack is formed (Figure 3.2.2). This crack will grow under an externally applied load such that it will reach a size at which it will continue to grow spontaneously and cause the denture to fracture.

The crazes may be formed in response to heat (due to polishing, for example), differential contraction around porcelain teeth, or attack by solvents such as alcohol.

CLINICAL SIGNIFICANCE

The introduction of cross-links in the polymer chains by the addition of diethylene glycol dimethacrylate has been found to reduce the potential for craze formation.

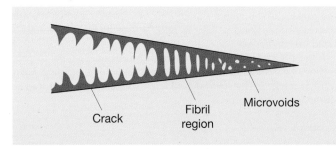

Figure 3.2.2 Crack formation resulting from a craze

Crack | Fibril region | Microvoids

PROPERTIES

Dimensional stability and accuracy

Given that the denture is placed on an adaptable cushion of soft tissues, one may wonder why it is so important that the denture does not change its shape. In fact, it is a matter of great concern to the *retention* of the denture, where retention can be defined as the resistance to forces that tend to displace the denture in an occlusal direction. This is distinct from *stability*, which is the resistance to movement in a horizontal direction.

The factors that determine the retention of dentures in the mouth are essentially physical in nature. Anatomical factors such as undercuts are a nuisance rather than an advantage, as the denture is rigid and cannot engage them. In some instances preprosthetic surgery may be required to remove the undercut.

The most appropriate explanation of the factors that govern the retention of a denture is the viscous flow model (as discussed in Chapter 1.9), which is based on the relationship

$$F = 3\pi\eta R^4 / 2h^3 \delta h / \delta t$$

for a disc with radius R, and a thickness of saliva h.

Adhesion of the denture to the mucosa is provided by saliva, and the greater the surface area, the better the adhesive bond (i.e. R should be as large as possible). At the same time, it is important that the cohesion of the saliva film is not destroyed, and this is best guarded against by having as thin a film of saliva between the mucosa and denture as is possible (i.e. h should be small), so the denture should fit as accurately as possible.

The establishment of a peripheral seal around the edge of the denture is very important for retention. The tighter the seal, the more difficult it is for additional saliva to enter the space between the denture and the mucosa, and this means that more force needs to be applied to separate the denture from the mucosa. Anything that may upset the peripheral seal, such as over-extension, interferences (e.g. a frenal notch) and occlusal imbalance, will impair the retention of the denture.

As patients get older, the rate of production and the consistency of their saliva may change. The saliva becomes less adhesive to the denture, due to poor wetting of the surface by an inadequate supply of saliva, and it also becomes less viscous. Denture retention can then become a particular problem, and denture fixatives may have to be employed.

CLINICAL SIGNIFICANCE

For a denture to have the optimum retention it should (1) cover the maximum area of mucosa compatible with the functional muscular activity and (2) be a close fit, so as to minimize the thickness of the saliva film and retain a good peripheral seal.

Mechanical properties

The tensile strength of acrylic resins is typically no more than 50 MPa. The elastic modulus is low, the flexural modulus being in the region of 2200–2500 MPa. When this is combined with a lack of fracture toughness, it is perhaps not surprising that dentures are prone to fracture. Some 30% of denture repairs carried out by dental laboratories involve midline fractures, which are most prevalent among upper dentures.

Most fractures are associated with some traumatic incident to the denture, although this may not be easily recognized. If dropped on the floor, a denture does not necessarily break instantly, but the chances are that a crack will have formed that will continue to grow unnoticed until the denture fails suddenly and catastrophically. Thus, eventual failure of the denture occurs due to flexural fatigue.

Some fractures may be associated with poor-quality processing. Lack of bonding between the resin and the acrylic teeth is such a possibility, and gives rise to a weak interface from which a fracture is likely to be initiated. The formation of crazes due to processing faults or exposure to solvents is another possibility.

For those patients who fracture their dentures on a regular basis, it is possible to consider a high-impact-resistant denture base resin. These resins are formulated with a rubber toughening agent, such as a fine dispersion of butadiene styrene. The rubbery inclusions stop cracks developing, showing a higher degree of resistance to fracture as a consequence. However, they also cause a lowering of the flexural modulus, and long-term fatigue failure due to excessive flexure can be a problem.

An alternative approach to the strengthening of acrylic dentures is the incorporation of fibres so as to produce a fibre-reinforced composite. These include:

- *Carbon fibres*, which have not proved popular due to difficult handling characteristics and poor aesthetics.
- *Aramid fibres* (polypara-phenylene terephthalamide), which have not proved effective due to the lack of bonding between the fibres and the resin matrix.
- *UHMPE* (ultra-high molecular weight polyethylene), which are neutral in colour, have low density and known biocompatibility, and can be surface-treated to enhance bonding to the resin, but fabrication is time-consuming.
- *Glass fibres*, which have shown the most promise and can be either incorporated in the resin as short fibres or embedded in cloth or loose form.

None of these has as yet evolved into an effective replacement of the unfilled acrylic resins due to unacceptable processing characteristics, and the rubber-reinforced resins are preferred, as these have handling properties similar to those of the conventional PMMA resins. Research to develop a successful method of producing a fibre-reinforced denture base is ongoing.

CLINICAL SIGNIFICANCE

The lack of strength and toughness of acrylic resin dentures is a serious problem and can result in fractures of up to 10% of dentures within 3 years of use.

Creep is a problem with acrylic resins (particularly the cold-cured resins), as they are viscoelastic materials. The addition of a cross-linking agent reduces the amount of creep, but it cannot be totally eliminated.

Physical properties

Thermal conductivity

The thermal conductivity of PMMA is approximately 6×10^{-4} cal·g^{-1}·cm^{-2}. This is very low, and can present problems during denture processing, as the heat produced cannot escape, leading to a temperature rise.

From the patient's point of view, the problem with a low coefficient of thermal conductivity is that the denture isolates the oral soft tissues from any sensation of temperature. This can lead to a patient consuming a drink that is far too hot without realizing it, which may lead to the back of the throat and possibly even the oesophagus being scalded.

Coefficient of thermal expansion

The coefficient of thermal expansion is approximately 80 ppm/°C. This is quite high, as one might expect from a resin. In general, this does not present a problem, except that there is a possibility that porcelain teeth set in denture base resin may gradually loosen and be lost due to the differential expansion and contraction.

Water sorption and solubility

Due to the polar nature of the resin molecules, PMMA will absorb water. This water sorption is typically of the order of 1.0–2.0% by weight.

In practice, this helps to compensate for the slight processing shrinkage. However, given the low rate of diffusion of water through the resin, it would take the denture some weeks of continuous immersion in water to reach a stable weight.

Although PMMA is soluble in most solvents (e.g. chloroform), as it is only lightly cross-linked, it is virtually insoluble in most of the fluids that it may come into contact with in the mouth. However, some weight loss *will* occur, due to leaching of the monomer in particular, and possibly some of the pigments and dyes.

Biocompatibility

In general, PMMA is highly biocompatible and patients suffer few problems. Nevertheless, some patients will show an allergic reaction. This is most probably associated with the various leachable components in the denture, such as any residual monomer or benzoic acid.

The allergic reaction tends to be virtually immediate, and is more likely to occur with cold-cured resin dentures because of their higher residual monomer content. Sometimes it may be possible to overcome this problem by subjecting the denture to an additional curing cycle, but there is a danger that this will cause the denture to distort as internal processing stresses are relieved.

When a patient has a confirmed delayed hypersensitivity to methacrylate resins, then an alternative denture base material, such as a polycarbonate or polyamide, may have to be considered. Dentures manufactured from these materials have to be processed by injection moulding and, whilst precision is high, the costs are also more than those of a denture constructed from PMMA.

Nylon, which is the generic name of a thermoplastic polymer belonging to the class of polyamides, was first considered for dentures in the 1950s. Deterioration of the colour, excessive water sorption and a high flexibility due to the low elastic modulus were some of the problems encountered. However, during the 1970s, different polyamide-based polymers were developed, which are claimed to have overcome some of these problems, although little is published about their performance. It would appear that even less is known about polycarbonate as a denture base material, although the material is widely used in safety helmets because of its excellent impact resistance.

Summary

The advantages of the use of poly methyl methacrylate are that it:

- has excellent aesthetics
- is easy and cheap to process
- has a low density.

The disadvantages are that the material:

- has barely adequate strength characteristics
- is susceptible to distortion
- has a low thermal conductivity
- is radiolucent.

DENTURE-LINING MATERIALS

The denture-lining materials fall essentially into three groups, namely:

- permanent hard reline materials
- semipermanent soft liners
- tissue conditioners/temporary soft liners.

Hard reline materials

Although the expected mean life of a complete denture may be 4–5 years, the actual life will depend on the rate of resorption of the alveolar bone. If the fitting surface of a denture needs to be replaced to improve the fit of the denture, a *hard reline* material can be employed. Relining a complete denture may be required due to soft-tissue changes arising from bone resorption. This tends to be more of a problem with mandibular than maxillary dentures. The criteria for relining are:

- poor retention or stability
- collapse of vertical dimension of the occlusion
- degradation of the denture base
- lack of denture extension into mucobuccal fold areas
- in an elderly patient for whom habituation to a new denture may be difficult, if not impossible.

The reline either can be achieved with a cold-cure acrylic resin at the chair side, or the denture is sent to a dental laboratory for relining with a heat-cured acrylic.

The heat-cured acrylics used by laboratories are identical to those used for the construction of dentures.

The cold-cured resins come in two types, with constituents as listed in Table 3.2.3. The reason for the second type of reline material is that MMA can be very irritant to soft tissues and can sensitize the patient. The poly ethyl methacrylate (PEMA) and butyl methacrylate are less irritant to the patient, but have the disadvantage that they cause a reduction in the Tg, and this increases the possibility of dimensional instability.

One of the most serious drawbacks with attempting a chair-side reline is that there is little control over the amount of denture material removed and the thickness of the reline material that replaces it. Other problems include high exothermic reactions, unacceptable taste and poor colour stability over time.

CLINICAL SIGNIFICANCE

At best, a reline should be considered only as a long-term temporary expedient, with laboratory relines being the preferred option.

Semipermanent soft liners

Occasionally, a patient will complain of persistent pain and discomfort from a denture, even though the denture would appear totally satisfactory in all other respects. This problem is seen most commonly in the lower jaw, where there is a smaller surface area over which to distribute the load, and where patients may have a sharp, thin or heavily resorbed alveolar ridge. In such cases, the patient has difficulty in tolerating a hard denture. If the pain persists when all possible measures have been taken to minimize the occlusal load and redistribute the load over as large an area as is possible, the denture may be made more comfortable by the use of a soft liner. This provides a means of absorbing some of the energy involved in mastication, by interposing a highly resilient material between the denture and the mucosa.

Polymers with a glass transition temperature just above the temperature in the mouth will have a rubbery behaviour and are highly resilient.

Some polymers have a naturally low glass transition temperature (e.g. silicone polymers) and others (e.g. PMMA) can be modified by the inclusion of plasticizers to reduce their glass transition temperature (Table 3.2.4). The plasticizer acts as a lubricant for the polymer chains, making it easier for them to slide past one another, allowing the material to deform more easily and giving it a lower elastic modulus. In fact, soft liners are usually constructed from one or other of these two materials.

Silicone rubber

The silicone rubber consists of a poly dimethyl siloxane polymer to which filler is added to give it the correct consistency. The material solidifies by a cross-linking process rather than by a polymerization process, as the material is already a polymer. This cross-linking can be achieved either by heat, using benzoyl peroxide, or at room temperature, using tetraethylsilicate (see Chapter 2.7).

Silicone rubber does not bond readily to the acrylic resin of the denture, so an adhesive needs to be employed. This adhesion can be achieved using silicone polymer dissolved in a solvent, or by the use of an alkyl-silane coupling agent. In both cases, the bond is very weak, and usually fails within a relatively short time. Another drawback is that this material tends to support the growth of *Candida albicans*, which leads to denture stomatitis.

Table 3.2.3 Two types of cold-cured resin

	Type I	Type II
Powder	Poly methyl methacrylate Benzoyl peroxide Pigments	Poly ethyl methacrylate Benzoyl peroxide Pigments
Liquid	Methyl methacrylate Di-n-butylphthalate Amine	Butyl methacrylate Amine

Table 3.2.4 Glass transition temperatures for polymethacrylate esters

Group	Transition temperature (°C)
Methyl	125
Ethyl	65
Propyl	38
Butyl	33

Acrylic soft liners

These soft liners have the advantage that they bond well to the PMMA denture. They can be subdivided into those containing leachable plasticizers and those containing polymerizable plasticizers.

Leachable plasticizer systems

PEMA has a glass transition temperature of only 66 °C, compared with 100 °C for PMMA. A combination of these two polymers, with a small amount of plasticizer (such as dibutylphthalate) is highly resilient. Thus, the powder is a mixture of PEMA and PMMA, and the liquid is MMA, containing 25–50% plasticizer.

Unfortunately, the plasticizer gradually leaches out and the liner becomes stiff as it loses its resilience. How rapidly this transition takes place depends to some extent on the patient's regime for cleaning the denture. In general, high temperatures and strong bleaching agents should be avoided.

Polymerizable plasticizer systems

New plasticizers have been developed that polymerize, and thus resist dissolution, but which maintain their lubricating effect.

Exact formulations of this new material are not known, but some use alkyl-maleate or alkylitaconate, while for one experimental system the liquid component is known to be a mixture of tridecyl methacrylate, 2-diethylhexyl maleate and ethylene glycol dimethacrylate. The liquid is mixed with either PEMA or copolymers of n-butyl and ethyl methacrylate.

The material is fairly hard at room temperature, which makes it easy to finish, and softens when taken up to mouth temperature.

Relative merits of soft liners

The relative merits of the silicone and acrylic soft liners are outlined in Table 3.2.5. Although the use of soft liners is perceived as a long-term solution to poor load distribution, their clinical life is generally no more than 6 months due to the problems described above. Hence they are described as semipermanent soft liners.

Table 3.2.5 Relative merits of soft liners

Silicone rubber	Acrylic
Highly resilient	Less resilient
Retain softness	Go hard with time
Requires bonding agent	Self-adhesive
Susceptible to growth of *Candida albicans*	More resistant to bacteria
Weak bond	Permanent bond
Poor tear strength	Acceptable tear strength
No permanent deformation	Susceptible to creep

CLINICAL SIGNIFICANCE

Soft liners are contraindicated in patients with poor saliva flow, as the subsequent friction between the mucoperiosteum and the soft liner can gives rise to painful friction.

Tissue conditioners/temporary soft liners

In some instances, the denture can give rise to inflammation or ulceration of the load-bearing soft tissues. A simple solution would be for the patient to stop wearing the denture until the inflammation has subsided. This is generally not acceptable to the patient, and a tissue conditioner can be employed to overcome the problem.

A tissue conditioner is a soft material that is applied temporarily to the fitting surface of the denture for the purpose of allowing a more even stress distribution. This permits the mucosal tissue to return to its normal shape, and to resolve any inflammation of the denture-bearing tissues. Once the inflammation has receded and the tissue has recovered, an impression can be taken for a new denture.

Such a material must be exceptionally soft, yet not so soft as to squeeze out from between the denture and the mucosa. These materials typically consist of a powder such as PEMA, which, when mixed with a solvent such as ethyl alcohol and an aromatic ester such as a plasticizer (e.g. butyl phthalylbutylglycolate), produces a gel-like substance. Its consistency will depend on the initial powder-to-liquid ratio and the relative amounts of each of the components. When the powder and liquid are mixed together, the solvent readily penetrates the polymer beads, and this allows the plasticizer to enter the polymer very rapidly so as to create gel structure.

The alcohol and plasticizer will leach out quickly, and, therefore, the tissue conditioner needs to be replaced *every few days* if the traumatized tissue is to revert to a healthy state as soon as possible. For some patients, the tissue conditioner may be maintained for up to 3 weeks; hence the frequently used term 'temporary soft liner'.

One suggestion to improve the short lifespan of the tissue conditioners is to coat them with a thin surface layer of semiset methyl methacrylate resin so as to reduce the rate at which the solvent and plasticizer leach out.

CLINICAL SIGNIFICANCE

Tissue conditioners/temporary soft liners should not be used without giving the patient an appointment for review.

Tissue conditioners are susceptible to colonization by microorganisms. Unless the tissue conditioner is replaced regularly, it will act as a reservoir for microorganisms. This can cause serious complications such as respiratory infections, especially in elderly patients. Although mechanical and chemical cleaning can keep the microorganisms at bay, the cleaning methods can cause considerable damage to the tissue conditioner. Another approach being explored is the incorporation of anti-microbial agents, such as silver-zeolite or itraconozole, which appear to be efficacious.

The tissue conditioners are sensitive to denture cleansers and are best cleaned with plain soap and water.

FURTHER READING

Braden M, Wright PS, Parker S (1995)
Soft lining materials – a review. Eur J
Prosthodont Rest Dent **3**: 163

Chow CK, Matear DW, Lawrence HP (1999)
Efficacy of antifungal agents in tissue
conditioners in treating candidiasis.
Gerodontology **16**: 110

Diaz-Arnold AM, Vargas MA, Shaull KL (2008)
Flexural and fatigue strengths of denture
base resin. J Prosthet Dent **100(1)**: 47–51

Garcia LT, Jones JD (2004) Soft liners. Dent
Clin N Amer **48**: 709

Gronet PM, Driscoll CF, Hondrum SO (1997)
Resilience of surface-sealed temporary soft
denture liners. J Prosthet Dent **77**: 370

Hamanaka I, Takahashi Y, Shimizu H (2011)
Mechanical properties of injection-molded
thermoplastic denture base resins. Acta

Odontol Scand **69(2)**: 75–79. Epub 2010
Sep 27

Jagger DC, Harrison A, Jandt KD (1999)
Review: the reinforcement of dentures.
J Oral Rehab **26**: 185

Lamb DJ, Ellis B, Priestley D (1983) The
effects of processing variables on levels of
residual monomer in autopolymerizing
dental acrylic resin. J Dent **11**: 1

McCabe JF (1998) A polyvinylsiloxane denture
soft lining material. J Dent **26**: 521

Parvizi A, Lindquist T, Schneider R (2004)
Comparison of the dimensional accuracy of
injection-molded denture base materials to
that of conventional pressure-pack acrylic
resin. J Prosthodont **13**: 83

Pronych GJ, Sutow EJ, Sykora O (2003)
Dimensional stability and dehydration of a

thermoplastic polycarbonate-based and two
PMMA-based denture resins. J Oral Rehab
30: 1157

Shim JS, Watts DC (2000) An examination of
the stress distribution in a soft-lined acrylic
resin mandibular complete denture by
finite element analysis. Int J Prosthodont
13: 19

Stafford GD, Huggett R, MacGregor AR,
Graham J (1986) The use of nylon as a
denture-base material. J Dent **14**: 18

Ueshige M, Abe Y, Sato Y (1999) Dynamic
viscoelastic properties of antimicrobial
tissue conditioners containing silver-zeolite.
J Dent **27**: 517

Yunus N, Rashid AA, Azmi LL (2005) Some
flexural properties of a nylon denture base
polymer. J Oral Rehab **32**: 65

Chapter | **3.3** |

Casting alloys for metallic restorations

INTRODUCTION

The production of metallic restorations, such as crowns, bridges, inlays, cast posts and cores and partial dentures, in the dental laboratory is carried out by the *lost wax casting* technique. This method of casting has been around for a considerable time, and is much used by craftsmen to produce intricate jewellery and ornaments. Its history can be traced back beyond 3000 BC, but it was not used in dentistry until the 1890s.

The basic principles are simple. A wax model is produced of the desired shape, and this model is invested in a material resistant to high temperatures. The wax is then removed by melting and burning, leaving behind a cavity of the desired shape. This can now be filled with molten metal, so that the metal assumes the shape of the original wax carving. The stages in the production of a dental casting are therefore as follows:

- preparation of the dentition
- production of an impression
- pouring of a model
- waxing of the desired shape
- investing the wax pattern
- burn-out and heating
- melting and casting the alloy
- finishing and polishing
- heat treatments.

Thus, it can be seen that many different materials are involved in the production of a metal casting. These include impression materials, model and die materials, waxes, investment materials and casting alloys. Some of these have already been discussed in previous sections.

A detailed account of the various practical stages involved in the production of a metal casting will not be provided here, as this process is the prerogative of the dental technician. Instead, attention will be focused on the alloys that are used and the requirements that are placed on them for their applications in restorative dentistry.

When the lost wax casting technique was first developed by Taggart in the early 1900s, the alloys of choice were gold alloys. For the construction of removable partial dentures, the gold alloys were gradually replaced by cobalt–chromium (Co–Cr) alloys during the 1950s and, to a lesser extent, Co–Cr–Ni alloys. In the latter part of the 20th century, titanium made its appearance as a fixed and removable partial denture-casting alloy.

It is the responsibility of the dentist to request the most suitable alloy for a particular application when instructing a dental laboratory to produce a prosthesis. This choice should not be left to the dental technician. After all, it is the dentist who will be placing these materials in the patient's mouth.

CLINICAL SIGNIFICANCE

It is the dentist's responsibility to know what metals they are providing for their patients. This requires a knowledge of the types of alloys available, and their composition and properties.

DESIRABLE PROPERTIES

The choice of alloy is governed by a number of factors. *Cost* is a serious consideration due to the increased price of gold today. Other considerations are the *biocompatibility* of the alloy and its resistance to corrosion and tarnish. It is these factors that particularly limit the range of alloys available for dental applications.

Suitability for a specific application, be it a low-stress-bearing inlay or a posterior bridge, is determined primarily by the *mechanical properties* of the alloy, such as its stiffness, strength, ductility and hardness. Stiffness is a consequence both of design and of the elastic modulus of the alloy. The higher the elastic modulus, the stiffer the structure will be for the same shape. This is an important consideration, especially for long-span bridges, cast posts, partial dentures and denture clasps. These restorations are also likely to be subjected to fairly high loads and therefore need to be resistant to permanent deformation. This requires the alloy to have a high yield stress or proof stress.

However, for such things as clasps, high strength needs to be balanced against ductility, since it is important that the alloy is not so brittle as to fracture when small adjustments are made.

In the case of inlays, where marginal adaptation is usually improved by burnishing, ductility is even more important. Alloys for these applications need to be very ductile and soft if they are not to fracture during this procedure.

The *ease of casting* of the alloy is an important consideration for the dental laboratory technician. The dental technician will want to know what the melting range and casting temperature are for the alloy as, in general, the higher these are, the more problems the alloy presents in handling. Another important consideration in this context is the quality of fit of the restoration, which is a function of the casting shrinkage and cooling contraction of the alloy. These have to be accounted for if the casting is not to be too small. The higher the shrinkage, the more of a problem this becomes.

The *density* of the alloy is also important. Most castings are carried out in a centrifugal force-casting machine, and the higher the density of the alloy, the easier it is to force the air out of the mould space and to fill the space completely with alloy.

Thus, alloys with a wide range of properties are needed to satisfy these varied requirements. The main alloys that are employed in dentistry are noble and precious metal alloys and various base-metal alloys such as Co–Cr alloys and titanium.

CLINICAL SIGNIFICANCE

It is important for the dentist to have a close working relationship with the dental laboratory, and to take into account their views when choosing an alloy.

NOBLE AND PRECIOUS METAL ALLOYS

The noble and precious metals consist of eight elements that have a number of features in common. They are very resistant to corrosion (noble) and expensive (precious). The noble metals are considered to be made up of gold, platinum, rhodium, ruthenium, iridium and osmium, whereas silver and palladium are generally referred to as the precious metals.

High-gold alloys

This is a group of alloys that have been around for some considerable time and that can be distinguished from other alloys used in dentistry by their high precious metal content, which must not be less than 75% and a gold content in excess of 60%. The precious metal content is usually made up of gold, silver, platinum and palladium. These alloys can be classified into four distinct groups, as indicated in Table 3.3.1.

The amount of gold in an alloy is defined in one of two ways:

- *Carat*. Pure gold has a carat value of 24, and an alloy's carat is expressed in terms of the number of 24th parts of gold within it. Thus, an alloy with 50% gold would be designated as a 12-carat gold alloy. Much jewellery is 9-carat gold (37.5%) or 18-carat gold (75%).
- *Fineness*. Pure gold has a fineness rating of 1000, so that 18-carat gold is 750 fine, and 9 carat gold is 375 fine.

Thus, the dental gold alloys in Table 3.3.1 vary from 21.6 to 14.4 carat, or 900 to 600 fine.

Alloying elements in dental gold alloys

The largest fraction by far of these alloys is gold, with lower amounts of silver and copper. Some formulations also contain very small amounts of platinum, palladium and zinc.

The silver has a slight strengthening effect and counteracts the reddish tint of the copper.

The copper is a very important component, as it increases the strength, particularly of the type III and IV gold alloys, and reduces the melting temperature. The limit to the amount of copper that can be added is 16%, as amounts in excess of this tend to cause the alloy to tarnish.

Platinum and palladium increase both the strength and the melting temperature.

Zinc acts as a *scavenger* during casting, preventing oxidation, and improves the castability.

A variety of other elements, such as iridium, ruthenium and rhenium (<0.5%), may be present. These have very high melting temperature and act as nucleating sites during solidification, thus helping to produce a fine grain size.

Strengthening mechanism

Although all of the alloying elements give rise to some increase in the yield strength of the gold alloy by forming a solid solution, the most effective strengthening mechanism is the addition of copper, in what is known as *order hardening*.

This hardening heat treatment is carried out after the homogenizing anneal at approximately 700°C, which is performed to ensure a uniform composition throughout the casting. It involves reheating the alloy to 400°C and holding it at that temperature for approximately 30 minutes. Rather than being randomly distributed, the copper atoms arrange themselves in little ordered clusters.

This ordered structure prevents slippage of the atomic layers, which has the effect of raising the yield stress and the hardness of the alloy. There must be at least 11% copper in the gold alloy for order hardening to occur, so it cannot occur in type I and type II gold alloys. Type III gold alloys have just enough copper, and a small improvement in strength is observed. For type IV gold alloys, the improvement in strength is quite significant.

Table 3.3.1 Composition of high-gold alloys

Type	Description	Au%	Ag%	Cu%	Pt%	Pd%	Zn%
I	Soft	80–90	3–12	2–5	–	–	–
II	Medium	75–78	12–15	7–10	0–1	1–4	0–1
III	Hard	62–78	8–26	8–11	0–3	2–4	0–1
IV	Extra hard	60–70	4–20	11–16	0–4	0–5	1–2

Table 3.3.2 Range of mechanical properties of high-gold alloys

Type	Condition	σ_y (MPa)	UTS (MPa)	Elongation (%)	VHN
I	As cast	60–140	200–310	20–35	40–70
II	As cast	140–250	310–380	20–35	70–100
III	As cast	180–260	330–390	20–25	90–130
	Hardened	280–350	410–560	6–20	115–170
IV	As cast	300–390	410–520	4–25	130–160
	Hardened	550–680	690–830	1–6	200–240

UTS, ultimate tensile strength; VHN, Vickers hardness value.

The effect of this strengthening process is shown in Table 3.3.2. The addition of copper, combined with the hardening heat treatment, can result in a tenfold increase in the yield strength. The importance of the hardening heat treatment for the type III and IV gold alloys is also indicated. However, there is a price to pay in terms of a reduction in the ductility of the alloy, as shown by the lower percentage elongation at which failure occurs. Thus, excessive bending may give rise to brittle fracture, a problem that may arise when producing partial denture clasp arms out of a type IV gold alloy.

For some alloys, the hardening process is to allow the alloy to cool slowly on the bench rather than quenching it immediately on casting. This technique is commonly known as *self-hardening*. The disadvantage with this approach is that it is not as well controlled as when the alloy is first given a homogenizing anneal and then a hardening heat treatment. It is important that the dentist stipulates to the dental technician that a hardening heat treatment is to be carried out if a type III or IV gold alloy is chosen. If a self-hardening alloy has been selected, then it should be allowed to cool slowly on the bench and should not be quenched.

Other features

As the alloying elements form a solid solution readily with the gold, the difference between the liquidus and the solidus is small. This makes these alloys relatively easy to cast and produces a reasonably homogeneous result. The addition of platinum and palladium gives a larger gap between the liquidus and the solidus. The larger this gap, the more compositional segregation occurs on solidification, making a homogenizing anneal more desirable for the type III and IV gold alloys.

Due to their low casting temperature, the casting shrinkage (~1.4%) is readily compensated for by the use of a gypsum-bonded investment.

The low Vickers hardness values (VHN) make these alloys easy to polish to a smooth surface finish, although, in the case of the heat-hardening alloys, this is better done in the as-cast condition.

In general, it can be said that the use of these alloys does not present a major problem to the dental technician, and good-quality, well-fitting castings can be produced. Their corrosion and tarnish resistance is excellent, as is their biocompatibility.

Applications

Given their different mechanical properties, the recommended applications for the use of these alloys is as follows.

Type I alloys

These are best used for single-surface inlays in low-stress situations. As they are relatively soft and easily deformed, they need plenty of support to prevent deformation under occlusal loading. The low yield stress of these alloys allows the margins to be burnished easily. Given the high ductility, they are unlikely to fracture.

Type II alloys

These can be used for most inlays. However, those with thin sections should be avoided, as deformation is still a possibility.

Type III alloys

These can be used for all inlays, onlays, full-coverage crowns and short-span bridges, cast posts and cores because of their greater strength compared with type I and type II alloys. However, they will be more difficult to burnish, and have a higher potential for localized fracture if they are burnished excessively.

Type IV alloys

These are used for cast posts and cores, long-span bridges and, in partial denture construction, particularly clasp arms. Clasp arms can be adjusted in the as-cast state and then heat-hardened. Of course, this will not be possible when using a self-hardening alloy. The low elastic modulus and high yield strength of the gold alloy provide a high degree of flexibility to clasp arms, which allows them to be withdrawn over quite severe undercuts without danger of permanent deformation. These alloys cannot be burnished in their hardened state and are therefore unsuitable for inlays.

Medium- and low-gold alloys

The rapid rise in the prices of noble metals in the 1970s stimulated manufacturers to produce many new alloys with reduced gold contents. Compositions of a few representative commercial examples are presented in Table 3.3.3.

Some of these may be classed as *medium-gold alloys*, with the gold content varying from 40 to 60%. These medium-gold alloys were introduced in the early 1970s, and have become very popular. The palladium and silver contents were increased to compensate for the reduced gold content, while the copper content is in the range of 10–15%. Palladium is added to counteract the tendency of silver to tarnish.

The palladium, silver and copper readily form substitutional solid solutions, with the gold producing a single-phase structure

Table 3.3.3 Composition of medium- and low-gold alloys

Alloy	Type	Colour	Au%	Pd%	Ag%	Cu%	In%
Solaro 3 (Metalor)	Medium-gold	Yellow	56	5	25	11.8	–
Stabilor G (Degussa)	Medium-gold	Yellow	58	5.5	23.3	12.0	–
Mattident E (Johnson Matthey)	Medium-gold	Yellow	55	8.0	24.0	11.5	–
Palaginor 2 (Metalor)	Low-gold	White	12.5	18.9	53.7	14.2	–
Palliag MJ (Degussa)	Low-gold	White	12.5	20.9	55.0	8.5	–
Mattident B (Johnson Matthey)	Low-gold	White	11.0	20.0	54.5	12.5	–
Realor (Degussa)	Low-gold copper-free	Yellow	20.0	20.0	39.0	–	16.0
Selector 3 (Metalor)	Low-gold copper-free	Yellow	20.0	21.0	38.7	–	16.5
Mattieco J (Johnson Matthey)	Low-gold copper-free	Yellow	20.0	20.0	40.1	–	17.8

Table 3.3.4 Comparison of some properties of medium- and low-gold casting alloys compared to a type IV gold alloy*

Alloy	Type	VHN	Elastic modulus (GPa)	0.2% proof stress (MPa)	Elongation (%)	Solidus–liquidus temperature (°C)	Casting temperature (°vC)
Aurofluid 3	Type IV	255	80	480	10	885–920	1070
Solaro 3	Medium-gold	285	90.5	600	10	870–920	1070
Stabilor G	Medium-gold	275	–	830	6	–	1000–1100
Mattident E	Medium-gold	269	–	685	7	885–945	1045–1145
Palaginor 2	Low-gold	170	82	340	12	875–970	1200
Palliag MJ	Low-gold	265	–	630	4	940–1010	1100–1200
Mattident B	Low-gold	256	–	645	3.5	945–1000	1100–1200
Realor	Low-gold Cu-free	185	–	405	6	860–1035	1200
Selector 3	Low-gold Cu-free	180	75	370	8	875–1035	1200
Mattieco J	Low-gold Cu-free	200	–	740	5	870–940	1080–1150

*Data taken from manufacturers' data sheets.

throughout the entire compositional range. The presence of copper allows order hardening, just as with the type III and IV gold alloys.

There are also a number of *low-gold alloys*, which have gold contents typically of the order of 10–20%. The other elements are silver (40–60%) and palladium (up to 40%); these alloys could thus be described as Ag–Pd alloys, but we will leave that description for those alloys containing minor amounts of gold (<2%) or no gold at all.

Due to the reduced gold content, these alloys are white in appearance; they are less attractive to the patient who prefers the appearance of the yellow gold alloys. In order to overcome this disadvantage, there are also a number of copper-free low-gold alloys, which contain high levels of indium. These have a two-phase structure consisting of a face-centred cubic (FCC) matrix with islands of a body-centred cubic (BCC) phase due to the high indium content. The matrix phase is essentially a Ag–Au solid solution with minor additions of palladium, indium and zinc. The BCC phase consists of Pd–In with substantial amounts of gold, silver and zinc, giving the alloy its yellow colour. Thus, the colour seems to be related to the presence of the indium rather than the absence of copper.

Properties and applications

Some of the properties of these alloys are compared in Table 3.3.4. The medium-gold alloys are recommended for the same applications as type III and IV gold alloys. Their ductility tends to be lower than that of the type IV gold alloys and their high yield stress makes them difficult to burnish. There is even a danger of fracture on burnishing, due to the localized work hardening that occurs and further reduces their ductility. However, they are very suitable for long-span prostheses and may be used for implant-supported prostheses and posts and cores.

The low-gold content alloys tend to have lower mechanical properties than the medium-gold alloys, and are recommended as an alternative to type III gold alloys. However, their white colour makes them less popular than they might otherwise be. These alloys are extensively used for posts and cores, where the white colour does not present a problem, as the casting will be covered with another material.

The removal of the copper and the addition of the indium again produce alloys with properties similar to those of the type III gold alloys, but with the advantage of the yellow colour. However, the gap

Table 3.3.5 Composition and properties of silver/palladium alloys*

Alloy	Ag%	Pd%	Cu%	Zn%	VHN	0.2% proof stress (MPa)	Elongation (%)	Solidus–liquidus temperature (°C)	Casting temperature (°C)
Palliag W (Degussa)	70.0	27.5	–	–	55	80	33	1080–1180	–
Mattieco 25 (Johnson Matthey)	68.5	25.0		3.0	199	500	31	1050–1110	1210–1290
Palliag M (Degussa)	58.5	27.4	10.5	–	310	940	3	950–1040	1100–1200
Palliag NF IV (Degussa)	52.0	39.9	–	4.0	270	595	6	1070–1145	1200–1250
Mattident P (Johnson Matthey)	46.6	33.4	19.0	–	290	780	3	1005–1040	1140–1240

*Data taken from manufacturers' data sheets.

between the solidus and the liquidus is greater, which can result in a less homogeneous structure, and their melting temperature is considerably higher, making the casting process more difficult.

Although, in general, the medium-gold alloys are a suitable alternative to the type IV gold alloys, and the low-gold alloys for type III gold alloys, one problem with these alloys is that their properties are more variable from alloy to alloy than for each of the four types of high-gold alloys (see Table 3.3.4).

The biocompatibility of these alloys appears to be excellent, and corrosion does not seem to be a problem, even with the two-phase, low-gold, copper-free alloys.

CLINICAL SIGNIFICANCE

The dentist must examine carefully the properties of each alloy and, if necessary, seek advice from the manufacturer or dental laboratory in order to determine the suitability of an alloy for a particular clinical application.

Silver–palladium alloys

As the name implies, Ag–Pd alloys contain predominantly silver with significant amounts of palladium.

The palladium improves the resistance to corrosion and helps to prevent tarnish, which is usually associated with the silver. These alloys were introduced in the 1960s as an alternative to the high-gold alloys, and are commonly called 'white golds'.

The composition and the properties of some representative alloys after their heat-hardening treatment are presented in Table 3.3.5. Although there is some self-hardening with these alloys if they are left to bench cool, the properties are generally inferior when compared to a carefully controlled hardening heat treatment.

There are two notable features of the data presented in Table 3.3.5. First, there is the wide range of properties in the different alloys, which again highlights the need to select the alloy for the application in mind very carefully. The low strength and hardness and the high ductility of one of the alloys shown (Palliag W) suggests that this alloy is suitable only for low-stress-bearing inlays. The other alloy with a similar composition (Mattieco 25) has superior mechanical properties, being more comparable to a type III gold alloy, and could be used for crowns, short-span bridges, and post and cores.

However, those alloys with reduced silver content and increased palladium content have properties similar to those of the type IV gold alloys. Nevertheless, their use for long-span prostheses is generally

contraindicated. This may be associated with the high casting temperatures for these alloys, which is the second most notable feature of these materials.

These high casting temperatures require the use of phosphate-bonded investments and high-temperature casting techniques, and it is well recognized that accurate casting at high temperatures is a problem for the dental technician.

The alloys have a tendency to work-harden rapidly, which precludes excessive adjustment and any burnishing. Although they are highly biocompatible, tarnishing does occur with these alloys. These disadvantages have resulted in this group of alloys being considerably less popular than the medium- and low-gold alloys.

BASE METAL ALLOYS

Cobalt–chromium alloys

Co–Cr alloys were first introduced to the dental profession in the 1930s, and since then have effectively replaced the type IV gold alloys for the construction of partial denture frameworks, primarily due to their relatively low cost, which is a significant factor with these large castings.

Composition

The alloy consists of cobalt (55–65%) with up to 30% chromium. Other major alloying elements are molybdenum (4–5%) and, in at least one case, titanium (5%) (Table 3.3.6).

The cobalt and chromium form a solid solution for up to 30% chromium, which is the limit of solubility of chromium in cobalt; additional chromium would produce a highly brittle second phase.

In general, the higher the chromium content, the better the corrosion resistance of the alloy. Therefore, the manufacturers try to maximize the amount of chromium without introducing the brittle second phase. Molybdenum is present in order to refine the grain size by providing more sites for crystal nucleation during the solidification process. It has the added benefit that it produces a significant solid solution hardening effect, an effect shared by the addition of iron. Nevertheless, the grains are very large, although grain boundaries are difficult to identify due to the coarse dendritic structure of the alloy.

Carbon, which is present only in small quantities, is nevertheless an extremely important constituent of the alloy, as small changes in the carbon content can significantly alter the strength, hardness and ductility of the alloy. Carbon can combine with any of the other

Table 3.3.6 Properties of some Co–Cr alloys*

Alloy	Co%	Cr%	Mo%	VHN	0.2% proof stress (MPa)	Elongation (%)	Solidus–liquidus temperature (°C)	Casting temperature (°C)
Biosil H (Degussa)	65.7	28.5	4.5	360	600	8	1320–1380	1500
Vitallium (Nobelparma)	60.6	31.5	6.0	428	616	3	1300–1370	1550
Wisil (Krupp)	65	28	5.0	390	580	7	1355–1375	1535

*Data taken from manufacturers' data sheets.

alloying elements to form carbides. The fine precipitation of these can dramatically raise the strength and hardness of the alloy. However, too much carbon will result in excessive brittleness. This presents a problem for the dental technician, who needs to ensure that no excess carbon is absorbed by the alloy during melting and casting.

The distribution of the carbides also depends on the casting temperature and the cooling rate, with discontinuous carbide formation at the grain boundaries being preferable to continuous carbide formation.

Properties

For the dental technician, these alloys are considerably more difficult to handle than the gold alloys because they must be heated to high temperatures before they can be cast. Casting temperatures are in the region of 1300–1400°C and the associated casting shrinkage is ~2.0%.

This problem has largely been overcome with the introduction of induction casting equipment and high-temperature-resistant phosphate-bonded refractory investments. Accuracy is compromised at these high temperatures, which effectively limits the use of these alloys to partial dentures.

The high hardness of these alloys makes them difficult to polish mechanically. Electrolytic polishing is used for the fitting surfaces, so as not to compromise the quality of fit, but non-fitting surfaces are still mechanically polished. The benefit is that the highly polished surface is retained for a very long time, which is a distinct advantage with a removable prosthesis.

The lack of ductility so easily exacerbated by carbon contamination *does* present problems, especially as these alloys are also prone to casting porosity. These limitations combine to give rise to a common problem with partial dentures: clasp fractures. This problem becomes even more pronounced when an attempt is made to adjust a clasp arm, and excessive or frequent adjustments will invariably lead to a clasp-arm fracture.

Nevertheless, there are some features of these alloys that make them ideally suited to the construction of partial denture frameworks. The modulus of elasticity of a Co–Cr alloy is typically 250 GPa, whereas, for the alloys previously discussed, the modulus is in the range 70–100 GPa. This high modulus of elasticity has the advantage that the denture, and particularly the clasp arms, can be made thinner in cross-section whilst maintaining adequate rigidity. This, combined with a density of about half that of the gold alloys, means that the castings are considerably lighter. This is of great benefit to the comfort of the patient.

The addition of chromium makes this a highly corrosion-resistant alloy, as can be emphasized by the fact that the alloy also forms the basis of many surgically implanted prostheses, such as hip and knee joints. It can be said, therefore, that these alloys have an excellent history of biocompatibility.

Some of the commercially available alloys also contain nickel, which is added by the manufacturer in order to increase the ductility and reduce the hardness. However, nickel is a well-known allergen, and its use in the mouth may trigger an allergic reaction. Therefore, for patients known to have a propensity for allergic reactions, it is advisable to use a nickel-free Co–Cr alloy.

Titanium alloys

The interest in titanium-based castings for removable and fixed prosthodontics came about at approximately the same time as the development of titanium dental implants. Titanium has a number of attractive features, such as high strength with low density and excellent biocompatibility. In addition, however, there were concerns that, if a metal different from the titanium used in dental implants were used to produce the crowns and bridges, this might lead to galvanic effects.

The discovery of the element titanium has been attributed to the Reverend William Gregor in 1790, but it was not until 1910 that the first pure form of titanium was produced and, even now, titanium is still very expensive compared with, for example, stainless steel. Pure titanium is produced by the Kroll process, which involves heating titanium ore (e.g. rutile) in the presence of carbon and chlorine. The resultant $TiCl_4$ is reduced with molten sodium to produce a titanium sponge, which is subsequently fused under vacuum or in an argon atmosphere to produce an ingot of the metal.

Composition

Clinically, two forms of titanium have received the most interest. One is the commercially pure form of titanium (cpTi) and the other is an alloy of titanium–6% aluminium–4% vanadium.

Commercially pure titanium

Titanium is allotropic, with a hexagonal close-packed (HCP) structure (α) at low temperatures and a body-centred cubic (BCC) structure (β) above 882°C. Commercially pure titanium (cpTi) is, in fact, an alloy of titanium with up to 0.5% oxygen. The oxygen is in solution, so that the metal is single-phase. Elements such as oxygen, nitrogen and carbon have a greater solubility in the HCP structure of the α-phase than in the cubic form of the β-phase. These elements form interstitial solid solutions with titanium and help to stabilize the α-phase. Transition elements, such as molybdenum, niobium and vanadium, act as β-stabilizers.

Titanium–6% aluminium–4% vanadium

When aluminium and vanadium are added to titanium in only small quantities, the strength of the alloy is much increased over that of cpTi. Aluminium is considered to be an α-stabilizer, with vanadium acting as a β-stabilizer. When these are added to titanium, the temperature at which the α–β transition occurs is depressed, such that both the α and β forms can exist at room temperature. Thus, Ti–6% Al–4% V has a two-phase structure of α and β grains.

Properties

Pure titanium is a white, lustrous metal, which has the attraction of low density, good strength and an excellent corrosion resistance. It is ductile and constitutes an important alloying element with many other metals. Alloys of titanium are widely used in the aircraft industry and military applications because of its low density, high-tensile strength (~500 MPa) and ability to withstand high temperatures. The elastic modulus of cpTi is 110 GPa, which is half that of stainless steel or Co–Cr alloy.

The tensile properties of cpTi depend significantly on the oxygen content and, although the ultimate tensile strength, proof stress and hardness increase with increased oxygen concentration, this is at the expense of the ductility.

By alloying titanium with aluminium and vanadium, a wide range of mechanical properties superior to the cpTi are possible. Such alloys of titanium are a mixture of the α- and β-phase, where the α-phase is relatively soft and ductile while the β-phase is harder and stronger but also less ductile. Thus by changing the relative proportions of α and β, a wide variety of mechanical properties can be achieved.

For the Ti–6% Al–4% V alloy, considerably higher tensile properties (~1030 MPa) are achievable than for pure titanium, which makes it attractive for use in high-stress-bearing situations such as partial dentures.

An important feature of these materials is the fatigue resistance of titanium alloys. Both cpTi and Ti–6% Al–4% V have a well-defined fatigue limit, with the S–N curve levelling out after 10^7–10^8 cycles of stress reversal at a tensile strength reduced by 45–50%. Thus, cpTi should not be used in situations where the tensile stress may exceed 175 MPa. In contrast, for the Ti–6% Al–4% V, the fatigue limit is approximately 450 MPa.

Corrosion of alloys can be a serious problem, both in terms of degradation of the prosthesis and the release of potentially toxic or allergenic compounds. Titanium has become popular because it is one of the most corrosion-resistant metals known to man and this applies equally to the alloys. Although titanium is a highly reactive metal, this is also one of its strengths because the oxide formed on the surface (TiO_2) is extremely stable and this has a passivating effect on the metal. The potential for corrosion of titanium in the biological environment has been studied and has confirmed its excellent corrosion resistance.

Castability does present a serious problem with these alloys. Titanium has a high melting point (~1670°C), which creates problems with regard to compensation of the cooling contraction. Because the metal is very reactive, all castings need to be carried out in a vacuum or an inert atmosphere, which requires special casting equipment. Thus only few dental laboratories will be set up for the casting of titanium alloys. The other problem is that the molten alloy has a propensity to react with the refractory investment mould, leaving behind a surface scale, which can compromise the quality of fit of the restoration. When constructed for implant-supported superstructures, very tight tolerances are required in order to achieve a passive fit on the implants. If this is not the case, the retention of the implant in the bone may be compromised. Internal porosity is also often observed with titanium castings. Hence, other forms of processing titanium for dental prostheses are also used, such as milling by computer-aided design–computer-aided manufacture (CAD–CAM) or electrical discharge machining.

Some of the properties of the base metal alloys discussed above are presented in Table 3.3.7 for comparison.

Table 3.3.7 Comparison of some properties of base metal casting alloys

Property	Co–Cr alloy	Titanium	Ti–6% Al–4% Va
Density (g/cm³)	8.9	4.5	4.5
Casting temperature (°C)	~1500	~1700	~1700
Casting shrinkage (%)	2.3	3.5	3.5
Tensile strength (MPa)	850	520	1000
Proportional limit (MPa)	550–650	350	920
Elastic modulus (GPa)	190–230	110	85–115
Hardness (Vickers)	360–430	200	–
Ductility (%)	2–8	20	14

SUMMARY

A rapidly growing variety of casting alloys are used in dentistry. In order to make a rational choice from the current spectrum of high-gold alloys and their alternatives, the dentist needs to have more knowledge about their appearances and their physical and mechanical properties than ever before.

Although the cost of the alloy is an important consideration, one generally finds that the cost savings on the prostheses are lower than might be expected. This is because the lower cost of the alloy is often offset by the increased cost of production. Also, in general, it can be said that the higher the gold content of the alloy, the better the quality of fit of the restoration.

When the dentist wishes to use alternative alloys to the precious metal alloys, it is important to liaise closely with the dental laboratory and find out what alloys are regularly used there, and what the laboratory's recommendations are, because of the wide range of properties obtainable.

CLINICAL SIGNIFICANCE

The ultimate responsibility for the materials used in the patient's mouth rests with the dentist, and not the dental technician.

FURTHER READING

Asgar K (1988) Casting metals in dentistry: past – present – future. Adv Dent Res 2: 33

Au AR, Lechner SK, Thomas CJ (2000) Titanium for removable partial dentures (III): 2-year clinical follow-up in an undergraduate programme. J Oral Rehab 27: 978

Bates JF (1965) Studies related to the fracture of partial dentures. Brit Dent J 118: 532

Besimo C, Jeger C, Guggenheim R (1997) Marginal adaptation of titanium frameworks produced by CAD/CAM techniques. Int J Prosthodont 10: 541

CDMIE (1985) Report on base metal alloys for crown and bridge applications: benefits and risks. J Am Dent Assoc 111: 479

Cruickshank-Boyd DW (1981) Alternatives to gold 1: Non-porcelain alloys. Dental Update 8: 17

Cunningham DM (1973) Comparison of base metal alloys and type IV gold alloys for removable partial denture frameworks. Dent Clin N Am **17**: 719

Huget EF (1978) Base metal alloys. In: O'Brien WJ, Ryge G (eds) An outline of dental materials and their selection. W. B. Saunders, London: ch. 23, p. 284

Karlsson S (1993) The fit of Procera titanium crowns: an *in vitro* and clinical study. Acta Odontol Scand **51**: 129

Landesman HM, de Gennaro GG, Martinoff JT (1981) An 18-month clinical evaluation of semiprecious and nonprecious alloy restorations. J Prosthet Dent **46**: 161

Leinfelder KF (1997) An evaluation of casting alloys used for restorative procedures. J Am Dent Assoc **128**: 37

Mezger PR, Stols ALH, Vrijhoef MMA, Greener EH (1989) Metallurgical aspects and corrosion behaviour of yellow low-gold alloys. Dent Mater **5**: 350

Russell MM, Andersson M, Dahlmo K (1995) A new computer-assisted method for fabrication of crowns and fixed partial dentures. Quintessence Int **26**: 757

van Noort R, Lamb DJ (1984) A scanning electron microscope study of Co–Cr partial dentures fractured in service. J Dent **12**: 122

van Roekel NB (1992) Electrical discharge machining in dentistry. Int J Prosthodont **5(2)**: 114–121

Watanabe I, Watkins JH, Nakajima H (1997) Effect of pressure difference on the quality of titanium casting. J Dent Res **76**: 773

Watanabe I, Kiyosue S, Ohkubo C (2002) Machinability of cast commercial titanium alloys. J Biomed Mat Res **63**: 760–764

Chapter |3.4|

Dental ceramics

INTRODUCTION

It could be said that the ceramic material known as porcelain holds a special place in dentistry because, notwithstanding the many advances made in composites and glass–ionomers, it is still considered to produce the most aesthetically pleasing result. Its colour, translucency and vitality cannot, as yet, be matched by any material except other ceramics.

CLINICAL SIGNIFICANCE

Ceramic restorations are indicated where aesthetics is needed and when the size of the preparation exceeds the limit for the use of direct composite resins.

Traditionally, its use is in the construction of artificial teeth for dentures, crowns and bridges. From the 1980s onwards, the use of ceramics has been extended to include veneers, inlays/onlays, anterior crowns and short-span anterior bridges. The construction of such restorations is usually undertaken in dental laboratories by technicians skilled in the art of fusing ceramics. In recent years, the advent of computer-aided design–computer-aided manufacture (CAD–CAM) in dentistry has opened up new opportunities to use new materials and the potential to extend the use of ceramics to posterior crowns and bridges.

As people retain their teeth for much longer than in the past, the need for aesthetically acceptable restorations is continuing to increase. This is reflected in the growing use by dentists of restorative procedures using ceramics.

CLINICAL SIGNIFICANCE

The demand for ceramic crowns has been increasing at the rate of 50% every 4 years. Therefore, ceramics will continue to be important restorative materials for many years to come.

HISTORICAL PERSPECTIVE

Pottery in Europe up to AD 1700

The achievement of making usable pottery was a considerable feat, and involved many trials and tribulations for the early potters. The raw material used for pottery is clay, and this presented the potter with two major problems.

The first problem the primitive potter met was how to transfer the clay into a form that provided the best consistency for manipulation and firing. Clay is usually too sticky to handle when simply mixed with water, and this problem was overcome by the addition of sand and ground seashells. In addition, clay shrinks as it dries out and hardens. If this shrinkage is non-uniform, either in rate or in overall amount, the pots will crack even before they have been fired. Again, the addition of a coarse-grained filler went some way towards overcoming this problem.

It was during the firing of the pots that the problems really began to be serious. Gases present in the mixture, whether air bubbles or gases formed during heating (such as water vapour and CO_2), create voids in the clay and may even cause it to fracture during firing. Early potters overcame this problem by beating the clay prior to moulding to get rid of the air. (*Wedging* is the term often used by craftsmen to describe this process.) Another development was the technique of raising the temperature very gradually during the firing process, as then, the steam and gases could diffuse out of the clay slowly, rather than bursting out and causing the pot to crack.

The most serious obstacle during this phase in the development of ceramic technology was the temperature at which the pottery could be fired. The conversion of clay from a mass of individual particles loosely held together by a water binder to a coherent solid relies on a process known as *sintering*. In this process, the points at which the individual particles are in contact fuse at sufficiently high temperatures (Figure 3.4.1).

The process relies on diffusion, which is greatly accelerated by elevated temperatures. The demand for high uniform temperatures could not be met by the traditional open fires, and this led to the invention of the *kiln*. The earliest of these was the *up-draught kiln*, in which higher temperatures and greater uniformity of temperature were obtained by

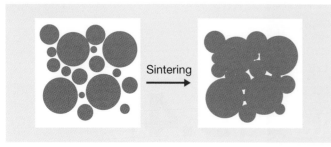

Figure 3.4.1 Sintering of ceramic particles

drawing air through the fire and putting the pots in the rising hot gases.

Early kilns were able to reach temperatures of up to 900°C, and pottery fired at this temperature is called *earthenware*. The resultant pottery is porous, as the sintering process has only just managed to fuse the particles of clay where they touch. Such pots were suitable for the storage of solid foods but could not hold any liquids. This problem was overcome eventually by fusing a thin layer of a glassy material, i.e. a glaze, over the surface of the pot. This technology was used as far back as 5500 BC in various places, including Turkey.

Gradual progress was made towards higher kiln temperatures, so that many more clays could be partially melted. The liquid phase would invariably solidify as a glass, resulting in impervious pottery that is generally known as *stoneware*. Stoneware appeared in Europe in the 15–16th centuries AD.

Chinese porcelain

In contrast to what was happening in Europe, stoneware had been produced in China by 100 BC, and, by the 10th century AD, ceramic technology in China had advanced to such a stage that Chinese craftsmen were able to produce:

A ceramic so white that it was comparable only to snow, so strong that vessels needed walls only 2–3 mm thick and consequently light could shine through it. So continuous was the internal structure that a dish, if lightly struck would ring like a bell.
   This is porcelain!

As trade with the Far East grew, this infinitely superior material came to Europe from China during the 17th century. Until then, there had been a distinct lack of interest in tableware. The majority of the population ate off wooden plates and the nobility were satisfied with eating off metal plates. For special occasions, gold and silver tableware would be used.

This all changed with the introduction of Chinese porcelain, which stimulated demand for high-quality ceramic tableware. There was no way in which the trade with the Far East could possibly satisfy this demand, so strenuous efforts were made by the European pottery industry to imitate the Chinese porcelain.

Passable imitations were made by using tin oxide as a glaze (producing the white appearance of porcelain), but it was found impossible to reproduce the translucency of Chinese porcelain. For example, Meissen in Germany in 1708 managed to produce what they called 'white porcelain', but their product more closely resembled northern Chinese stoneware. Many other manufacturers, now well-established names, were unable to produce genuine porcelain but still made a name for themselves with high-quality stoneware, such as Majolica from Italy, Wedgwood from England and Delft's Blue from Holland.

In the up-draught kiln, the technology existed to produce high temperatures, although the Chinese down-draught kiln was somewhat superior at controlling the temperature. The problem of reproducing Chinese porcelain was essentially one of selecting the material and the method of processing. Many, such as John Dwight of Fulham, who was granted a patent by Charles II in 1671, claimed to have discovered the secret of Chinese porcelain, but really only managed to make white stoneware.

In order to produce porcelain, the material has to remain or to become white on firing, and must be so strong that vessels with walls less than 3 mm thick can be produced. If the product needs to be made with walls thicker than 3 mm, even porcelain appears opaque. So, the major differences between stoneware and porcelain are that porcelain is white and can be made in such thin sections that it appears translucent. Stoneware could be made to look white, but had to be used in such a thickness that it was invariably opaque.

This situation prevailed for some time, until, in 1717, the secret was leaked from China by a Jesuit missionary, Father d'Entrecolles. He performed his missionary work in a place called King-te-Tching, which, at that time, was the porcelain centre of China. Going amongst the people in their place of work, he managed to acquire samples of the materials used. He sent the samples to a French friend of his, together with a detailed account of how the porcelain was manufactured. The samples and the description were passed on to M. de Réaumur, a scientist, who was able to identify the components used by the Chinese, such as kaolin, silica and feldspar.

Kaolin, known as china clay, is a hydrated alumino-silicate. The silica is in the form of quartz, and remains as a fine dispersion after firing; the feldspar is a mixture of sodium and potassium–aluminium silicates. These were mixed in proportions of 25–30% feldspar, 20–25% quartz and 50% kaolin. It should be said that, by the early 1700s, the Meissen factory in Dresden was already producing a very passable porcelain based on kaolin, silica and alabaster.

In a way, it is a little surprising that it took so long before the composition of the Chinese porcelain was unravelled. The art of making porcelain involves no complex chemistry, since the process is one of taking three rather common minerals (kaolin, feldspar and flint) and firing them at high temperatures. Once the mystery had been unravelled, however, it did not take long for new porcelains to be developed in Europe. Soon it was possible to make it in any shade or tint, and its translucency gave such a depth of colour that it was not long before the dental potential of this material was recognized.

The dental application of porcelain dates from 1774, when a French apothecary named Alexis Duchateau considered the possibility of replacing his ivory dentures with porcelain. Ivory, being porous, soaks up oral fluids and eventually becomes badly stained, as well as being highly unhygienic. Duchateau, with the assistance of porcelain manufacturers at the Guerhard factory in Saint Germain-en-Laye, succeeded in making himself the first porcelain denture. This was quite a feat, since the porcelain shrinks considerably on firing. This shrinkage had to be taken into account if the denture was going to fit at all well in the mouth. Since then, other materials such as vulcanite and, more recently, poly methyl methacrylate have helped to replace porcelain for denture applications.

Porcelain teeth, in conjunction with an acrylic denture base, are still extensively used. However, the most important application of dental porcelain is in the construction of veneers, inlays, crowns and bridges, where the aesthetic qualities of the porcelain are still superior to that of any other substitute for enamel and dentine.

Porcelains were the first materials used in the construction of the porcelain jacket crown. Many new materials have appeared on the market over recent years that are described as porcelains, but are, in fact, very different forms of ceramic when compared with the early porcelains.

COMPOSITION OF DENTAL PORCELAIN

The earliest dental porcelains were mixtures of kaolin, feldspar and quartz, and were quite different from earthenware, stoneware and domestic porcelain, as indicated in Figure 3.4.2. It was not until 1838 that Elias Wildman produced dental porcelain with a translucency and shades that reasonably matched those of the natural teeth. The compositions of domestic and dental porcelain are shown in Table 3.4.1.

Kaolin is a hydrated aluminium silicate ($Al_2O \cdot 2SiO_2 \cdot 2H_2O$) and acts as a binder, increasing the ability to mould the unfired porcelain. It is opaque, however, and its presence, even in very small quantities, meant that the earliest dental porcelains lacked the adequate translucency. Thus, for dental porcelains, the kaolin was omitted and they could thus be considered to be a feldspathic glass with crystalline inclusions of silica.

The quartz remained unchanged during the firing process and acted as a strengthening agent. It is present as a fine crystalline dispersion throughout the glassy phase that is produced by the melting of the feldspar. The feldspar fuses when it melts, forming a glass matrix.

The feldspars are mixtures of potassium alumino-silicate ($K_2O \cdot Al_2O_3 \cdot 6SiO_2$) and sodium alumino-silicate, also known as albite ($Na_2O \cdot Al_2O_3 \cdot 6SiO_2$). Feldspars are naturally occurring substances, so the ratio between the potash (K_2O) and the soda (Na_2O) will vary somewhat. This affects the properties of the feldspar, in that the soda tends to lower the fusion temperature and the potash increases the viscosity of the molten glass.

During the firing of porcelain, there is always the danger of excessive pyroplastic flow that may result in rounding of the edges and loss of tooth form. It is important that the right amount of potash is present to prevent this. These alkalis either are present as a part of the feldspars, or they may be added as carbonates to ensure the correct ratio. The typical oxide composition of a dental porcelain is presented in Table 3.4.2.

The porcelain powder used by the dental technician is not a simple mixture of the ingredients in Table 3.4.2. These powders have been fired once already. The manufacturer mixes the components, adds additional metal oxides, fuses them and then quenches the molten mass in water. The resultant product is known as a *frit*, and the process is known as *fritting*. One consequence of the rapid cooling is the build-up of large internal stresses in the glass, resulting in extensive cracking. This material can be ground very easily to produce a fine powder for use by the dental technician.

During the firing of a porcelain jacket crown, for example, there is no chemical reaction taking place; the glass is simply melted above its glass transition temperature when the particles fuse together by liquid-phase sintering and cooled down again. Thus, all that has happened is that the individual particles have fused together by sintering to produce a coherent solid.

The particle size distribution is critical in ensuring that the particles pack together as tightly as possible, in order that the shrinkage on firing is minimized. The average particle size is generally in the region of 25 µm, with a wide distribution of other particle sizes, such that the smaller particles fill in the spaces in between the larger particles. Some porcelain powders have a multimodal particle size distribution to increase the packing density.

A number of other ingredients will be present in the dental porcelain powders. These include metal oxides, which provide the wide variety of colours of the porcelain. For example, oxides of iron act as a brown pigment, copper as a green pigment, titanium as a yellowish-brown, and cobalt imparts a blue colour. A binder, consisting of starch and sugar, may also be present to help in the manipulation of the powders.

PROCESSING

The production of a porcelain jacket crown involves three technical stages:

* compaction
* firing
* glazing.

Compaction

In the construction of a porcelain jacket crown, the porcelain powder is mixed with water and made into a paste. This paste is applied to

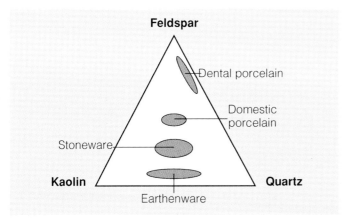

Figure 3.4.2 Relative composition of ceramic products based on feldspar, kaolin and quartz

Table 3.4.1 Composition of household and dental porcelains

Porcelain	% Kaolin	% Quartz	% Feldspar
Household	50	20–25	25–30
Dental	0	25	65

Table 3.4.2 Typical oxide composition of a dental porcelain

Material	Wt %
Silica	63
Alumina	17
Boric oxide	7
Potash (K_2O)	7
Soda (Na_2O)	4
Other oxides	2

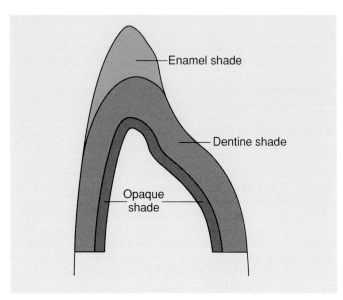

Figure 3.4.3 Porcelain build-up for a jacket crown

the die, which has been coated beforehand with a very thin platinum foil, to allow the porcelain crown to be separated from the die and transported to the furnace.

A porcelain jacket crown is made from a number of porcelain powders because it is impossible to recreate all of the aesthetic features of a tooth by the use of a single porcelain. Conventionally, three basic types of porcelain powder are used. These are an opaque shade to mask the colour of the underlying structure, which may be an amalgam or a metal post and core construction. Then a dentine shade is applied and finally an enamel shade. The exact enamel shade is selected from a guide that is used to compare with the shade of the natural tooth. The final construction is as shown in Figure 3.4.3.

The powder is mixed with water and a binder to form a slurry that can be applied to the die in a number of ways, such as spatulation, brush application, whipping or vibrating, all of which are aimed at compacting the powder. The objective of these condensation techniques is to remove as much water as possible, resulting in a more compact arrangement with a high density of particles that minimizes the firing shrinkage. The particle size and shape are extremely important, as they affect the handling characteristics of the powder and have an effect on the amount of shrinkage on firing. The binder helps to hold the particles together, as the material is extremely fragile in this so-called *green state*.

Firing

Initially, the crown is heated slowly in the open entrance to the furnace. This is carried out in order to drive off excess water before it has a chance to form steam. If the water in the mix was allowed to turn into steam, it would cause the fragile powder-compact to crack as the steam tried to escape to the surface. Once the compact has been dried, it is placed in the furnace and the binders are burnt out. Some contraction occurs during this stage.

When the porcelain begins to fuse, continuity is only achieved at points of contact between the powder particles. The material is still porous, and is usually referred to as being at the *low bisque stage*. As the exposure to the elevated temperature continues, more fusion takes place as the molten glass flows between the particles, drawing them closer together and filling the voids. A large contraction takes place during this phase (~20%), and the resultant material is virtually

non-porous. The cause of the high shrinkage of porcelain on firing is therefore due to the fusion of the particles during sintering, as the powder particles are brought into close contact.

The firing of the porcelain must be carried out exactly according to the manufacturers' instructions. If the crown should remain in the furnace for too long, it will lose form due to *pyroplastic flow* (flow of the molten glass) and will become highly glazed.

A very slow cooling rate is essential in order to avoid the possibility of cracking or crazing. The furnaces available usually offer a considerable degree of automation, and can be used for air- or vacuum-firing. Vacuum-firing produces a denser porcelain than air-firing, as air is withdrawn during the firing process. Fewer voids are formed, resulting in a stronger crown with a more predictable shade. Areas of porosity in air-fired porcelain alter the translucency of the crown, as they cause light to scatter. An additional problem is that air voids will become exposed if grinding of the superficial layer should be necessary, giving rise to an unsightly appearance and a rough surface finish.

Glazing

There will always be some porosity in the porcelain, with small air voids being exposed at the surface. These will allow the ingress of bacteria and oral fluids, and act as potential sites for the build-up of plaque. To avoid this, the surface is glazed to produce a smooth, shiny and impervious outer layer. There are two ways in which this can be achieved:

1. Glasses that fuse at low temperatures are applied to the crown after construction, and a short period at a relatively low temperature is sufficient to fuse the glaze.
2. Final firing of the crown under carefully controlled conditions fuses the superficial layer to an impervious surface glaze.

PROPERTIES OF DENTAL PORCELAIN

Dental porcelain is chemically very stable, and provides excellent aesthetics that do not deteriorate with time. The thermal conductivity and the coefficient of thermal expansion are similar to those of enamel and dentine, so, in the presence of a good marginal seal, marginal percolation is less likely to be a problem.

Although the compressive strength of dental porcelain is high (350–550 MPa), its tensile strength is very low (20–60 MPa), which is typical of a brittle solid. The material, being primarily a glass, lacks any fracture toughness. The maximum strain that a glass can withstand is less than 0.1%. Glasses are extremely sensitive to the presence of *surface micro-cracks*, and this represents one of the major drawbacks in the use of dental porcelain. On cooling from the furnace temperature, the outside of the porcelain will cool more rapidly than the interior, particularly as the porcelain has a low thermal conductivity. The outside surface contracts more than the inside initially, resulting in a compressive load on the outside and a residual tensile stress on the inside as the interior is being prevented from shrinking by the outside skin.

CLINICAL SIGNIFICANCE

If the differential dimensional change is sufficiently high, the internal surface layer that is under tension will rupture to relieve the stresses. This will result in the fit surface of the crown containing a large number of minute cracks, and it is these that will ultimately cause the crown to fracture catastrophically (Figure 3.4.4).

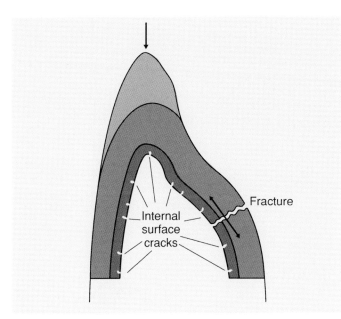

Figure 3.4.4 Palatal fracture of a porcelain jacket crown initiated from an internal surface flaw

The application of a glaze with a slightly lower coefficient of expansion would potentially fill in the cracks and also place the surface under compression. Unfortunately, this is not possible on the fitting surface of the crown, as it may result in the crown not seating properly. The porcelains were thus not strong enough to be used for the manufacture of multi-unit bridges, and problems even arose for anterior porcelain jacket crowns, especially when they were used in situations of heavy occlusion. The tiny surface flaws in the interior of the crown act as initiating sites for catastrophic failure. The inherently low tensile strength of feldspathic porcelains (<60 MPa) restricted their use to very low stress-bearing anterior applications. The answer is to provide a high-strength support for the porcelain, and nowadays a number of different systems are available.

CLASSIFICATION OF MODERN DENTAL CERAMICS

One of the most serious drawbacks with the early dental porcelains described above was their lack of strength and toughness, which seriously limited their use. As early as 1903, Land described, in an issue of *Dental Cosmos*, how to make porcelain crowns but came up against the problem that the crowns would break too easily. Similarly, Pincus described the concept of the ceramic veneer in an article in the

Californian Dental Association Journal of 1938, but was also frustrated by the lack of strength of the porcelains available at the time. By that time, for reasons of aesthetics, the porcelain used contained little or no kaolin and, strictly speaking, should no longer be referred to as a porcelain, as the essential ingredient was feldspar.

In order to overcome the problem of lack of strength and toughness of dental porcelains, there are two possible solutions. One solution is to provide the dental porcelain with support from a stronger substructure. The other option is to produce ceramics that are stronger and tougher. In this context, it is possible to consider dental ceramics as falling into three categories, based on the nature of the supporting structure:

* metal–ceramics
* reinforced ceramic core systems
* resin-bonded ceramics.

In each case, the philosophy is to provide a high-strength supporting structure for the ceramic providing the aesthetics finish. Obviously, the ideal ceramic would have both the strength and the aesthetics to perform both functions.

In the case of the metal–ceramic restoration, the aesthetic ceramic is supported by a strong and tough metal. This system is considered in detail in Chapter 3.5.

In the case of the reinforced ceramic core systems, the support for the aesthetic ceramic is provided by another ceramic material, which has the necessary high strength and toughness but may lack the desired aesthetics. The various options using this approach are explored in Chapter 3.6.

In contrast, in the case of the resin-bonded ceramic, the support of the ceramic is provided by the tooth structure itself by bonding the aesthetic ceramic directly to the enamel and dentine. In this instance, the ceramic provides the necessary aesthetics and the strength is provided by the ability to bond to the tooth tissues.

CLINICAL SIGNIFICANCE

For resin-bonded ceramic restorations, success depends on the quality of the bond, since bond failure will lead to a loss of support of the ceramic restoration and eventually result in fracture of the ceramic restoration.

This approach only became possible with the advent of enamel- and dentine-bonding procedures, discussed in Chapter 2.5, and resin–ceramic bonding, discussed in Chapter 3.7. A combination of aesthetics and high strength would be ideal, as this removes the high reliance on the bond and also provides the opportunity to develop resin-bonded ceramic bridges.

A detailed account of the procedures and materials for the cementation of the ceramic and metal–ceramic restorations can be found in Chapter 3.8.

FURTHER READING

Brodsky LJ (1933) Practical hints: porcelain inlays simplified. Dental Cosmos **95**: 1024

Calamia JR (1983) Etched porcelain facial veneers: a new treatment modality based on scientific and clinical evidence. NY J Dent **53**: 255–259

Land CH (1889) Porcelain restorations. Dental Cosmos **31**: 191

McLean JW, Hughes HT (1965) The reinforcement of dental porcelain with ceramic oxides. Brit Dental J **119**: 251

Pincus CR (1938) Building mouth personality. J Calif Dent Assoc **14**: 125–129

Rekow ED, Silva NR, Coelho PG et al. Performance of Dental Ceramics: Challenges for Improvement. J Dent Res 2011 **90(8)**: 937–952

Weinstein M, Katz S, Weinstein AB (1962) Fused porcelain-to-metal teeth. US Patent 3,052,982. 11 Sept

Wildgoose DG, Johnson A, Winstanley RB et al (2004) Glass/ceramic/refractory techniques, their development and introduction into dentistry: a historical literature review. J Prosthet Dent **91**: 136

Metal-bonded ceramics

INTRODUCTION

A major limitation of the aesthetic ceramics such as the feldspathic glasses was their lack of strength. For ceramic restorations, the presence of micro-cracks on the fitting surface is a major source of weakness, and their removal would significantly improve the strength of the crown. Glazing the internal fitting surface is one possibility but impractical. Another possibility is bonding the ceramic to a metal substrate, such that these microscopic cracks are effectively eliminated, with the consequence that the structure is considerably stronger. This is the basic premise behind the metal-bonded system (Figure 3.5.1). The significant breakthrough came with the publication of a patent by Weinstein, Katz and Weinstein in 1962, where they explained how it is possible to get a feldspathic glass to bond to an alloy surface by the inclusion of leucite crystals. The latter were added so as to ensure that the coefficient of thermal expansion of the ceramic closely matched that of the metal, as explained in more detail later.

The crown consists of a cast metal coping, on to which is fired a ceramic veneer. If a proper bond is created, then the internal cracks are eliminated, as the metal presents a barrier to the propagation of cracks by virtue of its high fracture toughness. One of the most likely modes of failure with this system is the separation of the ceramic from the metal due to an interfacial breakdown of the metal–ceramic bond. The success of the system depends on the quality of this bond.

CLINICAL SIGNIFICANCE

From a materials perspective, the most likely cause of failure of a metal–ceramic restoration is a breakdown of the metal–ceramic bond.

An important contributory factor to the ability to bond the ceramic to the metal is the degree of mismatch between the coefficients of expansion of the ceramic and the metal. If the mismatch is too great, then stresses will build up during the cooling process after firing. These stresses can be sufficient to result in crazing or cracking of the ceramic. The issues of the bond and the coefficients of expansion both require careful consideration.

THE BOND

The nature of the bond between the metal coping and the ceramic has been extensively studied and it is agreed generally that there are three mechanisms involved:

- mechanical retention
- compression fit
- chemical bonding.

Mechanical retention occurs as the ceramic flows into the microscopic spaces in the surface of the metal. The roughness of the surface is enhanced, often by applying an alumina-air abrasive or by grinding, so that the amount of interlocking is increased (Figure 3.5.2). This has the added benefit of producing a very clean surface that aids the wetting of the ceramic on to the metal.

Good bonding relies on an intimate contact between the ceramic and the metal coping, and any contaminants will jeopardize the quality of the bond. Before the ceramic is applied to the surface of the coping, the coping is subjected to a degassing cycle in the furnace, which burns off any remaining impurities and reduces the formation of bubbles due to trapped gases at the interface. The various stages in the surface preparation of the metal coping are described in more detail at a later stage. Most ceramics have a coefficient of thermal expansion that is considerably lower than that of metals (Table 3.5.1). On cooling, the metal will try to contract more than the ceramic due to its higher coefficient of expansion. This leaves the ceramic in a state of compression. Whilst this is potentially highly beneficial for this brittle material, it is important that the mismatch in the coefficients of thermal expansion is only small. If the mismatch is too big, internal stresses created during cooling could cause the ceramic to fracture, with the most likely place for failure being the interface between the metal and the ceramic.

There is now considerable evidence that a strong chemical bond is created between the ceramic and the oxide coating on the metal. During firing, the ceramic is taken above its glass transition temperature such that it can flow and fuse with the oxides on the metal surface by migration of the metal oxides into the ceramic. In the case of gold alloy copings, small amounts of oxide-forming elements are added to the alloy because gold does not naturally form an oxide. As a

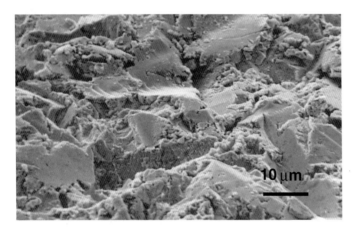

Figure 3.5.1 Construction of a metal–ceramic crown

Figure 3.5.2 Grit-blasted surface of a gold alloy

Table 3.5.1 Typical values of the coefficient of thermal expansion (α) of metals and ceramics

Material	α (ppm/°C)
Metals	
Aluminium	23.6
Gold	13.8
Nickel	13.3
Silver	19.0
Ceramics	
Alumina	8.8
Spinel ($MgAl_2O_4$)	7.6
Fused silica (SiO_2)	0.5
Soda–lime glass	9.0

consequence, the strength of the bond between the metal and the ceramic is increased manifold. This shows the importance of the presence of the surface oxides.

> ### CLINICAL SIGNIFICANCE
>
> The quality of the metal–ceramic bond is governed by the amount of micro-mechanical bonding, the thermal coefficient compatibility and the chemical interaction between the metal oxides and the ceramic.

PREPARATION OF THE METAL SURFACE

In order to obtain a good bond between the metal coping and the ceramic veneer, it is important for the metal surface to be carefully prepared. This involves a number of technical stages that warrant closer examination. The main reasons for the surface preparation of the metal are to ensure the removal of any contaminants and to produce a surface oxide layer of the correct composition and character to which the ceramic will fuse. The various stages can be identified as:

- surface grinding
- heating under partial vacuum
- acid pickling
- heating in air.

Surface grinding

When the metal casting is removed from the investment, there is always residual investment bonded to the surface of the casting. The surface is also contaminated with unwanted oxides, small porosities and fine projections, especially if the investment is susceptible to fracture of the surface layer.

The grinding process is carried out to remove all of these imperfections, and the increased surface roughness is believed to aid the retention of the ceramic by micro-mechanical interlocking.

However, the grinding process can itself suffer from the problem of debris, such as oils, waxes, bits of skin tissue or gases becoming trapped in undercuts. Even though the ceramic may be very effective in wetting the surface of the metal, it cannot always penetrate deep fissures.

> ### CLINICAL SIGNIFICANCE
>
> The presence of trapped air and contaminants that may decompose on firing results in the presence of gas bubbles at the interface between the metal and the ceramic, causing a marked degradation in the bond strength and the aesthetics of the prosthesis.

In general, methods of grinding that do not result in the formation of deep fissures, porosities or undercuts are preferred and, to this end, the use of fissure burs or carbide burs appears to be the recommended procedure.

Cleaning the casting in an organic solvent (e.g. carbon tetrachloride) in a sealed ultrasonic bath will remove surface contamination that has arisen during the handling of the casting.

Heating under partial vacuum

In the as-cast condition, the metal will not have the ideal oxide coating on its surface. Gold alloys will have virtually no oxide coating, given the noble nature of this metal. An oxide film can be formed by heating the casting at a temperature near to the firing temperature of the ceramic. This has the effect of allowing the metallic elements that are incorporated in the alloy (e.g. tin, indium, zinc or gallium) to migrate to the surface and form an oxide surface layer.

Great care must be taken to ensure that the correct heating cycle is used. Too brief a heat treatment could result in the formation of a thin or partial oxide coating, providing a poor substrate to which the ceramic can fuse. An excessively long heating cycle could result in the depletion of the oxidizing elements from the surface layer of the gold alloy.

No bond will form if all of the oxide formed is removed during the subsequent acid pickling process and none of the oxidizing elements are left sufficiently close to the surface to allow the formation of additional oxides.

Carrying out the heat treatment under reduced pressure aids the removal of gases that have been absorbed by the metal in great amounts during the casting process. The removal of these gases helps to prevent the formation of interfacial bubbles. For this reason, the heat treatment of the alloy prior to the ceramic firing cycle is often referred to as a degassing treatment.

In the case of base metal alloys, where nickel and chromium are commonly used, the metals oxidize very readily and the problem is generally the opposite of that for the gold alloys, in that too much of the oxide is formed.

Although oxides will naturally form during the firing of the ceramic, it has been found that it is better to preform the oxide coating, as this improves the wetting of the ceramic on the metal surface.

Acid pickling

The heat treatment of gold alloys will produce not only tin oxide but various other oxides on the surface as well.

The acid pickling procedure seeks to remove the unwanted oxides in preference to the tin oxide. There is the added advantage that the dark surface of the alloy is lightened from grey to white due to increased concentration of tin oxide on the alloy surface. Commonly used acids are 50% hydrofluoric acid or 30% hydrochloric acid, with the latter preferred because of the hazards associated with the use of hydrofluoric acid. Neither this nor the following procedure is generally required for base metal alloys.

Heating in air

A further heat treatment in air is frequently carried out in order to form an oxide coating of the correct thickness and quality.

The optimal oxide film on precious metal alloys should have a matt, greyish-white appearance, being composed mainly of base metal oxide. If the surface has a glossy appearance, this indicates a lack of oxide film and is usually the consequence of too many repeated surface treatments.

CLINICAL SIGNIFICANCE

The lack of an oxide film will result in a poor bond between the ceramic and the metal.

IMPORTANCE OF THERMAL EXPANSION

The composition of the ceramic for metal–ceramic restorations needs to be different from that of the ceramic used for all-ceramic restorations.

The coefficient of thermal expansion (α) of the feldspathic glasses used in the construction of the porcelain jacket crowns is 7–8 ppm/°C. This is far too low to be compatible with the alloys, which are typically in the region of 14–16 ppm/°C. This mismatch would give rise to serious problems due to excessive differential shrinkage on cooling. Depending on their composition, the coefficient of thermal expansion of the alloys and the ceramics can differ quite considerably.

CLINICAL SIGNIFICANCE

It is extremely important that the correct combination of metal and ceramic is used.

Thermally induced stresses

The ceramics used in the construction of metal–ceramic restorations lose their thermoplastic fluidity once they are cooled below their glass transition temperature, which is typically in the range of 600–700°C. From this point onwards, any difference in the coefficients of expansion between the metal and the ceramic will produce stresses in the ceramic as the ceramic attempts to shrink more or less than the metal substructure, depending on the type of mismatch. There are three possible scenarios that can be considered, namely:

$$\alpha_p > \alpha_m$$
$$\alpha_p = \alpha_m$$
$$\alpha_p < \alpha_m$$

where p is porcelain and m is metal. The stresses that result from each of the above conditions are shown in Figure 3.5.3.

When $\alpha_p > \alpha_m$, the ceramic will attempt to contract more than the metal (Figure 3.5.3a). As the metal prevents this from happening, the ceramic will be under a state of tension when it is cooled to room temperature, with the metal being in a state of compression. The surface tensile stresses cause the formation of surface cracks and a crazed surface.

When $\alpha_p = \alpha_m$, the two materials will shrink at the same rate and no differential stresses are generated (Figure 3.5.3b).

When $\alpha_p < \alpha_m$, the metal will attempt to shrink more than the ceramic and this places the ceramic in a state of compression (Figure 3.5.3c). This substantially reduces the potential for the ceramic to crack, since these compressive stresses have to be overcome before the ceramic is placed under tension. The metal will be in a state of tension but, since the tensile strength of the alloys used is quite high (500–1000 MPa), there is no danger of the metal failing. Thus it would appear that the best situation is one in which the coefficient of expansion of the metal is greater than that of the ceramic.

Whereas it would appear from the above discussion that the greater the mismatch, the better (as the ceramic will be under a higher compressive stress), this is in fact not the case. The mismatch should not be too great, as the stresses generated in the system may cause crazing or fracture of the ceramic, or debonding from the metal surface.

The reason for this is best explained by considering ceramic that is fused to a circular metal structure, especially as this is more akin to the real situation (shown in Figure 3.5.4). When the metal attempts to shrink more than the ceramic, radial tensile stresses and a circumferential compressive stress are generated. The latter are advantageous, but the former can be sufficient to cause debonding between the ceramic and the metal. If the mismatch is very large, the radial tensile stresses can cause the ceramic itself to fracture, with the fracture appearing circumferentially.

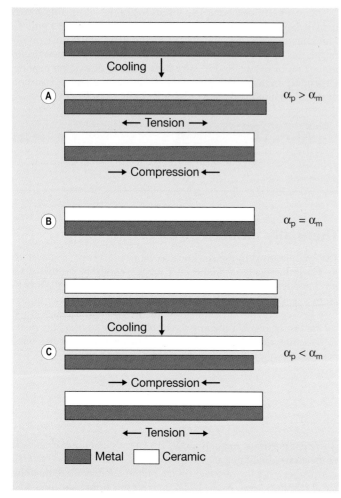

Figure 3.5.3 The effect of thermal mismatch on residual stress in the metal and the ceramic

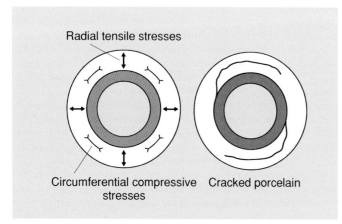

Figure 3.5.4 Cracking of metal-bonded-ceramic due to radial tensile stresses when $\alpha_p << \alpha_m$

CLINICAL SIGNIFICANCE

The best combination of metal and ceramic is one where the coefficient of expansion of the ceramic is only slightly lower than that of the metal.

Table 3.5.2 Typical compositions of metal-bonded ceramics as compared with a porcelain jacket crown (PJC) porcelain

| | PJC porcelain | Metal-bonded ceramics | |
		(a)	(b)
SiO_2 (%)	66.5	66.4	59.2
Al_2O_3 (%)	13.5	14.5	18.5
Na_2O (%)	4.2	6.2	4.8
K_2O (%)	7.1	10.2	11.8
Firing temp. (°C)	960	940	900

Effect of composition of the ceramic

The mismatch in the coefficient of expansion between the feldspathic ceramics used in the manufacture of porcelain jacket crowns and the metals available for ceramic bonding is normally far too great. To overcome this problem, the alkali content of the ceramic is increased, as indicated in Table 3.5.2. Both soda (Na_2O) and potash (K_2O) are added to push up the coefficient of expansion to be in the region of 14–16 ppm/°C.

Much more important is the fact that the addition of these oxides results in the formation of a crystalline phase in the glassy matrix. This crystalline phase is known as *tetragonal leucite*, which has a high coefficient of thermal expansion of 22–24 ppm/°C. The amount of precipitated leucite can be carefully controlled to provide a ceramic with the correct coefficient of expansion for a particular alloy, and can be 30–40% of the volume of the material (Figure 3.5.5). The associated reduction in firing temperature has the benefit of reducing the potential for distortion due to creep of the alloy.

After the ceramic frit is prepared by the manufacturer, it is held at an elevated temperature for a specific time to allow the formation of leucite crystals. Thus, this is a process identical to the ceraming of the glass ceramics described in Chapter 3.8. Hence the ceramics used for metal–ceramic restorations are perhaps best described as leucite-containing glass ceramics. These glass ceramics are, nevertheless, different for the leucite-reinforced glass ceramics described in Chapter 3.8, in that in this case the primary concern is to match its coefficient of thermal expansion with that of the metal and not to obtain the highest possible strength. In fact, the flexural strength of the ceramics used for metal–ceramic restorations is only of the order of 30–50 MPa. Hence the ceramic build-up on the metal framework should not be too thick, as this can lead to ceramic fractures when loaded in the mouth.

CLINICAL SIGNIFICANCE

The general recommendation is that the ceramic thickness should not exceed 1 mm.

An increase in the number and size of the leucite crystals can occur when firing the ceramic on to the metal. In the case of multiple firings, this will increase the coefficient of expansion of the ceramic. Such an increase can compromise the compatibility of the metal and the ceramic. Thus, excessive multiple firing of the metal–ceramic system is contraindicated. Slow cooling can also have the same effect as repeated firing, as can post-soldering, and the temperature should be

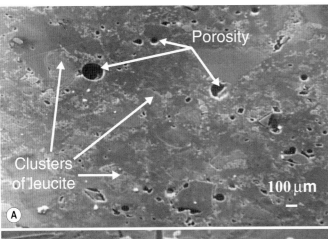

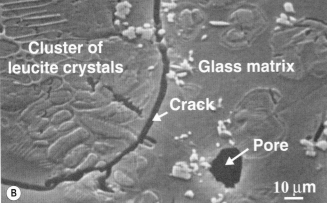

Figure 3.5.5 (a) The structure of a leucite-containing ceramic used in the construction of metal–ceramic restorations. Note the presence of residual porosity. (b) A close-up showing the detail of a leucite cluster and an associated crack, often seen in these ceramics due to the large mismatch in the coefficient of expansion of the leucite and the glass matrix

raised and lowered as quickly as possible without giving rise to thermal shock effects.

The opaque shade of the ceramic when it is first laid down on the metal coping tends to contain larger amounts of metallic oxides that help to mask the colour of the coping.

Great care must be exercised during the firing process, since the ceramic has a tendency to devitrify by a process of recrystallization. This results in cloudiness of the ceramic, as the small crystals that are formed act as scattering sites for light.

CHOICE OF METAL–CERAMIC ALLOYS

The requirements for alloys used in the metal-bonded ceramic system are somewhat different from those for the all-metal constructions (Table 3.5.3). As it is necessary to fire ceramic on to the surface of the metal, its high melting temperature must be higher than the sintering temperature for the ceramic. If the melting temperature of the metal is too close to the firing temperature of the ceramic, partial melting of thin sections of the coping may occur, or the coping may deform.

Especially in the construction of long-span bridges, the metal must have a high elastic modulus and high yield stress. The resultant high stiffness of the bridge structure will prevent the occurrence of

Table 3.5.3 Requirements of a metal–ceramic alloy

Biocompatibility
Corrosion resistance
Ease of casting
Accurate fit
High bond strength to the ceramic
Absence of adverse reaction with the ceramic
Melting temperature > firing temperature of ceramic
High elastic modulus
Low creep
Low cost

excessively high strains (that the ceramic cannot cope with) on occlusal loading. In addition, a low stiffness of the metal framework can result in distortion due to the differential contraction stresses that are generated on cooling after porcelain firing.

At one time, only high-gold alloys were available but, with the rising cost of gold, a variety of alternative alloys have been developed, which may be classified as high-gold, gold–palladium, high-palladium, palladium–silver, nickel–chromium alloys or commercially pure titanium. The compositions of some of the alloys are shown in Table 3.5.4.

High-gold alloys

For the high-gold alloys, the melting temperature is raised by the addition of platinum and palladium, both of which have a high melting temperature.

An immediately obvious difference between the non-ceramic–gold alloy and the ceramic–gold alloy is the omission of copper in the latter. This is done because copper reduces melting temperature and also has a tendency to react with the ceramic, producing a green discoloration. This is another feature of the alloys: they must not react with the ceramic in such a way as to spoil the aesthetics of the restoration.

The high-gold alloys have the advantage that they have been around for some considerable time and clinical experience has shown that they are extremely successful. In particular, the bond between the ceramic and the metal is very strong and highly reliable.

The main disadvantages of high-gold alloys are their relatively low melting temperatures, their susceptibility to creep at high temperatures and their low elastic modulus. A minimum coping thickness of 0.5 mm is required with their use.

In situations of limited biological width, this can give rise to aesthetic problems and often results in over-contouring to mask the metal colour. In this respect, the Pd–Ag and base metal alloys are more attractive.

Gold–palladium alloys

One reason for the introduction of the Au–Pd alloys in the early 1970s was the rapidly rising cost of gold. Precious metal prices have proved very fickle over recent years and costs can swing wildly from one year to the next. Perhaps it should be remembered that the cost of the material will represent only a small component of the cost of the dental treatment.

The performance of Au–Pd alloys is comparable to that of the high-gold alloys in terms of castability, accuracy of fit and corrosion resistance. However, there are some alloy–ceramic combinations that should be avoided due to a mismatch in thermal expansion characteristics.

Table 3.5.4 Typical compositions of metal–ceramic alloys

Type	Au%	Ag%	Pd%	Pt%	Ni%	Cr%	Mo%	In%, Cu%, Zn%, Ga%
High-gold	88	1	6	4	–	–	–	Balance
Au–Pd	50	10	38	–	–	–	–	Balance
High-palladium	–	–	80	–	–	–	–	Balance
Pd–Ag	–	30	60	–	–	–	–	Balance
Ni–Cr	–	–	–	–	70	20	10	–

High-palladium alloys

These alloys are primarily palladium, with small additions of other elements, such as copper, gallium and tin; they became very popular in the middle to late 1970s, when the price of gold increased substantially. The price of palladium has since also increased and thus even these alloys are falling out of favour simply due to cost.

The copper, which can be present in amounts up to 15%, may be a surprising addition, since this might have been thought to cause porcelain discoloration. However, unlike gold alloys, the inclusion of copper in palladium alloys does not seem to have this effect.

Their sag resistance can be poor due to excessive creep on ceramic firing.

CLINICAL SIGNIFICANCE

These alloys are contraindicated for long-span bridges where this may present a particular problem.

Palladium–silver alloys

The Pd–Ag alloys have the most favourable elastic modulus of all of the precious metal alloys, producing castings with low flexibility and a reduced tendency to sag on porcelain firing. The alloys are somewhat less forgiving in terms of castability and fit, but as long as appropriate procedures are followed, results can be as good as with the gold alloys.

Due to the presence of high amounts of silver, there is concern that porcelain discoloration may occur. This problem appears to be more severe with certain alloy–porcelain combinations than others, and can be minimized by careful selection of the metal–porcelain combination.

Multiple firings should be kept to a minimum, and overheating of the alloy avoided.

Nickel–chromium–molybdenum alloys

The Ni–Cr–Mo alloys have a composition that is typically 77% Ni, 12% Cr and 3.5% Mo, although the Mo and Cr content can rise to 9% and 22% respectively at the expense of nickel. The Ni–Cr–Mo alloys are very stiff, as their elastic modulus can be some 2.5 times higher than that of the high-gold alloys. This has the advantage that the coping thickness can be reduced from 0.5 mm to 0.3 mm, which lessens the problem of over-contouring. It also means that this alloy is a better choice for resin-bonded bridges, especially those with a cantilever design, where the high elastic modulus helps to reduce stresses in the adhesive layer.

They would also be better for the construction of long-span bridges, as they provide greater rigidity and, because of the high melting temperature, there is less potential for sag during firing.

The disadvantages with these alloys are that casting is more difficult and the higher casting shrinkage can give rise to problems of poor fit. Also, clinical experience would indicate that the ceramic-to-metal bond is not as reliable as for the other alloys.

However, as more experience is gained with these alloys, so their performance may well improve. The low cost of the alloy is certainly very attractive.

The biocompatibility of Ni–Cr alloys has long been a matter of concern. Nickel is a recognized allergen, although reports of nickel allergy arising from intra-oral devices are rare. Beryllium (Be) (<0.9%) is added to some Ni–Cr alloys to improve the castability and improve the bond to the porcelain. However, Be can be a potential problem for the dental technician. The mechanical grinding and polishing process causes the release of Be, which is a known carcinogen. Also the release of Be is some 5–6 times that of the bulk composition.

CLINICAL SIGNIFICANCE

Nickel-containing alloys are contraindicated in patients with known nickel allergy.

Commercially pure titanium (cpTi)

The dental use of cpTi has already been dealt with in Chapter 3.3 on casting alloys. It has also become popular for metal–ceramic restorations because of its good corrosion resistance, excellent biocompatibility, low weight and relatively low cost compared to the precious metal alloys. However, there are some additional issues that it is appropriate to address here, relating to its use with ceramics.

When titanium is cast, a reaction layer with a thickness of 50–100 μm forms on the surface of the casting due to an interaction between the titanium and the refractory investment. This reaction layer can become even more pronounced during the subsequent ceramic firing cycle. This layer, if not removed, will interfere with the bonding of the ceramic to the titanium. A variety of suggestions have been put forward to deal with this problem and include sand blasting, silicon-nitride coating and immersion dissolution.

The casting problems can be avoided by producing the restorations using an alternative technique, consisting of spark erosion and copymilling. However, titanium has a high chemical reactivity and, if taken above 800°C, this gives rise to a thick oxide coating, with the consequence of a weak bond to the ceramic.

Unlike the alloys described above, titanium has a coefficient of expansion of 9.6 ppm/°C. Thus the leucite-containing ceramics developed for the metal–ceramic alloys are inappropriate and it is important that ceramics specially designed for use with cpTi are used.

The bonding of the ceramic to cpTi is problematic and the bond strength is not as good as that obtained to the alloys.

SUMMARY

Metal–ceramic restorations can produce a good aesthetic outcome. The presence of a metal framework that has to be masked by the ceramic is a limitation with this system, but if given sufficient space to work in, the dental laboratory technician can produce a very good result. However, this does mean that these restorations are inherently destructive of tooth structure.

The main advantage of the metal–ceramic restoration over the all-ceramic restoration is its resistance to fracture. Until very recently, only short-span bridges could be made out of ceramics, such that metal-bonded ceramic was the only option available for anything more than a small three-unit bridge. This situation is rapidly changing and new developments in high-strength core ceramic systems using new materials are challenging a clinical situation that, for the last 40 years, was dominated by the metal–ceramic restoration.

CLINICAL SIGNIFICANCE

The introduction of high-strength ceramic core restorations for crowns and bridges and resin-bonded ceramic restorations for crowns is challenging many of the situations where traditionally a metal–ceramic crown would have been used. However, the metal–ceramic crown has provided sterling service for many years, whereas the all-ceramic restorations are still relative newcomers.

Whatever the advantages and disadvantages of the different systems, the following recommendations should be followed:

- The responsibility for the choice of alloy rests with the dentist and should not be delegated to the dental laboratory technician.
- Ensure that the correct metal–ceramic combination is used by the dental laboratory.

FURTHER READING

Anusavice KJ (1985) Noble metal alloys for metal–ceramic restorations. Dent Clin N Am **29**: 789

Bagby M, Marshall SJ, Marshall GW (1990) Metal ceramic compatibility: a review of the literature. J Prosthet Dent **63**: 21

Betolotti RL (1984) Selection of alloys for today's crowns and fixed partial denture restorations. J Am Dent Assoc **108**: 959

Bumgardner JD, Lucas LC (1995) Cellular response to metallic ions released from nickel–chromium dental alloys. J Dent Res **74**: 1521

CDMIE (1981) Porcelain–metal alloy compatibility: criteria and test methods. J Am Dent Assoc **102**: 71

Clyde CS, Boyd T (1988) The etched cast metal resin-bonded (Maryland) bridge: a clinical review. J Dent **16**: 22

Creugers NHJ, Käyser AF (1992) An analysis of multiple failures of resin-bonded bridges. J Dent **20**: 348

Fischer J, Fleetwood PW (2000) Improving the processing of high-gold metal–ceramic frameworks by a pre-firing heat treatment. Dent Mater **16**: 109

Johnson AJ, van Noort R, Stokes CW (2006) Surface analysis of porcelain fused to metal systems. Dent Mater **22**: 330

Lawson JR (1991) Alternative alloys for resin-bonded retainers. J Prosthet Dent **65**: 97

Livaditis GJ, Thompson VP (1982) Etched castings: an improved retentive mechanism for resin-bonded retainers. J Prosthet Dent **47**: 52

Mackert JR Jr, Williams AL (1996) Microcracks in dental porcelain and their behavior during multiple firing. J Dent Res **75**: 1484

Murakami I, Schulman A (1987) Aspects of metal–ceramic bonding. Dent Clin N Am **31**: 333

Northeast SE, van Noort R, Shaglouf AS (1994) Tensile peel failure of resin-bonded Ni/Cr beams: an experimental and finite element study. J Dent **22**: 252

Pang IC, Gilbert JL, Chai J et al (1995) Bonding characteristics of low-fusing porcelain bonded to pure titanium and palladium–copper alloy. J Prosthet Dent **73**: 17

Peregrina A, Schorr BL, Eick JD et al (1992) Measurement of oxide adherence to silver-free high-palladium alloys. Int J Prosthodont **5**: 173

Rochette AL (1973) Attachment of a splint to enamel of lower anterior teeth. J Prosthet Dent **30**: 418

Sarkar NK, Verret M, Ever CS et al (1985) Role of gallium in alloy–porcelain bonding. J Prosthet Dent **53**: 190

Saunders WP (1989) Resin-bonded bridgework: a review. J Dent **17**: 255

Tomsia AP, Pask JA (1986) Chemical reactions and adherence at glass/metal interfaces. An analysis. Dent Mater **2**: 10

Wang RR, Welsch GE, Monteiro O et al (1999) Silicon nitride coating on titanium to enable titanium–ceramic bonding. J Biomed Mater Res **46**: 262

Wood M (1985) Etched castings – an alternative approach to treatment. Dent Clin N Am **29**: 393

Wuy Y (1991) The effect of oxidation heat treatment of porcelain bond strength in selected base metal alloys. J Prosthet Dent **66**: 439

All-ceramic restorations: high-strength core ceramics

INTRODUCTION

The work by Land in the early 1900s and others since then showed that one of the problems with the all-ceramic anterior crown was that the porcelain would fracture from the fit surface outwards. Some improvements in the strength of porcelain were achieved by the introduction of vacuum firing furnaces, which helps to minimize porosity, and raised the flexural strength of the porcelain from 20–30 MPa to approximately 50–60 MPa. However, this proved not to be adequate to produce reliable ceramic restorations and thus the search was on for a core material that would provide the necessary strength and toughness to prevent fractures arising from cracks propagating from the fit surface of the crown.

Since ceramics tend to fail at the same critical strain of ~0.1%, one means of achieving an increase in fracture strength is to increase the elastic modulus of the material. If, at the same time, the propagation of cracks is made more difficult such that a greater strain can be supported, a higher strength ceramic will result (Figure 3.6.1). The flexural strengths of a number of ceramics are shown in Table 3.6.1. As the tensile strength is a difficult property to measure (giving rise to a wide degree of scatter in the data), it is common practice to determine the flexural strength. Although the silicon nitrides and carbides are attractive from the viewpoint of strength, they are not suitable because of the difficulties associated with the manufacture of individual crowns: the colour differences and the mismatch in the coefficient of thermal expansion.

CLINICAL SIGNIFICANCE

Alumina and zirconia are white and strong, and therefore these ceramics are now used in a number of dental ceramic systems.

In the mid-1960s, McLean and Hughes developed a core material based on the reinforcement of a feldspathic glass with alumina, commonly referred to as the alumina-reinforced porcelain jacket crown (PJC). Since then, other systems have been developed. In the 1980s, the glass-infiltrated, high-strength ceramic cores were developed (In-Ceram, Vita) and, in the 1990s, the all-alumina core made its first appearance (Techceram, Techceram Ltd: Procera AllCeram, Nobel Biocare). Recent work has seen the introduction of ytrria-stabilized zirconia for the fabrication of cores for crown and bridge frameworks.

ALUMINA-REINFORCED PORCELAIN JACKET CROWNS

The alumina-reinforced feldspathic core was introduced in the early 1960s by Hughes and McLean. The material consists of a feldspathic glass containing 40–50% alumina (Figure 3.6.2). The alumina particles are far stronger than the glass, and are more effective at preventing crack propagation than quartz, acting as crack stoppers (Figure 3.6.3). Whereas the flexural strength of feldspathic porcelain is, at best, some 60 MPa, this is raised to 120–150 MPa for the aluminous core porcelains.

In the construction of a crown, the opaque shade shown in Figure 3.4.3 is made with an aluminous core porcelain. It is still necessary to use the weaker dentine and enamel shades of the feldspathic porcelains because it is not possible to produce aluminous porcelains with the required translucency; the alumina causes the porcelain to appear dull and opaque.

The main application of the alumina-reinforced PJC is for the restoration of anterior teeth. Although the improvement in strength is considerable, it is still insufficient to allow its use posteriorly and the construction of even a three-unit bridge is out of the question.

CLINICAL SIGNIFICANCE

Yet stronger core materials were needed if the use of ceramics was to be extended to the posterior teeth.

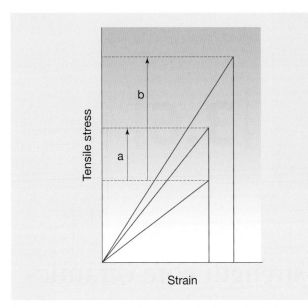

Figure 3.6.1 Improvements in the strength of ceramics by (a) raising the elastic modulus and (b) increasing the resistance to crack propagation

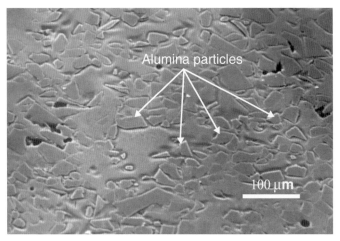

Figure 3.6.2 Scanning electron micrograph of an alumina-reinforced core material showing the alumina particles embedded in a glassy matrix composed of feldspar

Table 3.6.1 Typical strength values for high-strength ceramics

Type of ceramic	Flexural strength (MPa)
Hot-pressed silicon nitride	800–900
Hot-pressed silicon carbide	400–750
Partially stabilized zirconia	640
Alumina 98% pure	420–520

GLASS-INFILTRATED HIGH-STRENGTH CERAMIC CORE SYSTEMS

The addition of alumina to the feldspathic glass during the prefritting process limits the amount of alumina that can be incorporated to

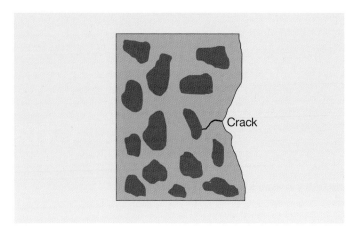

Figure 3.6.3 Alumina particles acting as crack stoppers

about 40–50 vol. %. An alternative approach has been adopted in a new system called In-Ceram (Vita Zahnfabrik, Bad Säckingen, Germany). This core material has an alumina content of ~85%.

A ceramic core is formed on to a refractory die from a fine slurry of alumina powder by a process known as slip-casting. After the die has dried, it is sintered for 10 hours at 1120°C. The melting temperature of alumina is too high to produce full densification of the powder by liquid-phase sintering and only solid-phase sintering occurs. Consequently, the coping thus created is only just held together at the contact points between the alumina particles and a porous structure is the result. The strength of this porous core is only about 6–10 MPa. The porous structure is then infiltrated with a lanthanum glass, which has a low viscosity when fired at 1100°C for 4–6 hours. The molten glass is able to penetrate into the pores, producing a dense ceramic. The aesthetics and functional form are then achieved by veneering the core with conventional feldspathic dental ceramics.

CLINICAL SIGNIFICANCE

Very high flexural strength values (400–500 MPa) have been claimed for this core ceramic, which makes this system suitable for anterior and posterior crowns, with excellent results.

Several attempts have also been made at producing anterior cantilever and posterior three-unit bridges, which is a highly ambitious use of ceramics but shows considerable promise.

A similar approach has been adopted with spinel ($MgAl_2O_4$) or zirconia replacing the alumina. The InCeram-Spinel offers superior aesthetics over the InCeram-Alumina at a slightly reduced flexural strength (~350 MPa) and is recommended for inlays and anterior crowns. The InCeram-Zirconia is based on the InCeram-Alumina, but with the addition of 33 wt % zirconia, and produces a ceramic core with a strength of some 700 MPa. Its drawback is that the combination of a glass, alumina and zirconia means that this core material is very opaque.

An alternative approach to the slip-casting route described above is now also available for the CAD–CAM (Computer Aided Design–Computer Aided Manufacture) production route, using either the CEREC system from Siemens or the Celay system from Vident. The CAD–CAM process involves three main steps:

1. the acquisition of data in a digital format
2. designing of the appropriate restoration on the computer
3. machining of the restoration from a prefabricated block of the material.

However, there are a number of variations on this theme, which are not possible to discuss here. The InCeram-Spinel/Alumina/Zirconia blocks from which the restorations are machined, are produced by dry-pressing the powder such that the open-pore structure is denser and more homogeneous, leading to a yet higher flexural strength after glass infiltration.

Pure alumina cores

It would seem a natural extension from the alumina-reinforced core systems described above to consider the possibility of a pure alumina core. There are at least two systems on the market that offer pure alumina cores, the Procera AllCeram (Nobel Biocare AB, Gothenburg, Sweden) and the Techceram system (Techceram Ltd, Shipley, UK). The potential advantages are increased strength and superior translucency compared with the glass-infiltrated core materials.

Production of the Procera AllCeram core involves producing a die from the impression, digitizing the geometry of the desired coping using specially designed computer software and transferring this information down a modem to a laboratory in Stockholm. This is all done by a designated dental laboratory that is a member of the Procera Network. The coping is produced by a special process, which involves sintering 99.5% pure alumina at 1600–1700°C such that it is fully densified. The coping is then returned to the dental laboratory for building on the crown's aesthetics using compatible feldspathic glasses. Turn-around time is approximately 24 hours. The flexural strength of the Al_2O_3 core materials is in the region of 700 MPa and thus similar to that achieved with the InCeram-Zirconia.

The Techceram system uses quite a different approach. In this system the impression can be sent to Techceram Ltd, who will produce a special die, on to which the alumina core is deposited using a thermal gun-spray technique. This process produces an alumina core with a density of 80–90%, which is subsequently sintered at 1170°C to achieve optimum strength and translucency. The alumina coping is then returned to the dental laboratory, where the ceramist will develop the final contour and aesthetics using conventional feldspathic glasses.

CLINICAL SIGNIFICANCE

One of the potential benefits of producing a pure alumina core is that the translucency is considered to be better than that of the glass-infiltrated alumina composite structures.

Zirconia core systems

The introduction of CAD–CAM technology to the dental laboratory manufacture of fixed partial dentures is having a profound influence on the choice of materials available. Until CAD–CAM, it was inconceivable to consider the use of zirconia (ZrO_2) as a material for the construction of crowns and bridges, largely because a zirconia powder would not densify until reaching a temperature in excess of 1600°C, making it impractical as a dental laboratory material. This has all changed and, with the aid of CAD–CAM technology, it is now possible to manufacture crown copings and bridge frameworks.

The reason that bridge frameworks are now considered is the high strength of this material, which is in excess of 1000 MPa. The actual material used is yttria-stabilized zirconia and the yttria has a very important function, although it is only present in a small amount (~3.0 mol %). Under normal circumstances, zirconia forms a stable monoclinic crystal structure at room temperature, but the addition of a small amount of yttria results in the formation of a metastable tetragonal crystal structure at room temperature. When a small defect such as a crack is present, it progresses through the material due to the localized stress at the crack tip being relieved by crack growth. As mentioned earlier, the way to improve ceramics is to prevent cracks from growing; in the case of yttria-stabilized zirconia, when the stress at the crack tip reaches a certain level, the metastable tetragonal crystal structure of zirconia transforms to the more stable monoclinic form. This stress-induced change in structure is accompanied by an expansion of the material, which causes the crack tip to close up and thus prevents it from advancing. Hence, it is very difficult for a crack to advance through an yttria-stabilized zirconia ceramic. In effect, the material is not only very strong but also very tough by comparison with other ceramics. It is this particular feature of zirconia that makes it possible to contemplate using this material not only as a core for crowns but also for bridge frameworks.

There is still the problem of manufacturing cores and bridge frameworks from this material and this is where CAD–CAM has made all the difference. A number of commercial CAD–CAM systems are now available in selected dental laboratories. The process followed is generally one of taking an impression, constructing a model, digitizing the model, designing the restoration on the computer and then machining the restoration. Because zirconia is so strong and tough, the most common approach used to deal with this is a technique often referred to as 'soft' machining. In this method, the restoration is machined from a porous blank, which is easy to machine; once the desired shape has been achieved, the item is fired in a furnace to cause the material to densify. The shrinkage that occurs, typically some 20 vol. %, is taken care of during the computer-aided design process. The result is a very close-fitting, semitranslucent to white core or bridge framework.

CLINICAL SIGNIFICANCE

The advent of CAD–CAM technology has opened up new opportunities to use materials not previously considered to be a viable option and thus new approaches to the construction of all ceramic crowns and bridges. However, clinical experience is very limited at this stage.

SUMMARY

One drawback with all the high-strength core systems described above is that none of them is amenable to acid etching to produce a micromechanically retentive surface, although some bonding with the cementing medium will arise due to the roughness of the surface from processing. Since the fit surface is made up largely of alumina and/or zirconia rather than silica, no coupling agents are currently available that can effectively bond the core to resins. Without an effective coupling agent or an ideal micro-mechanically retentive surface, these systems cannot be resin-bonded to the tooth tissues and will not derive the added benefit associated with resin bonded ceramic restorations.

CLINICAL SIGNIFICANCE

The reinforced core ceramic restoration must rely primarily on the strength and toughness of the core material and appropriate design to resist the forces of occlusion.

FURTHER READING

Andersson M, Razzoog ME, Odén A et al (1998) PROCERA: a new way to achieve an all-ceramic crown. Quintessence Int 29: 285

Banks RG (1990) Conservative posterior ceramic restorations: a review of the literature. J Prosthet Dent 63: 619

Duret F, Blouin J-L, Duret B (1988) CAD–CAM in dentistry. J Am Dent Assoc 117: 715

Lüthy H, Filser F, Loeffel O et al (2005) Strength and reliability of four-unit all-ceramic posterior bridges. Dent Mater 21: 930

May KB, Russell MM, Razzoog ME et al (1998) Precision of fit: the Procera Allceram crown. J Prosthet Dent 80: 394

Mörmann WH, Bindl A (1997) The new creativity in ceramic restorations:

dental CAD–CAM. Quintessence Int 27: 821

Odén A, Andersson M, Krystek-Ondracek I et al (1998) Five-year clinical evaluation of Procera AllCeram crowns. J Prosthet Dent 80: 450

Piconi C, Maccauro G (1999) Review of zirconia as a ceramic biomaterial. Biomaterials 20: 1

Pröbster L, Diehl J (1992) Slip-casting alumina ceramics for crown and bridge restorations. Quintessence Int 23: 25

Qualtrough AJE, Piddock V (1999) Recent advances in ceramic materials and systems for dental restorations. Dental Update 26: 65

Ritter A, Baratieri LN (1999) Ceramic restorations for posterior teeth: guidelines for the clinician. J Esthet Dent 11: 72

Rizkalla AS, Jones DW (2004) Mechanical properties of commercial high strength ceramic core materials. Dent Mater 20: 207

Spear F, Holloway J (2008) Which all-ceramic system is optimal for anterior esthetics? J Am Dent Assoc 139(Suppl): 19S–24S

Suttor D (2004) LAVA zirconia crowns and bridges. Int J Computerized Dent 7: 67

Tinschert J, Zwez D, Mark R et al (2000) Structural reliability of alumina-, leucite-, mica- and zirconia-based ceramics. J Dent 28: 529

Chapter |3.7|

All-ceramic restorations: resin-bonded ceramics

INTRODUCTION

One way in which the traditional approach of cemented restorations has been challenged is with the development of new adhesive techniques. These have extended the use of ceramics to areas not previously thought possible. The concept of the resin-bonded ceramic restoration could not become reality until techniques for bonding the ceramic to enamel and dentine had been discovered. The idea of bonding ceramics to enamel using a combination of the acid-etch technique and resins began to be developed during the 1970s, which led, in the 1980s, to the ceramic veneers restoration. Then, still in the 1980s, major progress was made in the development of dentine-bonding agents, which opened up the possibility of resin-bonded crowns. The combination of adhesion to enamel, dentine and ceramic, and the improved strength characteristics of the ceramics, has produced restorations with excellent mechanical integrity. In fact, the adhesive bond has the effect of eliminating the internal surface flaws and thus reduces the potential for fracture. This has led to a growth in the use of resin-bonded ceramics for crowns, veneers and inlays.

CERAMIC VENEERS

The concept of using ceramics as veneers is not new, and can be traced back to Dr Charles Pincus of Beverley Hills, who constructed porcelain veneers in the 1930s for actors in Hollywood, including Shirley Temple. The porcelain veneers were baked on platinum foil and retained on the teeth by denture powder. However, the veneers often broke because the thin porcelain was brittle and they were frequently removed from the teeth. When acrylic resin was introduced in 1937, Pincus switched to this material for the production of veneers for the acting profession. This eventually developed into the use of composite veneers, and ceramics were not used for a long time.

The advent of procedures for bonding resins to enamel using phosphoric acid etching of the enamel allowed the development of the resin-bonded ceramic veneer as a viable treatment option. This technique permitted bonding of resins to tooth enamel. In this situation, the fact that the thin ceramic material is bonded to the underlying tooth structure via a resin means that the tooth itself provides the support for the weak veneering material. An early reference to supporting a ceramic restoration by resin-bonding it to enamel was published by Rochette in 1975. This idea was then extended by Horn in 1983, who proposed the use of hydrofluoric acid as a glass etchant for veneers constructed from a leucite-containing feldspar, so as to enhance the bond between the ceramic and the resin. Thus, using the phosphoric acid-etch technique on enamel, he was able to bond the ceramic veneers permanently to the teeth with a resin-based composite. Bonding to ceramic has since been improved by the additional use of a silane coupling agent (see Chapter 3.8).

CLINICAL SIGNIFICANCE

Before the advent of resin-bonded ceramic veneers, the only options available were the composite veneer, the porcelain jacket crown and the metal–ceramic crown.

Ceramic veneers are considered superior to composites because of their improved aesthetics, colour stability, surface finish, abrasion resistance and tissue compatibility. They are also chemically very stable and have a coefficient of expansion similar to that of enamel. The finishing of porcelain veneers is more difficult than that of composites due to their high hardness. The thin feathered margins are more easily damaged than the margins of crowns, both in the laboratory and in the surgery. The ceramic veneers have the distinct advantage over crowns that improved aesthetics can be achieved with minimal tooth reduction, and the palatal surface of the tooth is unchanged so that incisal guidance is maintained. The material used for the construction of veneers is either a simple feldspathic glass or a leucite-containing feldspathic glass (see Chapters 3.4 and 3.5); these are the materials of choice for the construction of veneers due to their excellent aesthetics, especially from the point of view of colour and translucency, something which it is difficult for any other ceramic to match.

Although, in the time of Land and Pincus, the veneers were constructed on platinum foil, nowadays a variety of methods are available, which include:

- sintering on a refractory die
- hot pressing
- computer-aided design–computer-aided manufacture (CAD–CAM) machining from block.

Sintering process

In the sintering process, a slurry of the ceramic powder is applied to a refractory die (as opposed to a Pt-foil-coated die in the case of the porcelain jacket crown), dried and subsequently fired in a porcelain furnace. Multiple layers can be built up to develop characterization. Great skill is required by the dental laboratory technician to get the best aesthetics and appropriate contour. Examples of commercial leucite-reinforced ceramics using the sintering processing route are Fortress (Mirage Dental Systems, Kansas City, USA) and Optec-HSP (Jeneric/Pentron Inc, Wallingford, USA).

Hot-pressing

In order to surmount the problems of the inherent inaccuracies of fit of the sintered ceramics, which are due to the high firing shrinkage, attention has recently been paid to the possibility of using glass ceramics, which employ a casting process for the manufacture of crowns, veneers and inlays. Hot-pressing is one such approach and is a technique that involves the heating up an ingot of the ceramic. The ingot is a solid block of the material, which is made of a leucite-reinforced feldspar, as is the case with Empress I (Ivoclar-Vivadent, Schaan, Liechtenstein). This method utilizes parts of the lost wax casting technique. As in lost wax casting, a wax pattern is produced, which is then invested in a refractory die material. The wax is burnt out to create the space to be filled by the leucite-reinforced glass–ceramic. A specially designed pressing furnace is then used to fill the mould space from a pellet of the glass–ceramic using a viscous flow process at a temperature of 1180°C (Figure 3.7.1). When the ingot is heated to a sufficiently high temperature, it will become a softened mass such that under pressure it will flow into a refractory mould. This process is also often described as transfer moulding. It is distinctly different from the sintering technique since it does not rely on the fusion of powder particles.

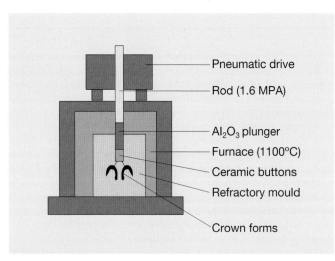

Figure 3.7.1 Schematic of the hot-pressing route for producing a leucite-reinforced glass–ceramic restoration

- Pneumatic drive
- Rod (1.6 MPA)
- Al$_2$O$_3$ plunger
- Furnace (1100°C)
- Ceramic buttons
- Refractory mould
- Crown forms

The final shading may be done by applying surface stains. For anterior restorations, the veneer is cut back and a powdered form of the leucite-reinforced glass–ceramic is bonded using the conventional sintering technique.

CAD–CAM

Since the feldspathic glasses and the leucite-containing feldspathic glasses can be prefabricated into blocks, the veneers can also be constructed using CAD–CAM technology. This can be done at the chair side with the CEREC system from Sirona using Vitablocks (Vita Zahnfabrik, Germany) or Procad (Ivoclar-Vivadent, Liechtenstein). The dental laboratory also has CAD–CAM technology for the construction of veneers, inlays and crowns.

PROPERTIES

The aesthetic results with the feldspathic glasses and the leucite-containing feldspathic glasses are excellent due to their high translucency, fluorescence and opalescence. When used in combination with resin bonding to enamel and dentine, these materials are very good for veneers and inlays and are also used for anterior crowns. However, the mechanical strength is insufficient for this class of ceramic to be used in the construction of posterior crowns and all-ceramic bridges.

Due to these limitations and a desire to produce ceramics suitable for use in the posterior part of the mouth, linked to a wish to extend their use to the construction of small three-unit bridges, there has been a major drive to develop new ceramics suitable for use as resin-bonded all-ceramic restorations. The focus of this development has been a class of materials known as glass–ceramics.

GLASS–CERAMICS

The majority of materials available for resin-bonded ceramic restorations are, in essence, varieties of a special group of ceramics known as glass–ceramics. The various dental glass–ceramics that have been developed for resin-bonded ceramic restorations will be described, along with some of the new processing techniques that have evolved at the same time.

Glass–ceramics were first developed by Corning Glass Works in the late 1950s. In principle, an article is formed while liquid, and a metastable glass results on cooling. During a subsequent heat treatment, controlled crystallization occurs, with the nucleation and growth of internal crystals. This conversion process from a glass to a partially crystalline glass is called *ceraming*. Thus, a glass ceramic is a multiphase solid containing a residual glass phase with a finely dispersed crystalline phase. The controlled crystallization of the glass results in the formation of tiny crystals that are evenly distributed throughout the glass. The number of crystals, their growth rate and thus their size are regulated by the time and temperature of the ceraming heat treatment.

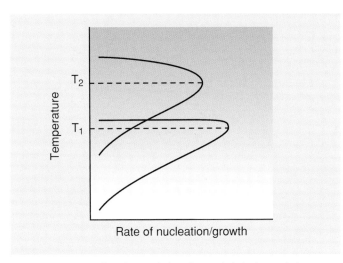

Figure 3.7.2 Rate of nucleation (T_1) and growth (T_2) of crystals in a glass–ceramic

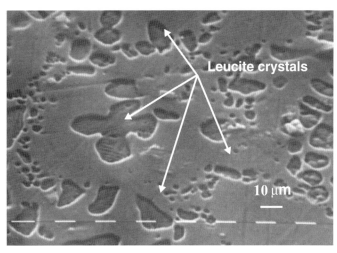

Figure 3.7.3 A scanning electron micrograph of the structure of a leucite-reinforced ceramic

There are two important aspects to the formation of the crystalline phase: crystal nucleation and crystal growth. The schematic in Figure 3.7.2 shows that the rate of crystal nucleation and the rate of crystal growth are at a maximum at different temperatures. The ceraming process consequently involves a two-stage heat treatment. The first heat treatment is carried out at the temperature for maximum nucleation of crystals, so as to maximize the number of crystals formed. The material temperature is then raised, after a suitable period of time, to the higher temperature to allow crystal growth. It is held at the higher temperature until the optimum crystal size is formed.

To ensure a high strength for the glass–ceramic, it is important that the crystals are numerous and are uniformly distributed throughout the glassy phase. The crystalline phase will grow during ceraming, and can eventually occupy from 50% to nearly 100% of the material.

Mechanical properties of glass–ceramics

The mechanical properties are believed to be greatly influenced by:

- particle size of the crystalline phase
- volume fraction of the crystalline phase
- interfacial bond strength between phases
- differences in elastic moduli
- differences in thermal expansion.

Fracture in brittle solids is nearly always initiated at a small internal or surface defect, such as a micro-crack, that acts as a stress raiser. If the crystalline phase is relatively strong, then the cracks will form in the glassy phase. The dimension of these micro-cracks can thus be limited to the distance between the crystalline particles. Therefore, the critical parameter is the mean free path, in the glassy phase, L_s, which is given by:

$$L_s = d(1 - V_f)/V_f$$

where d is the crystal diameter and V_f is the volume fraction of the crystalline phase.

Thus, the smaller the crystals and the larger the volume fraction of the crystals, the shorter the mean free path will be, and, consequently, the greater the strength of the material.

CLINICAL SIGNIFICANCE

A feature of glass–ceramics is that the size and the amount of the crystalline phase can be carefully controlled during the ceraming process.

Most glass–ceramics are opaque or cloudy and would not be suitable for dental use. The first glass–ceramic employed in dentistry was introduced by MacCulloch in 1968 for the construction of denture teeth, and was based on the $Li_2O \cdot ZnO \cdot SiO_2$ system. At the time, the use of acrylic denture teeth was becoming popular, and the idea of glass ceramics was not exploited further. Now we have a wide range of glass–ceramics and processing routes for the construction of resin-bonded ceramic restorations.

Leucite-reinforced feldspar glass–ceramics

The ceramic used in the original experiments of Horn was a leucite ($KAlSi_2O_6$)-containing feldspathic glass, which he used in the construction of metal–ceramic restorations (see Chapter 3.5). This ceramic was optimized with regard to being able to bond to the metal surface. The ceramics used now for resin-bonded ceramic restorations are a modified version of the ceramic used by Horn. They differ from the ceramic used in metal–ceramics primarily in that the composition and microstructure has been changed in order to produce the best leucite crystalline phase distribution from the point of view of strength, since compatibility with a metal framework is no longer a consideration.

Whereas the leucite-containing ceramic used in metal–ceramic restorations have a flexural strength of the order of 30–40 MPa, the leucite-reinforced glass–ceramics have flexural strengths of up to 120 MPa. A typical example of the structure of leucite-reinforced ceramic is shown in Figure 3.7.3. What is particularly noticeable is the uniform distribution of the leucite crystals and the lack of internal cracking that is so evident in the example of the leucite-containing feldspars used for veneering a metal framework (see Figure 3.5.5).

The construction of ceramic restorations using leucite-reinforced feldspars can be done either by sintering, using a modified version of the sintering process described earlier to construct the porcelain jacket crown, or by hot-pressing.

The mechanical properties of leucite feldspar glass–ceramics are considered to be sufficient for this material to be used for veneers, anterior crowns and posterior inlays. As yet, the use of this material for posterior crowns or any form of bridge is contraindicated, as the mechanical properties are too low to carry the loads involved.

Fluormica glass–ceramics

In order to be able to extend the possible use of resin-bonded ceramic restorations for posterior crowns, onlays and bridge construction, a glass–ceramic was developed that was based on the composition $SiO_2 \cdot K_2O \cdot MgO \cdot MgF_2 \cdot Al_2O_3 \cdot ZrO_2$. The addition of some fluorides imparts fluorescence in the prostheses in a way similar to that encountered in the natural dentition. These glass–ceramics are known as fluoromicas. For this composition, the ceraming process results in the nucleation and the growth of tetrasilicate mica crystals within the glass. The crystals are needle-like in shape and arrest the propagation of cracks through this material. Mechanical property measurements suggest that the flexural strength is in the region of 120–150 MPa, which, when combined with the adhesion to tooth tissues, may just be adequate for posterior crowns but is probably still insufficient for the construction of all-ceramic bridges.

The passage of light through the material is affected by the crystal size and the difference in the refractive indices of the glass phase and the crystalline phase. If the crystals are smaller than the wavelength of visible light (0.4–0.7 μm), the glass will appear transparent, such that the tendency for light to scatter is lower than for the aluminous porcelains.

CLINICAL SIGNIFICANCE

The refractive index of the small mica crystals is closely matched to that of the surrounding glass phase, which produces a translucency close to that of enamel.

The processing of this glass–ceramic involves the same principles as for the lost wax casting process of metallic restorations. The restoration is waxed up on a die, using conventional materials. The pattern is removed from the die and invested in a special phosphate-bonded investment. Then an ingot of the castable ceramic material is placed in a special crucible and centrifugally cast at a temperature of 1380°C. The casting then requires a further heat treatment to create the crystalline phase and develop the strength. The desired shade is achieved by firing self-glazing shading porcelains on the surface. The concept of producing ceramic restorations using a casting technique is by no means new, and was first attempted in the 1920s. It is only with the recent introduction of the castable glass–ceramics that this has become possible.

In recent years, the casting route (e.g. Dicor) has lost its popularity with laboratories and now the main application of fluormica glass–ceramics is in the CAD–CAM production of restorations (e.g. Macor).

Lithium disilicate and apatite glass–ceramics

Some versions of glass–ceramics have the strength and toughness to be considered suitable for the production of posterior crowns and possibly even short-span bridges. However, these materials do not have the necessary aesthetics to allow the production of the restoration as a single unit. The option then is to produce a high-strength core material and veneer it with an aesthetic ceramic. The difference with the high-strength ceramic-core systems discussed in the previous chapter is that these core materials are still based on silica glass and therefore can be bonded to the tooth structure using a combination

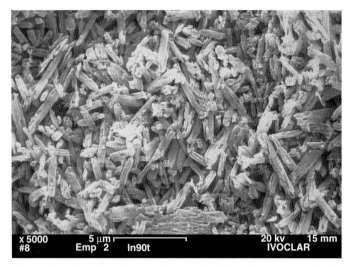

Figure 3.7.4 Scanning electron micrograph of the microstructure of a lithium disilicate glass–ceramic, showing the interlocking needle-like crystals (courtesy of Ivoclar-Vivadent UK Ltd, Leicester, UK)

of silane coupling agents and resins. One such system is a glass–ceramic based on an $SiO_2–Li_2O$, that has been developed recently (Empress II, Ivoclar-Vivadent, Schaan, Liechtenstein).

The crystalline phase that forms is a lithium disilicate ($Li_2Si_2O_5$) and makes up some 70% of the volume of the glass–ceramic. Lithium disilicate has an unusual microstructure in that it consists of many small, interlocking, plate-like crystals that are randomly oriented (Figure 3.7.4). This is ideal from the point of view of strength because the needle-like crystals cause cracks to deflect, branch or blunt. Thus, the propagation of cracks through this material is arrested by the lithium disilicate crystals, providing a substantial increase in the flexural strength.

A second crystalline phase, consisting of a lithium orthophosphate (Li_3PO_4) of a much lower volume, is also present.

The mechanical properties of this glass–ceramic are far superior to those of the leucite feldspar glass–ceramic, with a flexural strength in the region of 350–450 MPa and a fracture toughness approximately three times that of the leucite feldspar glass–ceramic.

CLINICAL SIGNIFICANCE

The high strength of lithium disilicate glass–ceramics creates the possibility of producing not only anterior and posterior crowns, but also all-ceramic bridges.

The glass–ceramic is claimed to be highly translucent due to the optical compatibility between the glassy matrix and crystalline phase, which minimizes the internal scattering of the light as it passes through the material. The processing route is the same as the hot-pressing route described earlier, except that the processing temperature, at 920°C, is lower than for the leucite glass–ceramic.

For the alumina-based core systems described earlier, it is possible to use feldspathic glasses to provide the aesthetic surface layer, as their coefficients of thermal expansion are closely matched at ~7–8 ppm/°C. For the leucite glass–ceramics, the layering ceramic is identical to the core ceramic and so a mismatch in coefficient of expansion does not arise. However, for the lithium disilicate glass–ceramic, the coefficient of expansion is greater than 10 ppm/°C and, consequently, a new compatible layering ceramic had to be developed. This new layering ceramic is an apatite glass–ceramic. The crystalline phase formed on ceraming is a hydroxyapatite [$Ca_{10}(PO_4)_6(OH)_2$], which is the same

Table 3.7.1 The relative merits of a number of ceramic crown systems

System	Aesthetics			Relative cost			Popularity			Strength		
	High	Medium	Low	High	Medium	Low	High	Medium	Low	High	Medium	Low
High-strength ceramic cores												
Alumina reinforced core		√		√			√					√
Glass-infiltrated alumina core		√		√				√		√		
Pure alumina core	√				√			√		√		
Resin-bonded ceramics												
Refractory die	√					√	√				√	
Casting system		√			√				√		√	
Hot-pressed leucite reinforced		√			√		√				√	
Hot-pressed lithium disilicate reinforced	√				√				√	√		

basic constituent from which enamel is made. Thus, it represents a material that, at least in composition, is the closest match to enamel that has been achieved so far.

CLASSIFICATION OF RESIN-BONDED CERAMICS

- Feldspathic glasses
  - Sintered: e.g. Vitadur
  - CAD–CAM: e.g. Vita Blocks
- Leucite-reinforced glass–ceramics
  - Sintered: e.g. Mirage, Fortress, Optec-HP
  - Hot-pressed: e.g. Empress I
  - CAD–CAM: e.g. Procad
- Fluormica glass–ceramics
  - Cast: e.g. Dicor
  - CAD–CAM: e.g. Macor
- Lithium disilicate glass–ceramics
  - Hot-pressing: e.g. Empress II
  - CAD–CAM: e.g. IPS Emax CAD.

SUMMARY

There has been a revolution in the provision of ceramics for dental restorations in the last 20 years, such that all-ceramic restorations can now be used both anteriorly and posteriorly. New materials have come along that have allowed the extension of the use of resin-bonded ceramic restorations from veneers to anterior and posterior crowns and inlays. It is even possible to consider the limited use of all-ceramic bridges. There is no doubt that new materials and processing routes will continue to be developed and that ceramics will play a growing role in the provision of aesthetic restorations. Deciding between different ceramic systems will be a difficult task; the relative merits that might be considered in the selection process are summarized in Table 3.7.1.

CLINICAL SIGNIFICANCE

There will be a growing need for dental practitioners to be aware of the rapidly changing field of dental ceramics so as to ensure that the correct choice is made for each patient.

FURTHER READING

Banks RG (1990) Conservative posterior ceramic restorations: a review of the literature. J Prosthet Dent 63: 619

Brodsky LJ (1933) Practical hints: porcelain inlays simplified. Dental Cosmos 95: 1024

Calamia JR (1983) Etched porcelain facial veneers: a new treatment modality based on scientific and clinical evidence. NY J Dent 53: 255–259

Cattell MJ, Chadwick TC, Knowles JC (2001) Flexural strength optimisation of a leucite reinforced glass ceramic. Dent Mater 17: 21

Chadwick B (2004) Good short-term survival of IPS-Empress crowns. Evid Based Dent 5: 73

Christensen G (1985) Veneering of teeth. Dent Clin N Am 29: 373

Clyde G (1988) Porcelain veneers: a preliminary review. Brit Dent J 164: 9

Duret F, Blouin J-L, Duret B (1988) CAD–CAM in dentistry. J Am Dent Assoc 117: 715

Grossman DG (1985) Cast glass ceramics. Dent Clin N Am 29: 725

Horn H (1983) Porcelain laminate veneers bonded to etched enamel. Dent Clin N Am 27: 671

MacCulloch (1968) Advances in dental ceramics. Brit Dent J 142: 361

Mörmann WH, Bindl A (1997) The new creativity in ceramic restorations: dental CAD–CAM. Quintessence Int 27: 821

Peumans M, Van Meerbeek B, Lambrechts P (2000) Porcelain veneers: a review of the literature. J Dent 28: 163

Pincus CR (1938) Building mouth personality. J Calif Dent Assoc 14: 125–129

Qualtrough AJE, Piddock V (1999) Recent advances in ceramic materials and systems for dental restorations. Dental Update 26: 65

Ritter A, Baratieri LN (1999) Ceramic restorations for posterior teeth: Guidelines for the clinician. J Esthet Dent 11: 72

Rochette AL (1975) A ceramic restoration bonded by etched enamel and resin to fractured incisors. J Prosthet Dent 33: 287

Toh CG, Setcos JC, Weinstein AR (1987) Indirect laminate veneers: an overview. J Dent 15: 117

Chapter |3.8|

Luting agents

INTRODUCTION

For the greater part of the 20th century, the only materials available for the retention and marginal seal of fixed prostheses such as veneers, inlays, crowns and bridges, were zinc oxide–eugenol and zinc–phosphate cements. Hence, the term cementation represented an appropriate description of the process of fixing a metallic or ceramic restoration to the teeth. However, in the last quarter of the 20th century, things began to change with the introduction of many more adhesive materials and procedures. A wide variety of new cements have become available, such as zinc–polycarboxylate cements, glass–ionomer cements (GICs) and resin-modified glass–ionomer cements (RMGICs). There is now also a growing market for resin adhesive technologies.

In this context, the term 'cementation' hardly does justice to the range of materials now in use. Another term for the process of fixing a restoration in place is luting. The word 'lute' means a cement or other material used as a protective covering or an airtight stopping. As this term is not specific to a cement, the term luting agent perhaps provides a more appropriate description of some of the materials that are used today, such as the resins.

Whatever the relative merits of the terminology used, this chapter is concerned with the materials used for the permanent retention of posts and indirect restorations, as outlined in Table 3.8.1.

GENERAL REQUIREMENTS FOR LUTING AGENTS

Biocompatibility

When luting agents are used in such situations as crowns and inlays, the material will inevitably be in contact with a relatively vast surface area of dentine. Hence, their susceptibility to producing postoperative sensitivity or pulpal inflammation is a very important consideration. Luting agents will also provide the main barrier to the ingress of bacteria, such that, besides a good marginal seal, possible antibacterial properties may prove to be highly beneficial.

Retention

The primary role of the luting agent is to provide retention of the restoration. With the water-based cements, such as zinc–phosphate cement, retention is governed by the geometry of the tooth preparation, the control of the path of insertion and the ability to provide mechanical keying into surface irregularities. This is not always ideal and lack of retention is a major cause of failure with fixed prostheses. If, in addition, an adhesive bond can be created, this can enhance the retention significantly and resin adhesive technologies have made this possible.

Mechanical properties

It is important that the thin layer of luting agent produced between the tooth and the restoration is able to withstand the large forces that are potentially transmitted through it. In order to resist fracture, a high tensile strength, fracture toughness and fatigue strength are very beneficial in this respect. The situation can be enhanced significantly by ensuring that the restoration produces a good marginal fit, such that a minimal amount of the luting agent is required.

Although only a small amount of the luting agent is exposed at the surface, it is important that the material is able to resist wear. Excessive wear can lead to sub-margination, which, in effect, means that a small groove is formed. Such a groove can become a site for marginal staining and plaque accumulation.

Marginal seal

The luting agent must also provide a good marginal seal in order to prevent recurrent caries. An ideal luting agent should not be susceptible to dissolution in the oral environment so as to maintain the marginal seal. A low solubility in neutral and acid environments is, therefore, important. If the luting agent is able to provide an adhesive bond to the tooth tissues and the restoration, then this will also help to maintain the integrity of the marginal seal. Recent developments in cementation have sought to achieve exactly that but, with the wide variety of materials to be bonded (enamel, dentine, metal, ceramic), a correspondingly wide variety of adhesion promoters have also become available.

Table 3.8.1 Range of procedures and luting agents provided for the cementation of indirect restorations

Restoration type	Procedure	Luting agents
Metal crowns, bridges, onlays and inlays	Conventional cementation	Zinc–phosphate cements
		Zinc–polycarboxylate cements
Metal–ceramic crowns and bridges		Glass–ionomer cements
		Resin-modified glass–ionomer cements
Metal and ceramic endodontic posts		Compomers
Base metal alloy restorations	Etching	Dark-cure luting resins
	Grit blasting	Adhesive resins
Precious metal alloy crowns and bridges	Tin plating	Dark-cure luting resins
	Silica coating	Adhesive resins
	Metal primers	
Porcelain jacket crown and other reinforced core all-ceramic systems	Conventional cementation	Zinc–phosphate cements
		Zinc–polycarboxylate cements
		Glass–ionomer cements
Resin-bonded ceramic veneers, inlays and crowns	Hydrofluoric acid etch + silane coupling agents	Aesthetic dual-cure luting resins
Composite inlays	Resin-to-resin bonding	Aesthetic dual-cure luting resins
Fibre-reinforced resin bridges		Dark-cure luting resins
Fibre-reinforced resin endodontic posts		

Low film thickness

The film thickness is important because a luting agent needs to be sufficiently thin both to fill the space between the crown or bridge and the tooth, and to ensure proper seating of the restoration. A thick film would be unacceptable, as the restoration may end up higher than was originally intended, causing occlusal problems and a need for it to be ground down. Also, a poor marginal fit would result in more cement being exposed at the surface than necessary. As some luting agents are soluble in the oral environment and prone to erosion, this will cause the loss of material at the margin, which can lead to plaque accumulation, staining and recurrent caries.

Ease of use

Many of the luting agents are provided as powder–liquid delivery systems and, as long as great care is exercised to make sure that the correct powder-to-liquid ratio is used on mixing, this should not present a problem. However, there is a tendency to produce a slightly more fluid mix to give rheological properties that allow the luting agent to flow more readily into the space between the tooth and the restoration and produce a very close adaptation. For some materials, changing the powder-to-liquid ratio can have a profound effect on its properties, especially working and setting times, and is therefore not generally recommended.

The working and setting times need to be such that sufficient time is allowed to place the restoration and yet it does not take too long to set once placed. The best way to ensure the correct powder-to-liquid ratio is to follow the instructions for use carefully or to avoid the whole issue by using encapsulated delivery systems.

Radiopacity

It is important for the practitioner to be able to distinguish between a luting agent and recurrent caries under a fixed prosthesis. In order to avoid possible misinterpretation, it is beneficial if the luting agent is more radiopaque than dentine. It also makes it easier to detect possible excess luting agent and marginal overhangs, especially in those difficult-to-see proximal areas.

Aesthetics

Although not a major consideration with metal and metal–ceramic restorations, aesthetics becomes very important when using all-ceramic restoration. For some of the core-reinforced ceramics, a luting agent that has a white/opaque appearance is acceptable, but as the ceramic restoration becomes more translucent, the optical properties become more important. This has meant that, for the highly translucent resin-bonded ceramics, such as those used in the construction of anterior veneers, new luting agents with comparable colour and colour stability, translucency and surface texture have had to be developed.

CLINICAL SIGNIFICANCE

No one material is capable of meeting all the stringent requirements for a luting agent, which is one reason why there is such a wide choice.

CHOICE OF LUTING AGENT

The oldest luting agent listed in Table 3.8.1 is zinc–phosphate cement, which provides nothing more than a space filler, sometimes referred to as a grout between the restoration and the tooth. Retention depends primarily on the careful design of the tooth preparation and the quality of fit of the restoration, as the cement has no bonding affinity for tooth tissue, metal or ceramic. The newer polyacrylic acid-based cements, such as zinc–polycarboxylate cement and GICs, go a stage further in being able to bond to enamel and dentine and also are claimed to have some affinity for metal and ceramic surfaces. The range of these tooth-adhesive cements has been extended to include the RMGICs. Although these water-based cements have some ability to bond to metals, in general it can be said that these materials do not provide an adequate bond to metal or ceramic restorations for some of the more demanding situations encountered. Hence, new ceramic and metal adhesives would need to be developed for it to impact on prosthetic dentistry to the same degree as new adhesive procedures and materials have changed operative dentistry. It is the advent of resin-bonding technology that most probably has had the biggest impact on the procedures used to retain indirect restorations.

In order to manage this wide diversity of water-based and resin luting agents and associated clinical procedures, for simplicity they will be considered under two categories, namely:

- water-based luting cements
- resin-based luting cements

WATER-BASED LUTING CEMENTS

The water-based cements include zinc–phosphate cement, zinc–polycarboxylate cement, GIC and RMGIC.

Zinc–phosphate cements

Zinc–phosphate cement is one of the oldest cements available and continues to be popular because of its long history of clinical success and favourable handling properties. These cements present as a white powder that is mixed with a clear liquid. The powder consists of mainly zinc oxide, with up to 10% magnesium oxide included, and the liquid is an aqueous solution of phosphoric acid of 45–64% concentration.

Presentation

Powder

The powder is fired at a temperature in excess of 1000 °C for several hours in order to reduce its reactivity and provide a suitable working and setting time for the cements; the material would set far too rapidly without this firing process.

The magnesium oxide is added, as it helps maintain the white colour of the cement. It has the additional advantages of making the pulverization process of the zinc oxide somewhat easier, and also increases the compressive strength of the cement. Other oxides (such as silica and alumina) have been added in small quantities of up to 5% to improve the mechanical properties of the set material and to provide a variety of shades.

Some formulations include fluorides (usually in the form of a few per cent of stannous fluoride), and are generally recommended for situations where fluoride release is going to be particularly beneficial, such as for the cementation of orthodontic bands.

Liquid

The liquid is buffered with a combination of the oxides that are present in the powder and with aluminium hydroxide, which acts to form phosphates in the liquid. The aluminium is essential to the cement-forming reaction, producing an amorphous zinc–phosphate, while the zinc helps to moderate the reaction, making sure that the cement has the appropriate working time. This control over the working time also helps to ensure that an adequate amount of the powder is incorporated into the liquid.

Setting reaction

When zinc oxide is mixed with an aqueous solution of phosphoric acid, the superficial layer of the zinc oxide is dissolved by the acid. In the case of pure zinc oxide mixed with phosphoric acid, the acid–base reaction first involves the formation of an acid zinc–phosphate:

$$ZnO + 2H_3PO_4 \rightarrow Zn(H_2PO_4)_2 + H_2O$$

This is followed by a further reaction, where, in this second phase of the process, a hydrated zinc–phosphate is produced:

$$ZnO + Zn(H_2PO_4)_2 + 2H_2O$$
$$\rightarrow Zn_3(PO_4)_2 \cdot 4H_2O \text{ (hopeite)}$$

This substance is virtually insoluble, and crystallizes to form a phosphate matrix, which binds together the unreacted parts of the zinc oxide particles. The reaction is slightly exothermic and some shrinkage of the cement takes place.

It is thought that, in the commercial materials, the presence of the aluminium prevents the crystallization process, so producing a glassy matrix in the form of an alumino-phosphate gel. This lack of crystallization is exacerbated by the presence of magnesium, which delays the development of any crystallinity. Some crystallization, resulting in the formation of hopeite, may occur with time.

Unbound water forms globules within the material and makes the cement highly permeable, resulting in a porous structure when the material is dry. The final structure is that of particles of unreacted zinc oxide in a matrix consisting of phosphates of zinc, magnesium and aluminium.

Properties

As a general observation, it is worth noting that zinc–phosphate cements have been around for some considerable time and have provided excellent clinical service. This may be related to the general ease with which the material can be used, as well as the wide range of applications available. They have a well-defined working time and a rapid setting time.

Working and setting times

The working time for most brands of zinc–phosphate cement, when used with the consistency of a luting agent, is usually within the region of 3–6 minutes. The corresponding setting time can vary from 5 to 14 minutes. Both of these times depend on the mixing procedure adopted.

Depending on the application, the material is mixed to either a thick consistency for cavity bases or a thinner consistency when used as a luting agent. The mixing process is carried out by the slow incorporation of the powder into the liquid. The recommended procedure is that, initially, only small increments are added to the powder, followed by a couple of larger increments. Finally, smaller increments are again added, as this will ensure that the desired consistency is not exceeded.

Extended working and setting times can be achieved by mixing the powder into the liquid in increments over a large area of the mixing slab. This helps to dissipate the heat of reaction that would otherwise speed up the setting process. Conversely, the rapid mixing of powder into the liquid will shorten both the working and setting times. This will have the result that a thick mix is obtained, with a low powder-to-liquid ratio, because of the early initiation of the setting process. The low powder content will mean that an inferior material is obtained.

By using a cooled glass slab for the mixing procedure, it is possible to extend the working time without simultaneously increasing the setting time. This also has the benefit of allowing more powder to be added to the liquid, so raising the strength and reducing the solubility. However, great care must be exercised when using this technique, as there is a danger of water contamination either from the slab not having been dried properly or due to condensation. Both will have the effect of reducing the working time. The combination of the cool glass and the incremental process ensures that an adequate working time is maintained. The mixing procedure should be completed within about 60–90 seconds.

The setting time can be extended by a process known as *slaking the fluid*, in which a small quantity of the powder is added to the liquid about a minute before the main mixing procedure is started.

The consistency of the paste depends on the powder-to-liquid ratio, and it is important that the correct powder-to-liquid ratio is used for the particular application.

For instance, too low a powder-to-liquid ratio would produce a weak and highly soluble material with an unacceptably low pH. Whilst the manufacturers suggest optimum powder-to-liquid ratios for their products, these are difficult to adhere to in practice since the dispensing system is not very accurate. Consequently, most dentists prefer to mix sufficient powder into the liquid until a consistency is obtained which is suitable for the particular application. This makes it all the more important that a consistent and reproducible procedure is adopted.

The liquid is kept in a stoppered bottle. If the top is kept off the bottle, the loss of water by evaporation will lower the pH of the liquid as it becomes more concentrated; this will slow down the setting process. If a lot of water is lost, the phosphoric acid will begin to separate out and the liquid will take on a cloudy appearance. Should this occur, the liquid must be discarded.

When the cement is used as a luting agent, it is important that the powder and liquid are not dispensed until just prior to when they are needed, as evaporation of the water may occur and will slow down the setting reaction. Neither should the material be left for any length of time once mixed because the setting reaction takes place virtually immediately on mixing. If the paste is left for too long, the viscosity will have increased to such an extent that the material will no longer have adequate flow characteristics.

Biocompatibility

A freshly mixed zinc–phosphate cement will have a pH in the region of 1.3–3.6. This low value tends to persist for some considerable time, and it can take up to 24 hours for the cement to return to a near-neutral pH.

When placed over a heavily prepared tooth, the initial pH is sufficiently low to induce an inflammatory response in the pulp. This is especially so if a pulpal micro-exposure is suspected. It is important to remember that the thinner the mix, the lower the pH will be, and the longer it will take for the cement to return to a neutral pH.

Zinc–phosphate cement has no anti-bacterial properties and this, combined with the slight shrinkage on setting, means that it does not provide an ideal barrier to the ingress of bacteria. Thus, the pulpal sensitivity associated with the material may be due to a combination of shrinkage, a lack of anti-bacterial behaviour and the high acidity when freshly mixed, rather than just the high acidity as is generally thought.

The patient may experience some pain during a cementation procedure. This can arise as a result of both the low pH of the cement and the osmotic pressure developed by the movement of fluid through the dentinal tubules. Such an experience is usually only transient and should subside within a few hours. If there is a persistent pulpal irritation, it may have been caused by using too thin a mix of the cement.

The hardening process for a zinc–phosphate cement takes a considerable time, and during the first 24 hours there is a significant release of magnesium with lower amounts of zinc. What biological effects the presence of these various ions might have on the surrounding tissues is not known.

Mechanical properties

As with all other properties, the mechanical properties are very much dependent on the powder-to-liquid ratio of the final cement. The compressive strength can vary from as low as 40 MPa up to 140 MPa. The relationship between the powder-to-liquid ratio and the compressive strength is virtually linear.

The cement shows an initially rapid rise in strength, reaching 50% of its final strength within the first 10 minutes. Thereafter, the strength increases more slowly, reaching its final strength after approximately 24 hours. The cement is extremely brittle, and this is reflected by its very low tensile strength, which is of the order of 5–7 MPa. The modulus of elasticity is approximately 12 GPa, which is similar to that of dentine.

Consistency and film thickness

To ensure the proper seating of the restoration when zinc–phosphate cement is being used as a luting agent, it is important that the cement is capable of forming a very thin film.

On mixing, the powder is partially dissolved in the acid, such that the final size of the remaining powder in the set structure ranges from 2 to 8 µm. As the mix flows readily, a film thickness of less than 25 µm can be achieved. This is adequate for cementation purposes, but the thickness of the layer is very much dependent on the procedure adopted.

The viscosity of the mix increases quite rapidly with time. Within a couple of minutes, the viscosity can already be quite high, although the material itself is still quite manageable. Nevertheless, it is recommended that no undue delay is allowed to occur when cementing a restoration, as the reduced viscosity can result in a significantly higher film thickness for the cement and thus a poorly seated restoration.

Solubility

The solubility of a cement is an important consideration, particularly when it is being used as a luting agent. Dissolution contributes to marginal leakage around the restoration and results in bacterial penetration. This may cause either loosening of the restoration or, what is more likely, the induction of recurrent caries, which may undermine the whole tooth.

The cement is highly soluble in water for the first 24 hours after setting, and the loss of material can range from 0.04 to 3.3%; an acceptable upper limit is 0.2%. After this time, the solubility is much reduced. The solubility is highly dependent on the powder-to-liquid ratio achieved for the cement, with a high ratio being desirable. Once the material has fully set, it remains only slightly soluble in water (with some release of zinc and phosphates), but is still susceptible to acid attack. As the final set takes some time to achieve, it is important that the cement is not unduly exposed to the oral fluids.

The fluoride-containing cements show a continuous release of fluoride over a long period. The fluoride uptake by the surrounding enamel should reduce the likelihood of decalcification, especially when used for the cementation of orthodontic bands.

Applications

The most common application for zinc–phosphate cements is as luting agents for the cementation of metal and metal–ceramic crowns and bridges, although it is also used in other applications such as the cementation of orthodontic bands and as a temporary restoration.

These cements exhibit several advantages in that they:

- are easy to mix
- have a sharp, well-defined set
- have a sufficiently high compressive strength to resist the forces of amalgam condensation
- are a low-cost product.

The easy handling characteristics and their adequate retentive properties have made zinc–phosphate cements highly popular with dental practitioners for over a century.

However, the disadvantages are that they:

- have a potential for pulpal irritation due to low pH
- have no anti-bacterial action
- are brittle
- have no adhesive qualities
- are relatively soluble in the oral environment.

These factors contribute to the incidence of recurrent caries associated with cast restorations.

CLINICAL SIGNIFICANCE

Zinc–phosphate cements have been around for over 100 years and, despite their limitations, will continue to be used for the cementation of metal and metal–ceramic restorations for many years to come.

Zinc–polycarboxylate cements

The zinc–polycarboxylate cements were first introduced to dentistry in 1968 when a Manchester dentist had the bright idea of replacing phosphoric acid with one of the new polymeric acids: namely, polyacrylic acid. These materials rapidly became popular with the dental profession, as they provided the first cement that was able to bond to enamel and dentine. The bonding mechanism is the same as that described for the GICs (see Chapter 2.5).

Presentation

These cements come as a white powder and a clear, viscous liquid. The constituents of the powder are zinc oxide and magnesium oxide, and the liquid is a 30–40% aqueous solution of polyacrylic acid.

Powder

The powder is based on the same formulation used for the zinc–phosphate cements, containing zinc oxide with approximately 10% magnesium oxide or, sometimes, tin oxide. In addition, there may be other additives such as silica, alumina or bismuth salts. The powder is fired at a high temperature to control the rate of reaction and is then ground to the appropriate particle size. Some brands also contain stannous fluoride to impart the benefits of fluoride release. Pigments may be present to provide a variety of shades.

Liquid

The liquid is usually a copolymer of polyacrylic acid with other unsaturated carboxylic acids, such as itaconic and maleic acid. (The structures of polyacrylic acid and itaconic acid were presented in Chapter 2.3.) The molecular weight of the copolymer is in the range of 30 000–50 000.

In more recent formulations, the acid is freeze-dried and then added to the powder, in which case the liquid component is distilled water. This method was developed in order to simplify the achievement of the correct ratio between the components, which was difficult beforehand because of the high viscosity of the liquid. The pH is adjusted by the addition of sodium hydroxide, and tartaric acid is added to control the setting reaction.

Setting reaction

The basic setting reaction of these cements involves a reaction between the zinc oxide and the ionized copolymer of acrylic acid and itaconic acid.

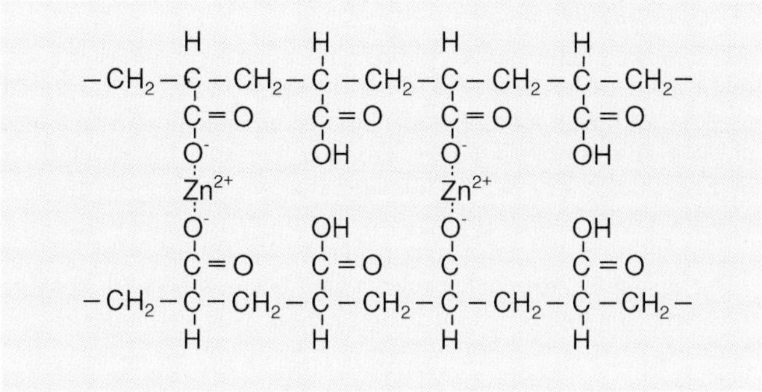

Figure 3.8.1 Zinc ions providing the cross-links between the carboxyl groups on the polyacrylic acid polymer chains

On mixing the powder and the liquid, the acid attacks the powder and causes a release of zinc ions. This is followed by the formation of cross-links (in the form of salt bridges), in the same way as occurs for the GICs, except that, in this case, the zinc provides the cross-links rather than calcium and aluminium, as shown in Figure 3.8.1.

The result of the reaction is a cored structure in which the unreacted powder particles are bound by a matrix of zinc–polyacrylate.

Properties

Working and setting times

When compared to the zinc–phosphate cements, the setting reaction proceeds rapidly; mixing should be completed within 30–40 seconds to ensure an adequate working time.

The viscosity of these cements does not rise as rapidly as for the zinc–phosphate cements. This has the effect that, after a couple of minutes, the viscosity of the zinc–polycarboxylate cement is less than that of the zinc–phosphate cement, even though the viscosity of the zinc–polycarboxylate cement was initially higher. In addition, the freshly mixed zinc–polycarboxylate cement has the property of being pseudoplastic, and shows shear thinning on mixing. This means that, although the material may appear to be too thick to flow properly whilst it is being placed, the pressure that is exerted makes it flow quite satisfactorily.

This property is not always appreciated by the dentist, who will be inclined to produce a thinner mix by reducing the powder-to-liquid ratio under the misapprehension that this will make the cement flow more readily. However, in doing so, the properties of the cement are considerably impaired.

In general, the higher the powder-to-liquid ratio or the higher the molecular weight of the copolymer, the shorter the working time will be. The recommended powder-to-liquid ratio for luting purposes is 1.5 : 1 by weight, which will give a working time at room temperature of 2.5–3.5 minutes and a setting time at 37°C of 6–9 minutes.

As with the zinc–phosphate cements, the working time can be extended by using a cooled glass slab or by refrigerating the powder. It is not recommended to refrigerate those liquids that still include the polyacrylic acid, as this leads to gelation of the polymer due to the hydrogen bonding.

The ability to extend the working time is particularly useful for mixes that have a higher powder-to-liquid ratio when they are being used as cavity bases. Nevertheless, the short working times of the zinc–polycarboxylate cements have been recognized as a potential problem.

This has been overcome with more recent formulations by optimizing the amount of tartaric acid in the material. Tartaric acid has the beneficial property of extending the working time without markedly affecting the setting time of the cement.

Biocompatibility

The presence of zinc–polycarboxylate in contact with either the soft or the hard tissues has been found to result in only a very mild response. Although it has a moderately low pH initially (in the range of 3.0–4.0), this does not appear to have the same adverse effect as the zinc–phosphate cements. It is suggested that this may be due to a combination of a rapid rise to neutrality of the pH on setting and a limited ability of the polyacid to penetrate the dentine.

The zinc–polycarboxylate cements have been found to have some anti-bacterial properties, which means that a better barrier to the ingress of bacteria is provided than by zinc–phosphate cements; this resistance to the penetration of bacteria is augmented by its adhesive quality.

It is probably these factors that are responsible for the lack of pulpal response, rather than the higher pH and the high molecular weight of the acid compared to the zinc–phosphate cements, although these latter factors *will* contribute to the blandness of the material.

Stannous fluoride is frequently incorporated into the cements, and this does not appear to affect the biological response. The fluoride release appears to be sufficient to have a genuinely beneficial effect on the neighbouring enamel and dentine.

Mechanical properties

When the cement is prepared to a consistency suitable for luting purposes, the compressive strength of the fully set cement is in the region of 55–85 MPa. This strength depends on the powder-to-liquid ratio achieved, and is somewhat lower than that of the zinc–phosphate cements.

The tensile strength is higher, however, being in the range of 8–12 MPa. The elastic modulus is around 4–6 GPa, which is about half that of the zinc–phosphate cement.

As already mentioned, the zinc–polycarboxylate cements set quite quickly, and this is reflected in the time it takes to reach its full strength; the cement will reach 80% of its final strength within 1 hour. Long-term storage in water does not appear to have an adverse effect on the mechanical properties.

Solubility

The solubility in water has been measured to be from 0.1 to 0.6% by weight, with higher values for solubility seeming to occur with the cements containing stannous fluoride.

As with the zinc–phosphate cements, these cements are susceptible to acid attack but, as yet, this does not appear to be sufficiently serious to be of any clinical significance, as indicated by the good clinical results obtained when using this cement. When failure has occurred, this is more often than not due to the improper handling of the material. This is usually related to the use of a powder-to-liquid ratio that is too low, possibly in an attempt to extend the working time.

Adhesion

A feature of the zinc–polycarboxylate cements that sets them apart from the zinc–phosphate and zinc oxide–eugenol cements is their ability to adhere to enamel and dentine.

The bonding mechanism is the same as that of the GICs, and has already been described in Chapter 2.3. The quality of the bond is such that it is maintained in vivo and can be good enough to exceed the cohesive strength of the cement. That being the case, the bond strength is, in fact, limited by the poor tensile strength of the cement, and is thus not likely to exceed 7–8 MPa.

Bonding to some metallic surfaces is possible with the zinc–polycarboxylate cements, and this can be very beneficial when it is used as a luting agent with cast restorations. This again involves specific ions binding to the metallic surface.

Bonding to gold alloys is not good, usually resulting in an adhesive failure of the interface due to the highly inert nature of the gold alloy's surface. This can be improved by sand-blasting or abrading the surface, thus providing some mechanical adhesion, but the benefit is very minimal.

Superior bond strengths are obtained with the base metal alloys (giving rise to cohesive rather than adhesive failures on testing the bond strength), and this is probably related to the presence of an oxide layer that provides the necessary metallic ions. Bond strengths are not especially high because of the low cohesive strength of the zinc–polycarboxylate cements.

Applications

The zinc–polycarboxylate cements can be used for the cementation of metal- or core-reinforced ceramic crowns etc., and have also been used for the cementation of orthodontic bands.

They have the following advantages:

1. They bond to enamel and dentine, as well as some of the metallic cast restorations.
2. They have a low irritancy.
3. Their strength, solubility and film thicknesses are comparable to that of zinc–phosphate cement.
4. They have an antibacterial action.

The disadvantages are that:

1. Their properties are highly dependent on handling procedures.
2. They have short working times and long setting times.
3. An exacting technique is required to ensure bonding.
4. Clean-up is difficult and timing is critical.

If removal of excess material is attempted too soon and the material is still in its rubbery state, the marginal seal may be compromised, while leaving it too long makes it difficult to remove due to the excellent bond to the tooth.

Although the potential advantage of fluoride release provided this cement with some popularity, the current use of zinc–polycarboxylate cements seems to be very limited and many dental practitioners prefer to use either zinc–phosphate or GICs. The perception amongst practitioners is that there is little to choose between the zinc–polycarboxylate and the GICs and this is supported by laboratory data on these products. If anything, the GICs described below are considered to be somewhat easier to use.

CLINICAL SIGNIFICANCE

Zinc–polycarboxylate cements are a viable alternative to the zinc–phosphate cements, with the added benefit of adhesion to enamel and dentine. Nevertheless, these cements appear not to be as popular as the other water-based cements.

Glass–ionomer cements and resin-modified glass–ionomer luting cements

Although many of the properties of glass–ionomer luting cements, such as fluoride release and adhesion to enamel and dentine, are the same as for the filling material described in detail in Chapter 2.3, some requirements are different. For example, since the space between the restoration and the tooth tissues is only of the order of 20–50 μm, it is important that the luting cement has a very thin film thickness. For this reason, the glass powder must have a smaller particle size than that for the filling materials. Since a change in the glass powder particle size changes the working and setting characteristics, different

Table 3.8.2 Physical and mechanical properties of two glass–ionomer luting cements

	Aqua-Cem (De Trey)	Ketac-Cem (3M/ESPE)
Radiopaque	No	No
Solubility in water		
7 minutes	0.90%	1.00%
1 hour	0.46%	0.40%
Solubility in lactic acid solution	–	0.57%
Compressive strength at 24 hours	82 MPa	105 MPa
Diametral tensile strength at 24 hours	7.6 MPa	5.3 MPa
Flexural strength at 24 hours	15.2 MPa	4.1 MPa
Creep at 24 hours	1.37%	0.63%

Table 3.8.3 Examples of commercially available resin-modified glass–ionomer luting cements

Products	Manufacturer
Protec-Cem	Ivoclar-Vivadent, Schaan, Liechtenstein
RelyX-Luting Cement	3M/ESPE, St Paul, USA
Fuji Plus	GC International Corp, Tokyo, Japan

formulations of the glass and polyacid have to be used from those used in filling materials in order to retain the optimum properties. It also means that it is not acceptable to use the restorative version of a GIC and modify its rheology by reducing the powder-to-liquid ratio.

The working time can affect the film thickness in that longer working times allow more flow and will aid seating of the restoration. Once the material begins to set, the viscosity rises rapidly and flow becomes impossible. Thus, it is extremely important that the mixing and placement of the cement is completed within 2–2.5 minutes, since, after this time, the material becomes stiff and a thicker film will result. It is a matter of preference and familiarity whether a short or slightly longer working time is desired.

It has been suggested that some of the newer formulations of the GIC luting cements do not need the protection of a surface coating because they have a more rapid set. The solubility, as measured by the water-leachable component at 7 minutes, has been reduced from approximately 2% to 1% in the transition from a conventional to a water-hardened cement. This solubility would appear to be even less for the maleic acid-based cements. Nevertheless, it may be as well to continue to offer some initial protection, since the dissolution due to acid erosion will continue to be a problem. In any case, it still takes some time for these materials to reach their final set.

CLINICAL SIGNIFICANCE

It is best to use a purpose-made cement for luting as changing the powder-to-liquid ratio of a glass–ionomer filling material in order to modify the working and setting times or film thickness will only result in a material with inferior properties.

Not only do the handling properties of different luting cements vary, but so do the physical and mechanical requirements. A comparison of a number of properties of two commercially available cements is presented in Table 3.8.2.

As far as the mechanical properties are concerned, the results would indicate that Aqua-Cem (Dentply Ltd, Weybridge, UK) has a lower stiffness (which would account for the higher diametral and flexural strength), but this is at the expense of the compressive strength and creep resistance. Ketac-Cem (3M/ESPE, Seefeld, Germany) is slightly more brittle than Aqua-Cem. In both instances, the materials have little resistance to fracture and need to be well supported by the surrounding structures. Clinically, it has been noted that it is easier to remove Ketac-Cem from the soft tissues than Aqua-Cem. This is probably because the former is more brittle immediately after placement.

Recently, the range of materials has been extended to include resin-modified glass–ionomer luting cements. These have all the potential advantages already discussed in relation to the restorative and lining cements. In particular, the low solubility and good adhesion to enamel and dentine should help to produce a durable marginal seal and aid retention. The main difference between these cements and the restorative and lining cements is that they have to rely on a chemical cure (dark cure) since it is not always possible to gain access with a light source. Examples of commercially available materials are shown in Table 3.8.3.

These cements have been recommended for use with cast metal crowns, bridges and inlays, metal–ceramic crowns and bridges, and reinforced-core ceramics.

When glass–ionomer luting cements were first used, there were some reports that the use of this material resulted in a higher incidence of postoperative sensitivity. However, it is generally agreed now that there is no significant difference in postoperative sensitivity between GICs and zinc–phosphate cements. In all other respects, there also seems to be no difference in the performance of GICs and zinc–phosphate cements when used for the cementation of crowns and bridges.

Clinical data on the use of RMGIC luting cements are few and far between. There have been reports of hygroscopic expansion associated with these materials and while such behaviour may be beneficial in reducing the marginal gap around a class V restoration, this expansion can also lead to fracture of all-ceramic crowns. The problem is made even more serious if RMGIC is also used as a core material. Metal posts with compromised mechanical retention may benefit from use of RMGIC. However, clinicians should be aware that, if the post is to be removed at a later date, the removal of posts cemented with an RMGIC can be extremely difficult.

CLINICAL SIGNIFICANCE

Glass–ionomer luting cements have become a popular alternative to zinc–phosphate cement, especially for reinforced-core all-ceramic restorations. The use of RMGICs for the cementation of all-ceramic restorations would appear to be contraindicated until such time that more clinical evidence is available.

RESIN-BASED LUTING CEMENTS

The resin cements can be divided into three subgroups:

1. Aesthetic light-/dual-cure composite resin cements
2. Adhesive chemical/dual-cure resin cements
3. Self-adhesive dual-cure resin cements

Table 3.8.4 Typical examples of aesthetic light-/dual-cure composite resin cements

Product	Manufacturer
Calibra	Dentsply, Konstanz, Germany
RelyX ARC	3M/ESPE, Seefeld, Germany
Nexus	Kerr Corp, Orange, CA, USA
Variolink	Ivoclar-Vivadent, Schaan, Liechtenstein

Aesthetic light-/dual-cure composite resin cements

These resins are based on conventional composite resin technology and have no intrinsic adhesive capabilities. They are used primarily for the cementation of resin-bonded ceramic restorations, where the aesthetic of the cementing medium is an important consideration. These luting resins need to be used in conjunction with adhesion promoters, requiring a dentine-bonding agent to ensure a bond to the dentine, as well as a silane coupling agent to provide a bond to the ceramic (see below). The luting resins provide the all-important means of bridging the gap between the silane-treated ceramic restoration and the prepared tooth structure. For the aesthetically demanding all-ceramic veneers, a composite luting resin is preferred because of the superior aesthetics and strength compared with the water-based cements, and the superior bond that is obtained to the etched and silanated ceramic surfaces. The composite luting resins are, in effect, lightly filled composites with small-sized filler particles to ensure thin film thickness. These luting resins are available in a wide range of shades and translucencies, which provides excellent marginal aesthetics.

Whereas the first luting resins were visible light-activated, the tendency is now towards the use of light and optional dual-cure resins. This makes the resins suitable for both veneers and inlays. The concern is that visible light curing resins may not cure properly when they are used to bond large inlays, as the light would be unable to penetrate to the full depth of the inlay. Similarly, the move towards resin-bonded all-ceramic crowns requires the use of a dual-cure resin in order to ensure that complete polymerization of the composite luting resin occurs. Typical examples are shown in Table 3.8.4.

Adhesive chemical/dual-cure resin cements

In order to improve the adhesive bond of resins to the metal surface, a variety of dual-cure composite luting resins have been developed in which the resin component has been modified to provide the ability to bond chemically to suitably prepared metal surfaces without the need for any adhesion promoter. These luting resins are generally referred to as chemically adhesive luting resins to differentiate them from the simple Bis-GMA type resins. In one such system, the active constituent is the carboxylic monomer 4-META (4-methacryloxyethyl trimellitate anhydride), and this is commercially available as C&B superbond (Sun Medical Co., Shiga, Japan). Another approach is to incorporate a phosphorylated methacrylate monomer, such as MDP (methacryloyloxydecyl dihydrogen phosphate); an example of this type of resin is Panavia 21 (Kuraray Co., Osaka, Japan). Resin bonding is facilitated by the high affinity of carboxylic acid or phosphoric acid derivative-containing resins for the metal oxide on base metal alloy (Figure 3.8.2). However these luting resins still require an adhesion promoter such as a dentine-bonding agent to bond to enamel and dentine, which brings us to the next group of luting resins.

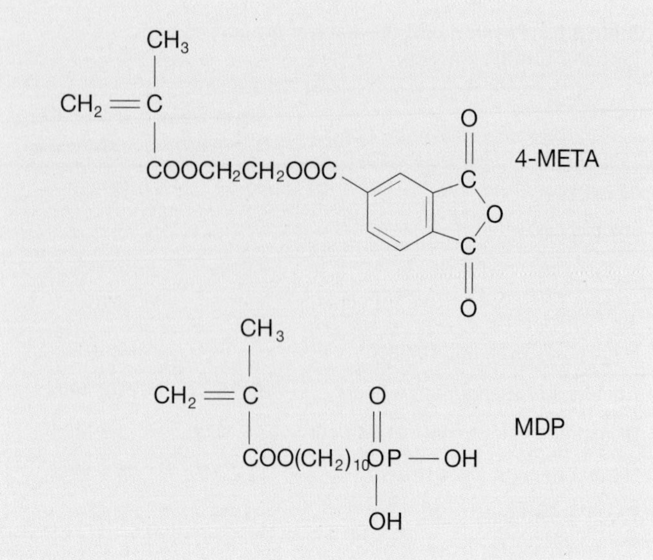

Figure 3.8.2 Structure of 4-META (4-methacryloxyethyl trimellitate anhydride) and MDP (methacryloyloxydecyl dihydrogen phosphate)

Self-adhesive dual-cure resin cements

This is a relatively new group of luting resins, which distinguishes itself from the other luting resins described above in that no pretreatment of the tooth surface is required, yet at the same time claiming to be able to establish a bond to base metal alloys and a range of ceramics. Thus the application is carried out in a single step similar to that of the water-based cements described earlier but with the added benefit of simultaneously providing adhesion to the tooth tissue and the restoration.

An example of these new self-adhesive luting resins is Rely-X Unicem (3M/ESPE), which contains a specially synthesized monomer having two phosphoric acid groups and two C=C double bonds (a methacrylated phosphoric ester), making the resin highly reactive with a very low pH of around 2.0. When the resin comes in contact with the tooth tissues, the negatively charged phosphoric acid groups react with the calcium ions (Ca^{2+}) in the enamel and dentine, and form an ionic bond. By the incorporation of a slightly acid-soluble glass filler that is able to react with the acidic monomer, the pH in the body of the resin cement rapidly increases to a neutral level, with the added benefit of fluoride ion release. Conceptually, this would appear to be not so dissimilar to the compomer resin (see Chapter 2.2), except that a more reactive phosphoric acid group is grafted on to a dimethacrylate, as opposed to an acrylic acid group.

A number of other systems with variations in composition have since come on to the market, such as MaxCem Elite (Kerr) and Smart-Cem2 (Dentsply). These systems are also based on the incorporation of a phosphoric acid monomer, but the acidic monomers used are ones that are commonly associated with the manufacturer's bonding agents, such as GPDM (glycerol dimethacrylate dihydrogen phosphate) in MaxCem or PENTA (dipentaerytritolpentacrylate phosphoric acid) in SmartCem2.

Unfortunately, it was not a simple case of adding an acidic monomer to a Bis-GMA- or urethane dimethacrylate (UDMA)-based dual-cure resin, as the acidic components interfere with the visible light and self-cure initiators. In particular, the alkaline amines used in self-cure systems become inactive in an acidic environment. In order to achieve a resin cement that would set either by curing with a visible light source or by chemical reaction, a new initiator system had to be developed. Therefore, one will find that each of the products will have their own proprietary acid-resistant amine/peroxide system.

Thanks to their simplicity of use and apparently univeral adhesive character, the self-adhesive resin cements have become very popular for the adhesive cementation of virtually all the indirect restorations, including metal and ceramic crowns, bridges and inlays. These luting resins have become particularly popular for the cementation of posts (including fibre posts), providing good retention due to the direct bond to the root dentine. One application for which the self-adhesive resins are not recommended is the bonding of ceramic veneers because of the need for high aesthetics. Also, whereas the bond to dentine is considered to be comparable to that of dentine-bonding agents, without the need for acid etching, the bond to enamel is not as good as can be achieved with the etch-and-rinse and self-etching dentine-bonding agents. For the same reason, these luting resins are not considered suitable for the bonding of orthodontic brackets.

RESIN-TO-CERAMIC BONDING

It was not all that long ago that all-ceramic restorations were cemented only with conventional cements, such as zinc–phosphate, zinc–polycarboxylate and glass–ionomer, and therefore relied on the strength of the ceramic core to withstand normal oral forces. This changed with the introduction of resin-bonded ceramics. As in the case of enamel, the aesthetic composite resins do not have a natural affinity for bonding to ceramic surfaces. Only with the advent of hydrofluoric acid etching of dental ceramics, introduced by Horn in 1983 for the construction of laminate veneers, did the direct bonding of resin composite to enamel become possible. The combination of adhesion provided by resin adhesion to phosphoric acid-etched enamel, dentine-bonding agents able to bond to dentine, hydrofluoric acid-etched and silane-treated resin bond to ceramic (Figure 3.8.3) and improvements in strength and toughness characteristics of dental ceramics has produced restorations with excellent mechanical integrity for both anterior and posterior use. The adhesive bond has the effect of eliminating surface flaws by replacing the surface with an interface and thus reduces the potential for fracture. However, the performance of the ceramic is crucially dependent on obtaining and maintaining a strong bond to the tooth structure, which requires a full appreciation of all the aspects of the principles of adhesion. A coupling agent is used to ensure a strong chemical bond between the composite luting resin and the ceramic. Hence, the resin-to-ceramic bond is based on an acid etchant creating a micro-mechanically

retentive surface and a coupling agent providing the chemical bond to the ceramic.

Hydrofluoric acid etching

The fitting surface of a ceramic, when constructed on a refractory die, is inherently rough due to the grit-blasting process used to remove the refractory. The application of hydrofluoric acid to the fitting surface of a ceramic, such as a leucite-reinforced feldspar, enhances the surface roughness even more, due to the preferential removal of either the crystalline leucite phase or the glassy phase. An example of this is shown in Figure 3.8.4, where the back-scattered image created under the scanning electron microscope reveals the heterogeneous composition of a leucite-reinforced ceramic. This heterogeneity can be made use of by preferentially etching one or other of the components with hydrofluoric acid. The effect of this etching is shown in Figure 3.8.5, which reveals a highly micro-mechanically retentive surface due to the preferential removal of the leucite phase. The resin is able to penetrate into these microscopic spaces and produce a very strong bond.

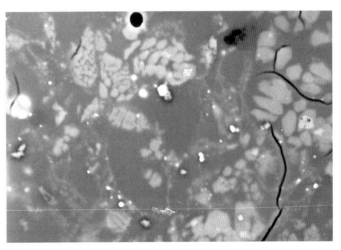

Figure 3.8.4 Back-scattered scanning electron microscope image of the surface of a leucite ceramic. The grey regions are the feldspathic glass, while the slightly lighter-shaded regions are the leucite crystals

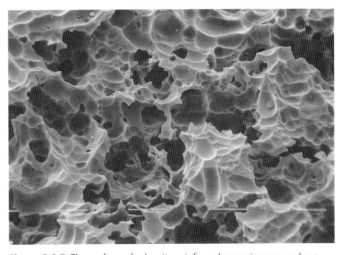

Figure 3.8.5 The surface of a leucite-reinforced ceramic seen under a scanning electron microscope after it has been etched with hydrofluoric acid. The re-entrant surface is a result of the more rapid dissolution of the leucite in the hydrofluoric acid than the glass matrix

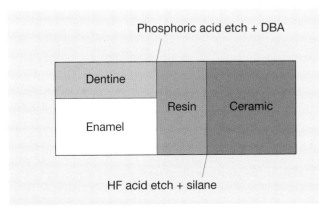

Figure 3.8.3 Schematic of the bonding interfaces when bonding a ceramic inlay. DBA, dentine-bonding agent

223

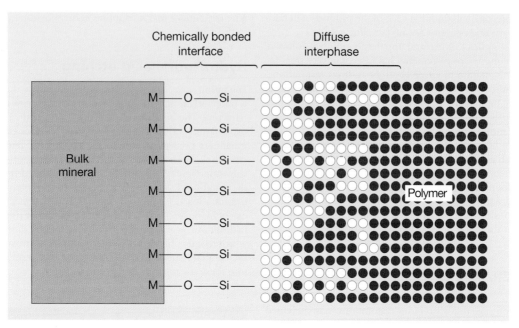

Figure 3.8.6 The interphase layer between the glass and the resin created by the application of a silane coupling agent
*(adapted from Chiang C-H, Koenig JL (1982) Spectroscopic characterization of the matrix–silane coupling agent interface in fiber-reinforced composites. J Polym Sci: Polym Phys Ed **20**: 2135–2143)*

In the case of an intra-oral ceramic fracture, the surface of the ceramic must first be etched in situ with hydrofluoric acid solution to create a micro-mechanically retentive surface. A fractured surface, even if roughened by a diamond bur, will not be as effective at providing micro-mechanical retention as an etched surface. The use of hydrofluoric acid in the mouth should be done with great care since it is a highly toxic material. Acidulated phosphate fluoride gels can also be used but the long etching time is prohibitive. Phosphoric acid is ineffectual as an etchant because the ceramic is totally resistant to attack from this acid, although it may sometimes be used as an effective surface-cleansing agent.

There are some general problems with hydrofluoric acid etching of which the dental practitioner should be aware:

- Hydrofluoric acid is a highly toxic substance and must be treated with great care.
- If the hydrofluoric acid is not neutralized completely, it may leach out and cause tissue damage at a later date.
- The hydrofluoric acid gel tends to slump, such that the lateral borders of particular veneers may not be fully etched. This can cause marginal leakage and chipping of the ceramic.
- Damage to the labial gingival margin of the veneer or inlay by the etchant can lead to plaque retention, inflammatory gingival response and secondary caries.

Silane coupling agents

When two materials are incompatible, it is often possible to bring about compatibility by introducing a third material that has properties intermediate between those of the other two. Resins do not have the ability to bond chemically to a ceramic surface and yet the interface between resin and ceramic has to be able to withstand stresses generated by loads applied to the structure and polymerization shrinkage stresses. Thus a coupling agent can be used to overcome this problem (see Chapter 1.9).

The coupling agent most commonly used in conjunction with ceramic restorations is a silane, γ-methacryloxypropyltrimethoxysilane (γ-MPTS). A detailed account of how this particular silane works is provided in Chapter 2.2.

In the case of resin-bonded ceramic restorations, the dental practitioner will be in a position to silanate the ceramic surface. Hence, one factor that deserves to be considered is the method of application of a silane to the ceramic surface. Whereas, under ideal circumstances, a monolayer of the silane is all that is required to convert the ceramic surface from an Si–OH appearance to a methacrylate appearance, in reality more than a monolayer is put down. In fact, what is formed is an *interphase*, consisting of a multiple layer of the silane containing many oligomers, which are not especially well bonded to the ceramic surface or to the resin (Figure 3.8.6); this can compromise the hydrolytic stability of the ceramic–resin bond. The simple procedure of washing the surface of the ceramic after silane treatment, in order to remove the weakly bound oligomers, helps to reduce the problem. This produces a bond that is much more hydrolytically stable than if the silane were simply applied and left to dry.

Many of the luting resin kits are now provided with a silane coupling agent that can be applied directly to the clean fitting surfaces of veneers or inlays as they are received from the dental laboratory, or that can be used for the repair of fractured ceramic restorations.

Thorough cleaning of the ceramic surfaces with isopropyl alcohol, acetone or phosphoric acid is needed after the veneer or inlay has been checked for satisfactory fit and prior to applying the silane. This is necessary in order to remove any surface contaminants, such as grease or saliva, that would interfere with the application of the silane coupling agent.

For some products, it is recommended that a phosphoric acid solution is added to the silane coupling agent to hydrolyse the silane prior to applying it to the fitting surface (Figure 3.8.7). Others are made up of a dilute solution of the activated silane in ethyl alcohol. In this case, the addition of phosphoric acid solution is therefore not necessary because the silane is already hydrolysed, although this will limit the shelf life of the silane coupling agent.

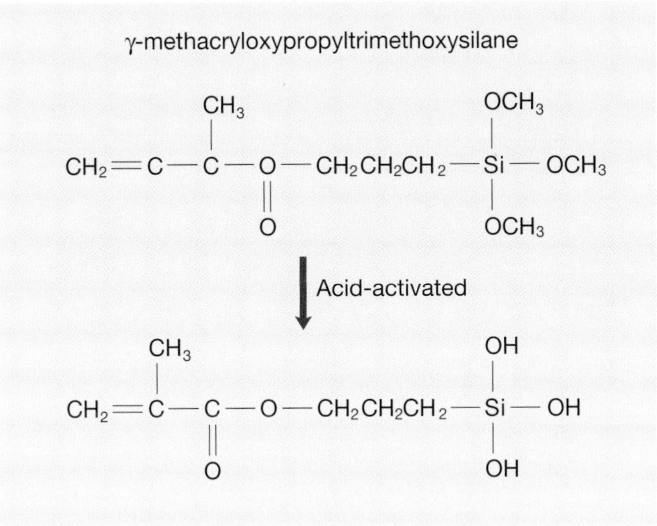

γ-methacryloxypropyltrimethoxysilane

Figure 3.8.7 Acid activation of a silane

CLINICAL SIGNIFICANCE

The ability to bond resins to ceramics with hydrofluoric acid etching and silane coupling agents has transformed the use of ceramics in restorative dentistry.

RESIN-TO-METAL BONDING

The ability to bond resins to metals is of growing interest as the range of applications continues to increase. These include:

- the use of resin instead of ceramics facings on metal substructures, especially for implant-retained prostheses
- bonding of minimal-preparation, resin-retained bridges
- resin bonding of conventional crowns and bridges where there is compromised retention
- intra-oral repair of ceramic fractures on metal–ceramic restorations.

The first three of these require adhesion of a resin to a well-defined alloy, whereas in the last case the alloy may not even be known. All represent a challenge and many new surface treatments and new resin adhesives have become available.

In order to improve the bond between the metal and the resin, a number of different approaches have been explored. Initially, these involved the use of macroscopic retentive features, but gradually, adhesive procedures involving micro-mechanical and/or chemical bonding were developed. The latter can be accomplished with a resin adhesive that has functional groups that can bond directly to the metal. Another approach is the use of adhesion promoters, such as silica coating, tin-plating, tribochemical coatings and metal primers, which have been developed in order to improve the bond between the metal and the more conventional Bis-GMA- or UDMA-based resins. There is an added complication since the efficacy of many of these procedures depends on whether one is seeking to bond to a base metal alloy or a precious metal alloy.

Macro-mechanical bonding

From the 1940s, dental laboratories were using resin facings on cobalt–chrome partial dentures. At that time, the resin was polymethyl methacrylate, which was attached to the metal framework by mechanical retention. Problems arose because the resin would not adapt well to the metal due to the large polymerization shrinkage of the methyl methacrylate, resulting in the formation of microgaps, discoloration, loosening and fracture. With the arrival of metal–ceramic restorations in the 1960s, many of these problems were overcome. It was not until the 1980s that there was a resurgence of interest in using resins as facings on metal substructures, which corresponded with the improved composite resins that had become available by then. At that time, bonding was still by mechanical retention. This mechanical retention required beads, wires or loops in the metal design. One problem was the bulkier framework needed to accommodate the macro-retentive features, and improved methods for bonding resin to metal were required.

In the dental clinic, the situation was no different. In 1973, Rochette first reported the use of metal structures that were bonded by resins to acid-etched enamel. He used thin, perforated metal castings, bonded with cold-cure acrylic resins, to splint mobile lower incisors that were affected by advanced bone loss. Following the successful retention of these devices, he had occasion to extract one of the incisors, and it was then that the idea of adding a pontic to the splint was first conceived. This provided a means of replacing a missing tooth that involved minimal tooth preparation. As resin technology improved, so the concept was explored in greater detail by other workers. One weakness of the Rochette bridge design was the use of small perforations for retention. These exposed the resin to wear and meant that the attachment was to a relatively small area of the metal retainer. Other macro-retentive features, as used on the metal frameworks produced in the dental laboratory, did not resolve the problem.

Micro-mechanical bonding

The problem of having to rely on macro-retentive features was overcome, to some degree, in the early 1980s, when a method of treating the Ni–Cr alloys was developed. With this method, the entire fitting surface of the retainer is rendered micro-mechanically retentive by either electrolytic or acid-gel etching. This technique is only applicable to Ni–Cr and Co–Cr alloys, which have a eutectic microstructure, as shown in Figure 3.8.8. The main alloy used for metal–ceramic restorations is Ni–Cr rather than Co–Cr alloy because of the greater difficulty of fusing ceramic to the latter. The etching process preferentially removes one of the phases, which results in a pitted and grooved surface appearance, as shown in Figure 3.8.9. This technique provides a highly retentive surface that adheres strongly to the composite luting resins due to the high degree of micro-mechanical interlocking introduced. It bonds the entire area of the retainer to the etched enamel and protects the underlying resin. Retainers can be made to a minimum thickness of 0.3 mm, and can be waxed directly on to investment models, resulting in a good accuracy of fit. The bridges made using the electro-etching method were called *Maryland bridges*, as it was there that this technique was developed. However, with the advent of other methods of achieving a resin-to-metal bond, other terms such as resin-bonded bridges or minimal-preparation bridges are now commonly used.

Since electro-etching requires a high degree of skill and specialist equipment, the gel-etching process has become the more popular of the two. The gel is a high-concentration solution of hydrofluoric acid, which is highly toxic and needs to be handled with great care.

The main advantages of these resin-bonded bridges are:

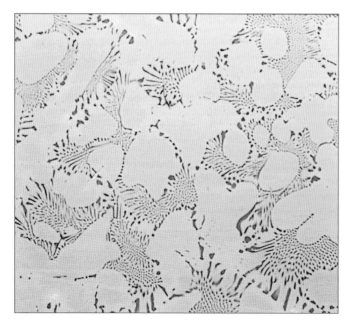

Figure 3.8.8 Eutectic microstructure of a Ni–Cr alloy as it appears under the scanning electron microscope using back-scattered imaging

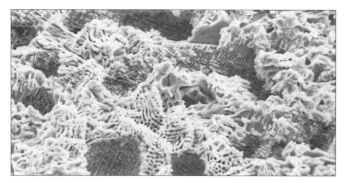

Figure 3.8.9 Scanning electron microscope view of the surface of a Ni–Cr alloy after etching with a gel etchant

- The minimal enamel preparation does not require local anaesthetics.
- The procedure leaves the teeth largely intact, such that traditional treatment options can still be used in the future.
- Possible irritation of the pulp is prevented, as usually there is no exposure of dentine.

Disadvantages include:

- There is a high debonding rate for the retainers.
- There are colour changes in anterior abutment teeth due to shine-through of the metal retainer.
- The process is only applicable to Ni–Cr alloys.

The aesthetic problem can be overcome, to some degree, by using opaque composite luting resins. The high rate of debonding is more difficult to resolve and may require careful reconsideration of design of the retainers and the properties of the resins available.

Since the prosthesis relies on the presence of enamel for its attachment, sufficient enamel is required on to which to bond the retainers. Short crowns, extensive restorations, congenital defects and tooth surface loss would prevent the use of these resin-retained castings. Also, for unsightly abutment teeth, conventional bridges would be a better proposition.

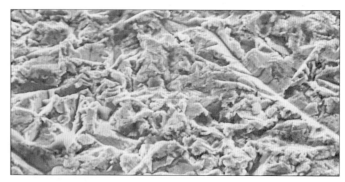

Figure 3.8.10 Scanning electron microscope view of the surface of a Ni–Cr alloy after grit-blasting with alumina

The composite luting resins are essentially very similar to composite restorative materials, consisting of a Bis-GMA or UDMA resin and glass filler. Where these resins differ from the restorative composites is that they are invariably two-paste chemical or dual-cure systems, since the access of light is restricted by the metal retainers. The filler particle size is less than 20 µm and the filler loading tends to be slightly lower in order to ensure a low film thickness. An optical opacifier, such as titanium oxide, may be added to prevent shine-through of the metal.

One of the drawbacks with this restorative technique is that there is a reluctance on the part of some clinicians to use Ni–Cr alloys, as nickel is a known allergen. Some of the alloys also contain beryllium (Be), which is highly toxic in its free state. Be is usually present in order to improve the castability of the Ni–Cr alloy and to provide a superior eutectic microstructure for effective etching. However, beryllium may be released during grinding and polishing of the castings, and therefore dental technicians are probably more at risk than either the dentist or the patient. Hence, the preference of dental laboratories is for Be-free alloys, which, unfortunately, do not etch so well.

Another constraint of this approach is that it is not possible to etch precious metal alloys since they have a relatively homogeneous microstructure. Hence, it is not possible to use the etching technique for resin bonding with precious metal alloys. In order to circumvent the wishes of dental laboratories that do not want to use Be-containing Ni–Cr alloys and want to avoid the etching process, some other means of bonding to the alloy had to be found. The difficulty here is that Bis-GMA- and UDMA-type resins do not adhere well to untreated metal surfaces, relying primarily on micro-mechanical and physical adhesion. The latter tends to be readily overcome by hydrolytic attack, as water is absorbed at the interface and displaces the resin. Grit-blasting of base metal alloys with 50-µm alumina grit produces some surface roughening for micro-mechanical adhesion, as shown in Figure 3.8.10. However, the surface does not have the re-entrant features associated with the etched surface and has therefore proved to be inadequate. Hence, the Bis-GMA- or UDMA-based composite luting resins cannot be used directly on grit-blasted Ni–Cr alloy surfaces, as the bond to a grit-blasted metal surface is not sufficiently strong for these luting resins. In these situations, the chemically adhesive luting resins are the material of choice.

Since these resins can provide a durable bond to the grit-blasted metal surface of a Ni–Cr alloy, there is no need for etching and thus no need for special laboratory equipment or the use of dangerous chemical reagents. With the advent of these resins, it is now possible to form a strong chemically adhesive bond between a grit-blasted base metal alloy and acid-etched enamel. However, whilst these chemically adhesive luting resins are excellent for bonding to base metal alloys, they have a relatively low affinity for precious metal alloys, such as gold and palladium alloys, due to the lack of a surface oxide coating.

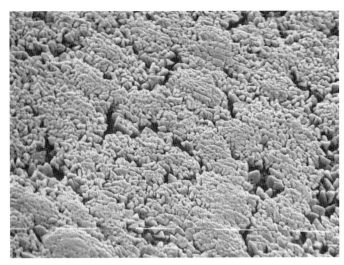

Figure 3.8.11 Scanning electron microscope view of the surface appearance of a precious metal after tin-plating

Chemical modification of the alloy surface

The poor quality of bonding between the precious metals and the chemically adhesive resins is a consequence of the low chemical reactivity of the surface of precious metals alloys as compared with that of base metal alloys. This problem may be overcome by surface modification of the precious metal so as to make it more amenable to forming a bond with a luting resin. Three popular options are available, namely:

- apply a coating to the surface that will create a micro-mechanical bond, e.g. tin plating
- change the surface chemistry by silica coating or tribochemical coating
- apply specially formulated metal primers.

Tin plating

Tin plating is based on an invention that offers a means of resin bonding to noble and precious metal alloys at the chair side. The procedure deposits a layer of tin on the alloy surface, which can be seen by the appearance of a grey discoloration. The surface layer produced is irregular in form and provides micro-mechanical retention for the resin, whilst also being chemically attracted to the tin oxide on the alloy surface (Figure 3.8.11). This chair-side system is indicated primarily for the intra-oral repair of fractured metal–ceramic restorations, where metal is exposed and is to be repaired in situ with a composite resin.

Although laboratory data suggest that there is an improvement in the bond strength of resin to a tin-plated precious metal alloy, some results suggest that the improvement is only marginal and better methods of bonding to precious metal alloys are required. Additionally, it has been suggested that the application of an excessively thick tin-plating layer can result in a low bond strength due to the oxide coating being too thick. Thus, the application of the tin coating is critical and open to error. In addition, there may be clinical situations, such as in the case of intra-oral repairs, when the alloy is unknown. If the exposed metal is a Ni–Cr alloy, then tin plating provides no benefit and may even be detrimental to obtaining a strong resin bond.

Silica coating

The use of silane coupling agents to enhance adhesion of dental ceramics to tooth structure via resin composite is well established (see

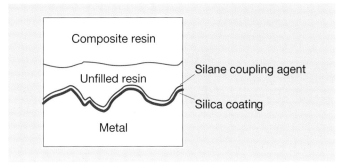

Figure 3.8.12 Metal surface with silica coating

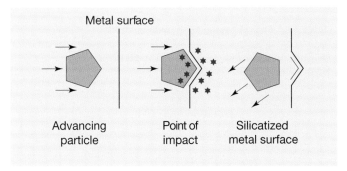

Figure 3.8.13 Tribochemical coating of metal surface

above). The possibility of silanating cast metal is limited due to the lack of appropriate binding sites on the alloy surface. In contrast, these are found in abundance on a silica-based ceramic surface, such as silanols, i.e. Si–OH. It is now possible to produce a silica coating on metal surfaces, making them amenable to silane coupling and successful resin bonding. Two techniques are available, one involving a special coating and heat treatment technique of the alloy, and the other involving a tribochemical approach.

Silicoater (Kulzer Co GmbH, Friedrichsdorf, Germany)

The Silicoater system requires the metal surface to be passed through a propane–air flame, in which tetramethoxysilane is decomposed. As a result, an intermediary layer of SiO_x is formed – providing Si–OH groups for silane bonding (Figure 3.8.12). A silane coupling agent is then applied to this silicoated surface, which is then able to bond with the resin.

Tribochemical coating

In this technique, the alloy surface is grit-blasted at high pressure with a special powder that contains fine alumina and colloidal silica particles. This is available as a laboratory-based system and a chair-side technique called Rocatec and Cojet respectively (3M/ESPE, Seefeld, Germany).

The objective is to form a thin layer of silica (SiO_x–C) which contains sufficient free hydroxyl (–OH) groups to allow coupling to resin via a silane (Figure 3.8.13). This technique is known as tribochemical silica coating, as it has been shown that high-energy colloidal silica particles impacting the alloy surface cause physical fusion of a silica layer to the metal, which is said to be stable. This pretreated surface is then silane-treated and is ready for resin bonding.

The chair-side coating system (Cojet, 3M/ESPE, Seefeld, Germany) has been promoted for the in situ repair of fractured metal–ceramic units with exposed metal surfaces requiring improved adhesion to

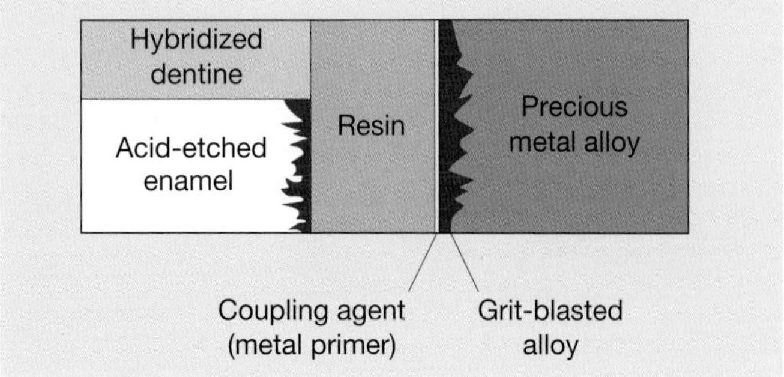

Figure 3.8.14 Schematic of metal-to-resin bond

Table 3.8.5 Typical examples of metal primers

Product name	Primer	Manufacturer
V-Primer	VBATDT in 95% acetone	Sun Medical Co., Kyoto, Japan
Alloy Primer	VBADT/MDP	Kuraray Co., Osaka, Japan
Metal Primer II	MEPS in MMA	GC Corp., Tokyo, Japan
Metaltite	Thiouracil in 96% ethanol	Tokuyama Inc., San Mateo, USA

MDP, methacryloxyethyl-phenyl phosphate; MEPS, methacryloyloxyalkyl thiophosphate derivatives; MMA, methylmethacrylate; VBATDT, 6-(4-vinylbenzyl-n-propyl)amino-1,3,5-triazide-2,4-dithiol.

resin composite. In addition, the system is also claimed to be effective as a surface treatment for the repair of fractured resin composite restorations.

One drawback with these techniques is the need to purchase laboratory or chair-side equipment. In addition, the high number of steps involved potentially increases the likelihood of errors.

Metal primers

What many dentists want is a simple adhesive liquid that they can apply directly to the metal surface, requiring nothing more special than a brush (Figure 3.8.14). The use of simple chemical pretreatment techniques of the alloy surface is therefore an area of increasing research. In particular, the use of coupling agents based on bifunctional monomers has gained interest because they have been shown to be effective yet simple alternatives to most of the surface modification techniques already described. They are usually supplied as single-liquid primers composed of a polymerizable monomer in a suitable solvent. (The products are invariably called primers despite them being, in fact, coupling agents.) The monomer has a bifunctional structure, with one end carrying a methacryl or similar functional group for resin bonding, and the other end carrying mercapto or thiol (–SH) groups for bonding to the precious metal alloy. When the metal primer is applied to a grit-blasted alloy surface, it is capable of enhanced adhesion to resin composite cement because of the ability of sulphur to react with precious metal alloys. Hence, the presence of the mercapto groups allows chemical adhesion to precious metal alloy surfaces. A number of commercial products, based on these bifunctional primers, are now available and include the products shown in Table 3.8.5.

The chemical structure of the primers is shown in Figure 3.8.15, from which it can be seen that these metal primers are, in fact,

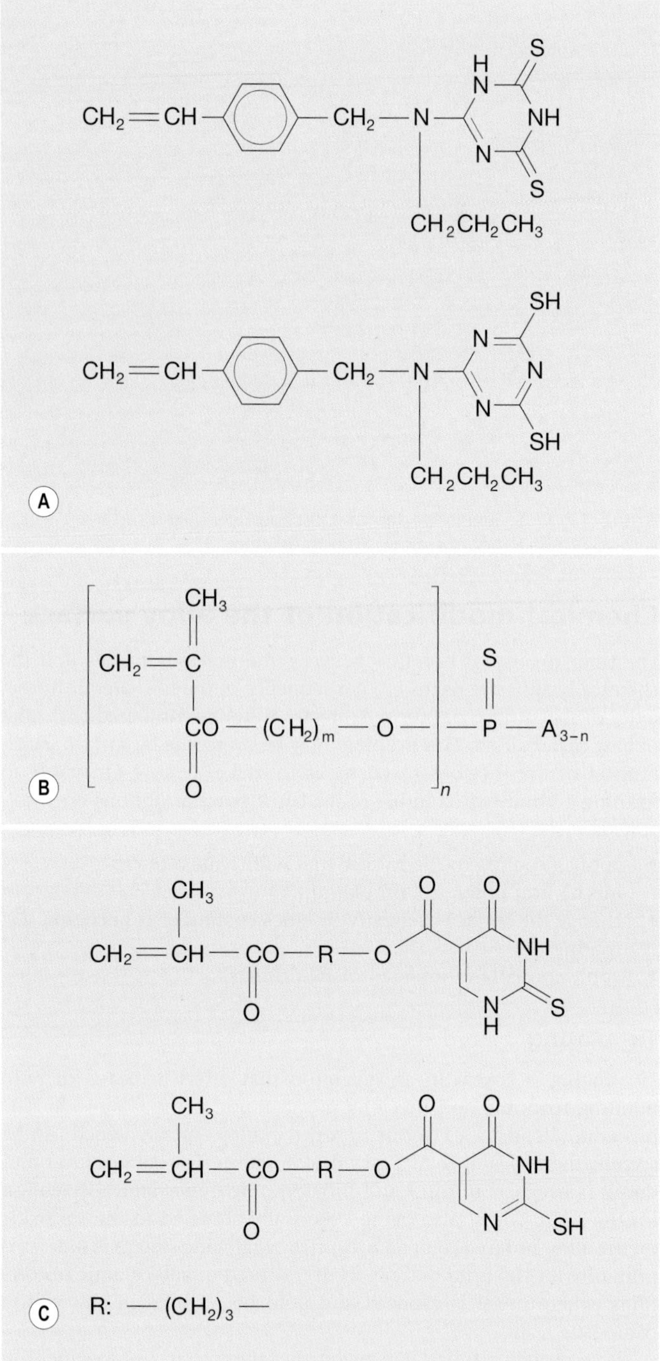

Figure 3.8.15 Chemical structure of three metal primers used in commercial products. (a) VBADT, 6-(4-vinylbenzyl-n-propyl)amino-1,3,5-triazide-2,4,dithiol; (b) MEPS, methacryloyloxyalkyl thiophosphate derivative; (c) metaltite primer based on a thiouracil derivative

coupling agents. The VBATDT-containing primer works well with 4-META-based luting resins, but does not work so well with the more conventional methacrylate resins, which is possibly associated with the fact that the VBATDT interferes with the polymerization reaction of the methacrylate resins. The combination of MEPS with 4-META-based resins is also deemed unacceptable. Thus there are still issues of resin-primer compatibility that need to be addressed.

CLINICAL SIGNIFICANCE

Resin-to-metal bonding will continue to be an area of development and the bond will continue to improve, bringing with it better clinical performance.

RESIN-TO-RESIN BONDING

There are a growing number of prefabricated resin prostheses, such as composite inlays and fibre-reinforced crowns, bridges and endodontic posts. Whilst one might imagine that resin-to-resin bonding should be free of problems, this is, in fact, not the case. In particular, with composite inlays, there have been problems of debonding between the luting resin and the composite inlay.

When increments of freshly placed composite resin restorative material are being built up, the bonding of one increment to the next is helped by the fact that, after light-curing, there is still a very thin resinous surface layer of some 10–50 μm thick that has not set due to oxygen inhibition of the cure. When one deals with prefabricated resin components such as inlay and posts, this uncured surface layer does not exist. Hence, the luting resin has to bond directly to fully cured resins. This situation is, in fact, similar to that encountered when considering the option of replacing the lost segment of a fractured composite restoration with new composite resin. It would seem that resins do not have any particular advantage when bonding to other resins, except that close adaptation can readily be achieved.

Various approaches to improve the resin-to-resin bond have been proposed, including grit-blasting with alumina or grinding the surface with a coarse instrument to increase the surface roughness and thus create a micro-mechanical bond. Although this helps, neither approach is particularly effective, as the retentive features created by grit blasting are not ideal, not unlike the situation encountered when bonding resins to grit-blasted metal surfaces. In the case of glass-particulate-filled composites, it may be possible to remove the glass particles near the surface by hydrofluoric acid etching and to introduce more retentive features on the micron scale. However, the experience with repairs of glass-particulate-filled composites is that the best quality of bond that can be achieved is only 50–75% of the cohesive strength of the composite resins.

Chemical bonding via a silane coupling agent has also been suggested on the basis that, for glass-particulate-filled composites, there will be a large amount of exposed glass at the surface after grit-blasting or grinding, which has not been silanated. However, the problem with this is that the silane will also coat the resin part of the surface and may well impair the resin-to-resin bond while improving the resin-to-ceramic bond. Another suggestion is to use the tribochemical technique described earlier, which would embed a layer of silica into the resin surface and then using the silane coupling agent to bond to the luting resin.

CLINICAL SIGNIFICANCE

The problem of bonding resins to resins has not yet been resolved satisfactorily and thus will continue to be an area of research interest.

FURTHER READING

Blum IR, Schriever A, Heidemann D (2003) The repair of direct composite restorations: an international survey of the teaching of operative techniques and materials. Eur J Dent Educ 7: 41

Jockstad A, Mjor IA (1996) Ten years' clinical evaluation of three luting cements. J Dent 24: 309

Kiatsirirote K, Northeast SE, van Noort R (1999) Bonding procedures for intraoral repair of exposed metal with resin composite. J Adhes Dent 1: 315

Knibbs PJ, Plant CG, Shovelton DS (1986) The performance of zinc polycarboxylate and glass-ionomer luting cements in general dental practice. Brit Dent J 160: 13–15

McLean JW, Wilson AD, Prosser HJ (1984) Development and use of water-hardening glass–ionomer luting cements. J Prosthet Dent 52: 175–181

Mitchell CA (2000) Selection of materials for post cementation. Dent Update 27: 350

Phillips RW, Lund MS (1987) In vivo disintegration of luting cements. J Am Dent Assoc 114: 489

Radovic I, Monticelli F, Goracci C (2008) Self-adhesive resin cements: a literature review. J Adhes Dent 10: 251–258

Rosenthiel SF, Land MF, Crispin BJ (1998) Dental luting agents: a review of the current literature. J Prosthet Dent 80: 280

Sindel J, Frankenberger R, Kramer N, Petschelt A (1999) Crack formation of all-ceramic crowns dependent on different core build-up and luting materials. J Dent 27: 175

Teixeira EC, Bayne SC, Thompson JY (2005) Shear bond strength of self-etching bonding systems in combination with various composites used for repairing aged composites. J Adhes Dent 7: 159

Yoshida K, Kamada K, Taira Y (2001) Effect of three adhesive primers on the bond strengths of four light-activated opaque resins to noble alloy. J Oral Rehab 28: 168

Stainless steel

INTRODUCTION

Most of us are familiar with stainless steel as a widely used quality product for both domestic and industrial applications. However, it is also extensively used in medical and dental applications, such as for the production of dental instruments, e.g. scalpel blades and forceps, orthodontic wires, denture bases and partial denture clasps, endodontic posts and as stainless steel crowns for the treatment of severely decayed primary molars. The material has generally been heavily worked to give it the desired shape and is therefore defined as a *wrought alloy*.

A wrought alloy distinguishes itself from the many casting alloys used for the construction of crowns and bridges in that it is *a cast alloy which has been formed by mechanical processing such as rolling, extrusion or drawing to give it a new desired shape*. When this is done at a low temperature, the mechanical processing is known as *cold working*, by which the metal is simultaneously shaped and strengthened (Figure 3.9.1). If the process is carried out at high temperatures, this is called *hot working* and generally involves shaping without strengthening. No strengthening occurs because the metal continually recrystallizes and the amount of deformation that can be performed is virtually limitless.

Many alloys besides stainless steel are available in wrought form, such as gold alloys for posts and denture clasps, Ni–Ti alloys for orthodontic wires and endodontic files, and Co–Cr–Ni alloys for denture clasps and orthodontic wires. However, only stainless steel will be considered in detail in this chapter.

Steels are available in a wide variety of compositions, with each having very specific properties that are carefully tailored to suit their particular application. One feature of steels that makes them such popular materials is the enormous range of mechanical properties that can be obtained with only small changes in composition. A comparison of steel to other products is shown in Table 3.9.1. The steel wires show a wide range of strengths, which the other materials cannot match.

Before the introduction of stainless steels in dentistry (generally in the early 1930s), the only metal that was felt to have good enough corrosion resistance to allow it to be used in the mouth was gold. Stainless steel possesses a high tensile strength, and is used to form springs in removable orthodontic appliances. It is also used in fixed appliances for construction of bands, brackets and arch wires. In fact, virtually all the components for fixed appliances used in orthodontics can be constructed out of stainless steel.

Orthodontic wire is made from what is known as austenitic stainless steel. This is a form of steel that can be readily shaped into a wire by rolling and subsequent extrusion through dies. This elongates the grains into long fibrous structures which run in the direction of the wire.

More specifically, the material used for orthodontic wires is known as a *stabilized austenitic stainless steel*. The best way of describing this material is to take the raw material, iron, and develop it, step by step, into the final product. Along the way, the different types of steel will be explored and their particular applications considered.

IRON

Iron is an allotropic material, i.e. it undergoes two solid-state phase changes with temperature. At room temperature, pure iron has a body-centred cubic (BCC) structure, known as the α-phase. This structure is stable up to a temperature of 912 °C, where it transforms to a face-centred cubic (FCC) structure, the γ-phase.

At 1390 °C the FCC iron reverts back to BCC, and retains this structure until it melts at 1538 °C. These changes are accompanied by changes in the volume of the iron (Figure 3.9.2).

STEEL

Steel is an alloy of iron and carbon, in which the carbon content must not exceed 2%. Iron with a carbon content greater than 2% is classified as a *cast iron* and will not be considered here.

Carbon steels

Carbon steel is an alloy of only iron and carbon. In its BCC form, when small amounts of carbon are dissolved in the iron, the material is known as α-iron or *ferrite*.

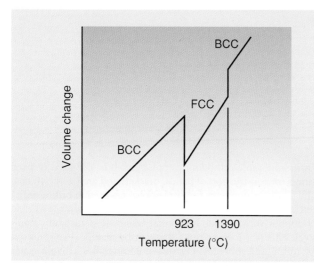

Figure 3.9.1 The effect of cold working on the mechanical properties of a metal. Note the reduction in ductility ($\leftrightarrow$) as the yield stress (σ_y) is increased

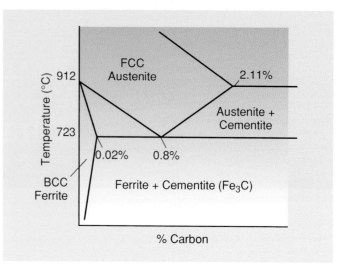

Figure 3.9.3 The Fe–Fe$_3$C system

Both of these forms of steel are relatively soft and ductile; in particular, the austenite is readily shaped at elevated temperatures by hot forging and rolling operations.

When the limit of solubility for the carbon is exceeded for either of these forms of steel, the excess carbon precipitates out as Fe$_3$C, which is a hard and brittle phase, given the name *cementite*. The various phases in the iron–cementite system are presented in the partial equilibrium phase diagram in Figure 3.9.3.

Hyper- and hypo-eutectoid steels

At a carbon concentration of 0.8%, the alloy shows a transformation at 723°C from the single-phase austenite to a two-phase structure consisting of ferrite and cementite:

$$\gamma \rightarrow \alpha + Fe_3C$$

austenite $\rightarrow$ ferrite + cementite

This solid transformation is defined as a *eutectoid*, as distinct from a *eutectic*, which is a transformation of a single liquid phase directly into two solid phases (see Chapter 1.4).

Steels with a carbon content of exactly the eutectoid composition are called *eutectoid steels*. Those with a carbon content of greater than 0.8% are *hyper-eutectoid steels*, and are used in the manufacture of burs and cutting instruments, while those with a carbon content of less than 0.8% are *hypo-eutectoid steels*, and are used in the manufacture of dental instruments such as forceps.

The eutectoid transformation is very important in the production of steels because a number of interesting things can happen when a carbon steel is cooled from its austenitic high-temperature condition to room temperature.

Slow cooling

On slow cooling, the changes in structure for a 0.8% carbon steel are as predicted from the equilibrium phase diagram. The austenite is converted into a mixture of ferrite and cementite, which is described as *pearlite* (Figure 3.9.4). However, cooling is not usually carried out slowly, but involves rapid cooling by immersing the object into cold water in a process that is known as *quenching*.

Rapid cooling

When austenite is quenched in water, the ferrite and cementite cannot form because there is not enough time for diffusion and

Figure 3.9.2 The volume change of pure iron with temperature. BCC, body-centred cubic; FCC, face-centred cubic

Table 3.9.1 A comparison of fracture or yield strengths of steels with other materials

Material	Fracture or yield strength (MPa)
Steel wire	300–2800
Bulk steel	300–800
Iron	150–200
Brass	200–400
Aluminium alloys	200–600
Copper alloys	300–600
Titanium alloys	600–1100
Glass	50–150
Carbon fibre	2200–2800

The solubility of the carbon in this BCC structure is very low compared with that in the FCC structure, being a maximum of 0.02 wt % at 723°C and only 0.005 wt % at room temperature. This is despite the greater unoccupied volume in BCC (packing factor 68%) compared to FCC (74%).

The FCC form of the material has a considerably higher solubility of carbon, of up to 2.11%. The reason for this is that the largest interstitial holes in BCC iron (diameter 0.072 nm) are smaller than those in FCC iron (diameter 0.104 nm). This FCC form of the steel is known as *austenite*.

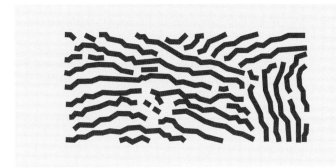

Figure 3.9.4 The structure of pearlite, which is a laminar mixture of ferrite and cementite

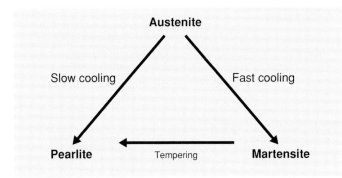

Figure 3.9.5 Heat treatment known as tempering of martensitic steels to control the mechanical properties

Table 3.9.2 Three forms of stainless steel that are used in dental applications

	Cr (%)	Ni (%)	C (%)
Ferritic	11.5–27	0	0.2 (max.)
Austenitic	16–22	7–22	0.25
Martensitic	11.5–17	0–2.5	0.15–0.25

manganese), the two of greatest importance for dentistry are chromium and nickel for the production of stainless steel.

Stainless steel is an alloy of iron that is resistant to corrosion. This was discovered accidentally in the UK during the early part of the First World War. At the time, a Sheffield metallurgist named Brearley was working on steels for armament construction. A rejected billet of a steel alloy was left out in the work's yard for some months, and he subsequently observed that the billet had not rusted in the wet weather. This turned out to be due to its high chromium content.

The possibilities presented by the alloy were recognized, and it was patented in 1917. The addition of chromium to the carbon steel improves the corrosion resistance of the metal by forming a protective surface coating of chromium oxide. For this to be fully effective, the chromium content of the alloy has to exceed 11%.

CLINICAL SIGNIFICANCE

The chromium content of a steel must exceed 11% for it to be designated as a *stainless steel*.

Austenitic stainless steel

The addition of 8% nickel prevents the transformation of austenite to martensite on cooling, such that the austenite becomes stable at room temperature when cooled rapidly. Slow cooling would again allow the formation of ferrite and cementite, but, since this is a diffusion-controlled process, the rapid cooling by quenching prevents these phases from forming.

There are essentially three forms of stainless steel used for dental applications (Table 3.9.2).

The ferritic steels are used mainly for the production of tools, whereas austenitic stainless steels have a very wide application and are used in orthodontic wires, autoclaves, table tops and cabinets. The martensitic steels are primarily used for cutting instruments.

The attraction of the austenitic stainless steel is that it is highly malleable and so can be readily shaped for a wide variety of purposes. The alloy cannot be heat-treated to change the properties in the way that martensitic and ferritic steels can, but it can be cold-worked to improve the yield stress (although this will be at the expense of the ductility). Nevertheless, it is this ability of austenitic stainless steel to be made with a wide variety of mechanical properties whilst maintaining its corrosion resistance in the mouth that has made it such an attractive material for orthodontic applications.

CLINICAL SIGNIFICANCE

For intra-oral applications, we are concerned almost exclusively with the austenitic variety of steel, and the alloy most used is 18/8 stainless steel, which is composed of 18% chromium, 8% nickel and 0.2% carbon.

rearrangement of the atoms. Instead, a very rapid transformation occurs to a body-centred tetragonal structure, which is rather like a distorted BCC. This form of steel is described as *martensite*, and is extremely hard and brittle. (In fact, it is far too hard and brittle for any practical purposes.) Nevertheless, this transformation can be put to good use because, by reheating to a temperature in the range of 200–450°C and then cooling rapidly, it is possible to transform the martensite into *pearlite* (ferrite + cementite). The degree of conversion can be carefully controlled by the temperature and duration of the heat treatment, a process known as *tempering* (Figure 3.9.5).

For cutting instruments, a hyper-eutectoid steel (carbon content >0.8%) is generally used because it combines the hard martensite with a large presence of the hard cementite, such that a cutting edge can be produced which does not blunt readily. For instruments such as forceps, the brittle nature of hyper-eutectoid steel would be unacceptable and a lower carbon content is present, as in the hypo-eutectoid steels (carbon content <0.8%). This allows the formation predominantly of the more ductile ferrite, while the hardness is controlled by the presence of martensite and much lower amounts of cementite.

CLINICAL SIGNIFICANCE

Excessive heating up of cutting instruments (e.g. cutting blades in a bunsen flame) will result in a loss of hardness due to changes in the microstructure.

STAINLESS STEEL

Although many other elements can be added to the basic carbon steels to improve the properties (e.g. molybdenum, silicon, cobalt,

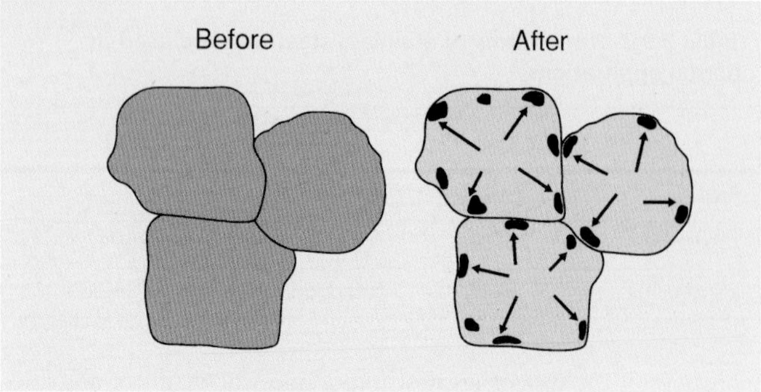

Figure 3.9.6 Weld decay due to overheating of the alloy

Stabilized austenitic stainless steel

Although it is common practice for most wrought alloys to be given a stress-relief anneal, this is not possible with the austenitic stainless steels due to microstructural changes that occur at the annealing temperature.

Formation of chromium carbides

At temperatures in excess of 500°C, chromium and carbon react to form chromium carbides, which precipitate at the grain boundaries, causing brittle behaviour. Also, the corrosion resistance is decreased due to depletion of the central regions of the crystals of chromium, which has migrated to the boundaries to form the carbides (Figure 3.9.6).

This process is known as *weld decay*, since it was first noticed as a problem when welding sheets of steel. The problem can be overcome by adding titanium to the alloy, which has the effect that the carbon preferentially reacts with the dispersed titanium such that the chromium remains where it is at its most effective. This produces what is known as *stabilized austenitic stainless steel*.

Transformation to ferrite and cementite

The austenite is formed by rapid cooling from elevated temperatures so as to prevent the formation of cementite and ferrite. Raising the temperature allows diffusion of the atoms, such that these other phases *can* form.

This formation of other phases is an irreversible process unless the material temperature is raised above the eutectoid and then quenched to room temperature to reform austenitic steel.

However, the annealing process allows recrystallization and the formation of the chromium carbides, which impairs the corrosion resistance.

Recrystallization

If the temperature is raised above the eutectoid temperature, recrystallization of the metal takes place, and the long, fibrous grains which are produced by rolling and drawing during fabrication of the wire become transformed into large, equiaxed grains.

If this happens, the material will have softened and the springy properties of the wire will have been lost and cannot be restored. The rate at which this occurs is controlled by time and temperature.

CLINICAL SIGNIFICANCE

Dental products made from stainless steel should not be heated above 500°C.

Table 3.9.3 Mechanical properties of a range of stainless steels used for orthodontic appliances				
	0.2% proof stress (MPa)	Young's modulus (GPa)	Elongation (%)	Hardness (BHN)
Soft	280	200	50	170
Hard	1050	200	6	250
Extra-hard	1450	230	1	350
BHN, Brinell hardness number				

Properties

Austenitic stainless steels are favoured for orthodontic applications because of their excellent corrosion resistance in the biological environment, the wide range of mechanical properties available and the ease with which they can be joined by soldering or electrical resistance welding.

Mechanical properties

Depending on the degree of cold working carried out by the manufacturer in forming the orthodontic wire, a range of mechanical properties are produced (see Table 3.9.3). It is important to select the appropriate type for the application in mind.

If little shaping, i.e. cold working by bending, is needed, a hard or extra-hard stainless steel wire can be selected. If, on the other hand, a lot of shaping is required, then one needs to start with a soft alloy, as it will work-harden on bending.

CLINICAL SIGNIFICANCE

If too hard a wire is selected to begin with, there is a danger that the wire will fracture on bending due to the loss of ductility.

Soldering and welding

Since the fabrication of appliances often requires the joining of separate components by soldering or welding, the heat produced can have an extremely detrimental effect on the properties of stainless steel. Therefore, techniques must be designed to avoid prolonged exposure of the components to high temperatures.

Hard soldering

Stainless steel components are generally joined by 'hard soldering' as distinct from 'soft soldering', the latter involving the use of low melting point alloys such as Sn–Pb alloys. Hard soldering may be carried out with gold or silver alloys, which are sufficiently corrosion-resistant. Since gold-alloy solders must contain at least 45% gold to ensure a low enough melting temperature, silver solders are preferred on cost grounds. The composition of silver solders used in orthodontics is approximately 50% silver, 16% each of copper, cadmium and zinc, and 3% nickel.

There are two basic methods of producing the heat that is necessary to melt the solder: the gas blow torch and electrical resistance welding. Gas soldering has the advantage of requiring only low-cost equipment. The apparatus for electrical resistance soldering is considerably more expensive and requires greater skill in its use, but has the advantage that the heat is much more localized.

Table 3.9.4 Relative merits of alloys for orthodontic applications

Material	Stiffness	Resilience	Ductility	Ease of soldering or welding
Stainless steel	High	Good	Adequate	Reasonable
Gold alloy	Medium	Adequate	Adequate	Easy
Co–Cr alloy	High	Good	Low	Difficult
Ni–Ti alloy	Low	Very high	Poor	Difficult
β–Ti alloy	Medium	High	Adequate	Difficult

It is important to realize that the interface between a silver solder and stainless steel is more mechanical than alloying. An adequate amount of solder must therefore be used, and excessive finishing and polishing should be avoided, as this will weaken the joint.

Spot welding

When an electrical current is passed through a metal, it causes the metal to heat up. Spot welding involves the localized application of heat to the component to be joined by the use of a high current at low voltage. If, at the same time, pressure is applied at the point where the two parts are to be joined, recrystallization occurs across the joint and the two parts are fused together.

Note that the metal does not melt. In fact, if the metal is excessively heated and melting does occur, the joint is considerably weakened. In order to avoid this problem, as well as that of weld decay, welding time is kept to 1/50th of a second.

Basically, a welder is a set of electrodes that are brought together under pressure, and which are directly connected to the secondary winding of a pulse transformer. A timer is used to limit the duration of the welding cycle.

Most of the separate components of fixed appliances are joined by spot welding, although the need for this has reduced in recent years with the introduction of complex prefabricated components. However, both spot welding and soldering are still extensively used for the repair and construction of appliances.

OTHER ALLOYS

Other alloys that may be used for orthodontic appliances include gold alloys, Co–Cr alloys, Ni–Ti alloys and β–Ti alloys. The relative merits of these varieties of wrought alloy wire used in orthodontics are presented in Table 3.9.4.

The stiffness is a function of both the wire diameter and the elastic modulus of the material, and determines the amount of force applied to a tooth. For materials with a high elastic modulus, thinner wires can be used than for materials with a low elastic modulus. However, the thinner the wire, the more likely it is to suffer from permanent deformation and loss of applied force to the tooth. A high stiffness is desirable when rapid large forces need to be applied to cause a tooth to move, whereas flexible wires applying a low force need to be used when slow movement of a tooth is desired.

The resilience of the wire is a measure of its ability to undergo large deflections without causing permanent deformation. It is given by the ratio of yield stress and modulus of elasticity such that a combination of low modulus and high yield strength would be ideal.

CLINICAL SIGNIFICANCE

Selection of the orthodontic wire with the correct stiffness is extremely important.

SUMMARY

Stainless steel is widely used for intra-oral appliances, particularly in orthodontics. The advantages with stainless steels are high tensile strength and good corrosion resistance, along with the ability to be readily formed into complex shapes. The material has some limitations in that it is rapidly work-hardened and detrimental changes in properties can occur if excessively high temperatures are applied.

FURTHER READING

Burstone CJ, Goldberg J (1983) Maximum forces and deflections from orthodontic appliances. Am J Orthodont **84**: 95–103

Cohen BI, Penugonda B, Pagnillo MK (2000) Torsional resistance of crowns cemented to composite cores involving three stainless steel endodontic post designs. J Prosthet Dent **84**: 38

Fayle SA (1999) UK National Clinical Guidelines in Paediatric Dentistry. Stainless steel preformed crowns for primary molars. Faculty of Dental Surgery, Royal College of Surgeons. Int J Paediatr Dent **9**: 311

Kapila S, Sachdeva R (1989) Mechanical properties and clinical applications of orthodontic wires. Am J Orthod Dentofacial Orthop **96**: 100

Oltjen JM, Duncanson MG Jr, Ghosh J (1997) Stiffness-deflection behaviour of selected orthodontic wires. Angle Orthod **67**: 209

Purton DG, Love RM (1996) Rigidity and retention of carbon fibre versus stainless steel root canal posts. Int Endod J **29**: 262

Soxman JA (2000) Stainless steel crown and pulpotomy: procedure and technique for primary molars. Gen Dent **48**: 294

Thompson A (2000) An overview of nickel-titanium alloys used in dentistry. Int Endod J **33**: 297

Vallittu PK (1996) Fatigue resistance and stress of wrought-steel wire clasps. J Prosthodont **5**: 186

Waldmeier MD, Grasso JE, Norberg GJ (1996) Bend testing of wrought wire removable partial denture alloys. J Prosthet Dent **76**: 559

Waters NE (1975) Properties of wire. In: Von Frauenhofer JA (ed.) Scientific aspects of dental materials, pp. 2–15. Butterworth, Sevenoaks, UK

Waters NE (1992) Superelastic nickel-titanium wires. Br J Orthod **19**: 319

Index

Index

Index

Index